Beyond Nightingale

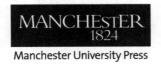

Manchester University Press

Nursing History and Humanities

Series editors: Christine E. Hallett and Jane E. Schultz

This series provides an outlet for the publication of rigorous academic texts in the two closely related disciplines of Nursing History and Nursing Humanities, drawing upon both the intellectual rigour of the humanities and the practice-based, real-world emphasis of clinical and professional nursing.

At the intersection of Medical History, Women's History and Social History, Nursing History remains a thriving and dynamic area of study with its own claims to disciplinary distinction. The broader discipline of Medical Humanities is of rapidly growing significance within academia globally, and this series aims to encourage strong scholarship in the burgeoning area of Nursing Humanities more generally.

Such developments are timely, as the nursing profession expands and generates a stronger disciplinary axis. The MUP Nursing History and Humanities series provides a forum within which practitioners and humanists may offer new findings and insights. The international scope of the series is broad. It embraces all historical periods and includes both detailed empirical studies and wider perspectives on the cultures of nursing.

Previous titles in this series:

Mental health nursing: The working lives of paid carers in the nineteenth and twentieth centuries
Edited by Anne Borsay and Pamela Dale

Negotiating nursing: British Army sisters and soldiers in the Second World War
Jane Brooks

One hundred years of wartime nursing practices, 1854–1953
Edited by Jane Brooks and Christine E. Hallett

'Curing queers': Mental nurses and their patients, 1935–74
Tommy Dickinson

Histories of nursing practice
Edited by Gerard M. Fealy, Christine E. Hallett and Susanne Malchau Dietz

Nurse Writers of the Great War
Christine Hallett

Who cared for the carers? A history of the occupational health of nurses, 1880–1948
Debbie Palmer

Colonial caring: A history of colonial and post-colonial nursing
Edited by Helen Sweet and Sue Hawkins

BEYOND NIGHTINGALE

NURSING ON THE CRIMEAN WAR BATTLEFIELDS

CAROL HELMSTADTER

Manchester University Press

Copyright © Carol Helmstadter 2020

The right of Carol Helmstadter to be identified as the author of this work has been asserted by her in accordance with the Copyright, Designs and Patents Act 1988.

Published by Manchester University Press
Oxford Road, Manchester M13 9PL
www.manchesteruniversitypress.co.uk

British Library Cataloguing-in-Publication Data
A catalogue record for this book is available from the British Library

ISBN   978 1 5261 4051 7 hardback
ISBN   978 1 5261 6048 5 paperback

First published 2020

The publisher has no responsibility for the persistence or accuracy of URLs for any external or third-party internet websites referred to in this book, and does not guarantee that any content on such websites is, or will remain, accurate or appropriate.

Typeset by Servis Filmsetting Ltd, Stockport, Cheshire

Contents

List of maps		vii
List of tables		viii
Acknowledgments		ix
Abbreviations		xi
Author's notes		xii
Maps		xiv
List of English names for Russian names		xix
	Introduction	1
1	The wider context of military nursing in the Crimean War	8

Part I Government-imposed nursing

2	British nursing at the beginning of the Crimean War	31
3	Nightingale's team of nurses	61
4	Lady nurses: myth and reality	80

Part II Religious nursing

5	Mother Francis Bridgeman and her Sisters of Mercy	103
6	The other British religious Sisters	131
7	The Daughters of Charity of St. Vincent de Paul	146
8	The financial costs of war	170

Part III Doctor-directed nursing

9	Turkish military hospitals: an absence of trained nurses and basic resources	193
10	The naval hospital at Therapia	202
11	The civilian hospitals	224

Contents

12	Russian nursing: Pirogov and the Grand Duchess	245
13	The Sisters take over	264
14	The reorganization of the community	290
15	Conclusion: transcending the limitations of gender	303
	Glossary	311
	References	313
	Index	326

List of maps

1. The war zone   xiv
2. The initial campaign, 1854   xv
3. Hospitals with female nurses   xvi
4. Allied occupied Crimea, 1855   xvii
5. The fall of Sevastopol, 8 September 1855   xviii

List of tables

4.1 Summary of reasons for nurses leaving 82
Source: WI Ms 8895, Letter 78

7.1 Outcomes for patients admitted to French medical
department hospitals, October 1854 (46,000 effectives) 159
Source: Scrive, *Relation*, p. 127

7.2 Outcomes for patients admitted to French medical
department hospitals, June 1855 (121,887 effectives) 161
Source: Scrive, *Relation*, p. 211

8.1 Outcomes for patients admitted to French medical
department hospitals, November 1855 (143,250
effectives) 176
Source: Scrive, *Relation*, p. 240

8.2 Outcomes for typhus patients admitted to French
medical department and regimental hospitals, December
1855 through March 1856 182
Source: Scrive, *Relation*, p. 278

Acknowledgments

This book has been a long time in the making and so many people have helped me with it that I hardly know where to start in thanking all those who gave their valuable time to assist me. Perhaps first I should thank Anna LaTorre of the University of Milan, who generously translated and sent me archival Piedmont-Sardinian material, and Jan Schallert, who did all the Pirogov translations. I am also most appreciative of the help Marie Smith and Martyn Bredehoeft gave me with my execrable German, and grateful to Defne Berkings for providing translations of Turkish books and correspondence with Turkish archives.

The archivists who helped me find my way through the rich resources for this project are far too numerous to name, but I would particularly like to thank Susan McGann, archivist of the Royal College of Nursing, who so kindly introduced me to archival research when I first started working on nineteenth-century nursing history. The archivists of all the sisterhoods were also exceptionally helpful and generous with their time. I am grateful to Professor Lynn McDonald for access to the electronic resources of the wonderful *Collected Works of Florence Nightingale* and I am indebted to Alan Gilliland who contributed his vast knowledge of historical cartography in his excellent maps. I also thank both the Canadian and American Associations for the History of Nursing. Without their networking opportunities I would never have found so many resources or so many helpful historians, both here in Canada and in Australia, the United States and United Kingdom.

I thank Professor Yves Saunier of Laval University, who gave me most valuable help with French sources, and I especially thank

Acknowledgments

Professor Trevor Lloyd of the University of Toronto, without whose advice and kind encouragement this book could not have been written.

I gratefully acknowledge the large grants from the Social Sciences and Humanities Research Council of Canada and Associated Medical Services (formerly the Hannah Institute for the History of Medicine) which made the research for this book possible. I am equally grateful for the numerous smaller grants I received from various bodies as diverse as the History Department of Wellesley College and the Nurses Alumnae Association of the Toronto hospital where I worked.

Abbreviations

BA   Bermondsey Annals in Convent of Mercy, Bermondsey Archives
BU   Boston University Nursing Archives
BL   British Library Additional Manuscripts
LMA   London Metropolitan Archives
PP   United Kingdom House of Commons: Sessional Papers 1854–55 (*Parliamentary Papers*)
WI   Wellcome Institute

Author's notes

1. The picture on the cover, showing a Sister of the Exaltation of the Cross tending a wounded soldier, is a detail from Franz Roubaud's panorama painting of the Russian victory on 18 June 1855 when the Sevastopol garrison repulsed the allied assault on the Malakhov.
2. All emphases in quotations are original.
3. The Russians used the Julian calendar (Old System or OS), which in the 1850s was roughly twelve days ahead of our Gregorian calendar or New System (NS). For example, when Tolstoy wrote 'Sevastopol in August' he was writing about the fall of Sevastopol on 27 August OS, which we date as 8 September. In order to avoid confusion between the two dating systems, the standard practice when using Russian texts is to give both dates: 27 August/8 September. When I do not give both dates, I am using the new or Gregorian dating.
4. Figures given for distances and numbers of troops are often very approximate. The armies issued official figures, but these are not completely reliable. Although the French army medical department kept good records, the French always under-reported the losses of the army as a whole. Figures given by individuals are usually very rough estimates and often wildly inflated. For example, the different British nurses reported the distance they had to walk from the Scutari Barrack Hospital to the Scutari General Hospital as anywhere from a half a mile to two miles. Lt. Colonel Hamley reported finding two thousand

Author's notes

wounded men in the Assembly of Nobles when in fact there were only 500. Some of Pirogov's numbers for troops involved in the trench battles are also guesses and undoubtedly too high.

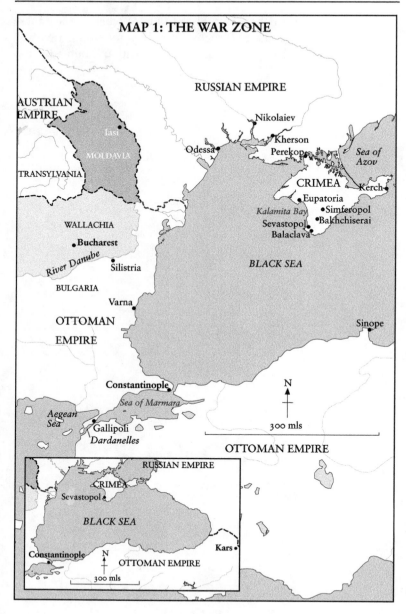

Map 1 The war zone

Maps

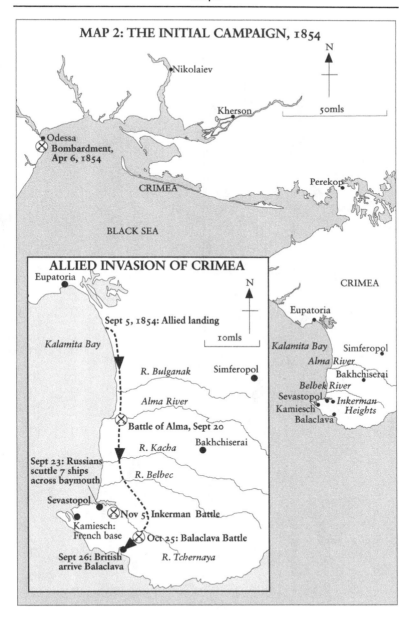

Map 2 The initial campaign, 1854

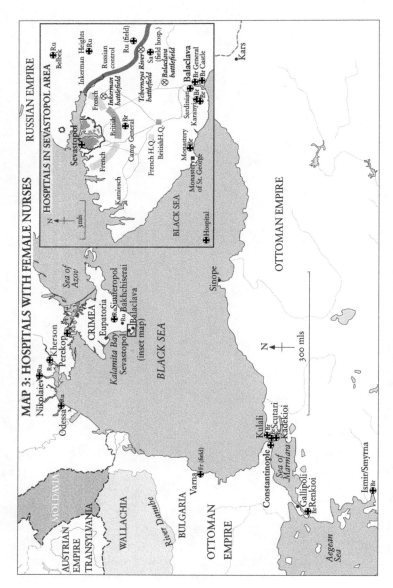

Map 3 Hospitals with female nurses

Maps

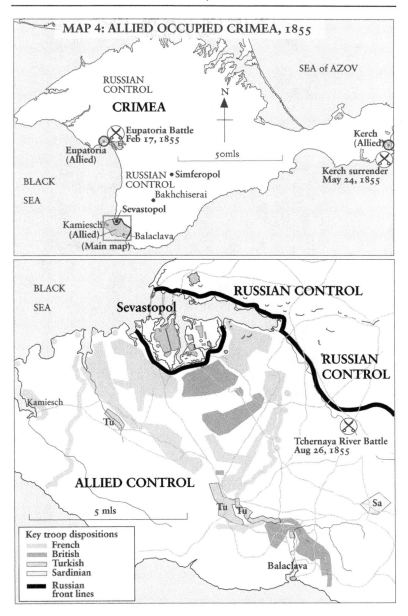

Map 4 Allied occupied Crimea, 1855

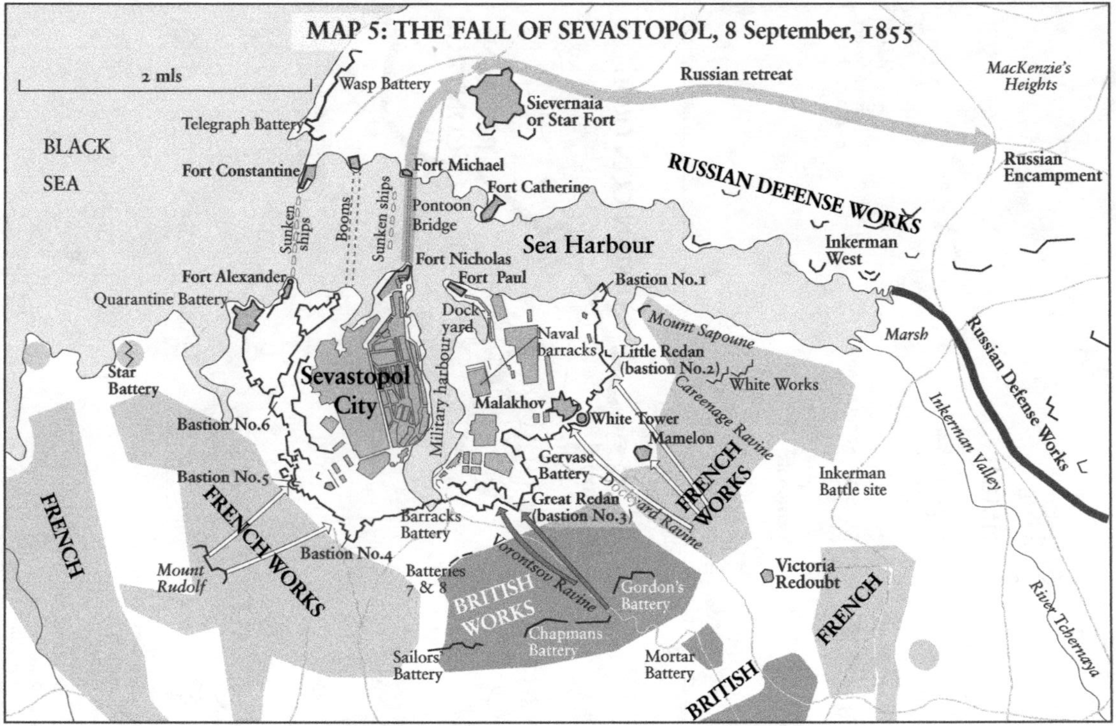

Map 5 The fall of Sevastopol, 8 September 1855

List of English names for Russian names

Russian name	English name
Bastion 1	There does not appear to be an English name for this bastion
Bastion 2	Little Redan
Bastion 3	(Great) Redan
Bastion 4	Flagstaff or Garden Battery
Bastion 5	Central Battery
Bastion 6	No English name
Kornilov Bastion	Malakhov
Seleginsk Redoubt	White Works
Volhynia Redoubt	White Works
Pavlosky Point	Paul Battery or Fort Paul
Aleksandrovsky Battery	Alexander Battery or Fort Alexander
Mikhaelevsky Battery	Michael Battery or Fort Michael
Nikholaevsky Battery	Nicholas Battery or Fort Nicholas

Introduction

When in the spring of 1854 British and French troops set off for the East to support the Turks in their war against the Russians, the allies expected the war to be over within three weeks. What came to be known later as the Crimean War lasted until March 1856 and resulted in a horrific bloodletting, a loss of life which would not be exceeded until World War I. The most famous siege of the war was fought in Sevastopol, the great Russian naval base in the Black Sea. Anyone who visits Sevastopol today is immediately struck by the numerous and very beautiful monuments commemorating the heroes of that siege. There is even a monument to the 'drowned ships', as the Russians call the battleships they sank at the entrance to the harbor in order to deny the allied fleet access. The harbor or bay of Sevastopol divides the city into a northern and a southern section. British, French, Turkish, and latterly Piedmont-Sardinian armies eventually captured the south side. The north side however never fell, and there, throughout the bitterly fought siege, the Russians buried 127,583 men who were killed defending the city. The ordinary soldiers lie in mass graves of fifty to a hundred; the officers have individual graves with their names and regiments written on them. It is a sobering sight. It is estimated that another 125,000 Russian soldiers, sailors, and civilians were killed in the long siege. The war was fought in many other places besides the Crimea, and for the whole war it is thought that Russian losses amounted to 500,000–600,000.

The allied losses were huge, but pale beside those of the Russians. There are no figures for the Turkish army but in round figures the French lost 100,000 out of 300,000 men, the British 20,000 out of 100,000, and the Piedmontese, who did not arrive in the Crimea

Introduction

until May 1855, 2,000 out of 18,000. Unlike the Russian memory of the war as one of brilliant, innovative, and heroic feats of arms, in France and Sardinia the Crimean War was unpopular from the beginning. By contrast, in Constantinople public opinion was eager for war. In Britain, people were keen on war with Russia. Still today, in English-speaking countries, the war is usually remembered as a rather senseless and unnecessary war which the British government stumbled into and the army bungled, most famously in the Charge of the Light Brigade. In popular memory Florence Nightingale's superhuman and successful efforts to improve military nursing were the war's only redeeming features. Indeed the massive blood loss provided many opportunities for improved medical and nursing practice, and, for the purposes of this book, it was the first war in which governments officially employed secular women to provide some of the nursing. It is a curiosity that Nightingale's mission is so well remembered and yet historians of nursing have largely ignored highly successful nursing in other British hospitals where she did not direct the nursing services. There are also no studies of the very different, but equally or even more successful, nursing in the Russian, French, and Piedmontese armies. This book seeks to redress these major omissions in the historiography of the Crimean War.

The way the war began and the way it was conducted had a major impact on how well army medical departments were able to function. The Russians did not expect the invasion to begin until the following summer and therefore their medical department was on a peacetime footing when the first two battles were fought. In Britain there was something to be said for the assessment that the war was senseless and unnecessary. Lord Aberdeen, Prime Minister from December 1852 through January 1855, was anxious to keep the peace and genuinely believed war was avoidable. On the other hand, Lord Palmerston, Home Secretary at the time, was violently anti-Russian and pro-war. He was also a vastly experienced and skillful politician, who understood the need to cultivate the press and how to appeal to the public in simple terms which they could understand. As the press took advantage of an underlying British Russophobia and inflamed it with stories of the horrible conditions under which British soldiers were fighting in the Crimea, Aberdeen lamented, 'An English Minister must please the newspapers. The newspapers are always bawling for

Introduction

interference. They are bullies and they make the government a bully.' Lord Clarendon, the British Foreign Secretary in 1854, thought the British were 'drifting' into war, and in a sense they were. When war was finally declared, Aberdeen told the Queen that Palmerston, with the support of the press and public opinion, had dragged him into it.[1] The British government habitually, at least until the twentieth century, found itself going into wars for which it had made very little preparation, but the results were not usually as spectacularly disastrous as was the case in the Crimean War. The medical department was ill-equipped to deal with what would be a new kind of war, one in which industrial power and more effective medical and nursing practice would make enormous changes. Adding to its lack of preparedness, the British army had not fought in a European war since 1815. By contrast, the French initially sent troops from Algeria who were hardened veterans of the contemporary colonial wars, and an efficiently functioning medical department. The Piedmontese were badly beaten by the Austrians in their first War for Independence in 1848–49, but nevertheless that war gave their army recent experience which it used well in the Crimea.

The war began ostensibly over religious issues between Russia and Turkey but what was really at stake was what was known as the Eastern Question – the long-standing international problem of the disintegrating Ottoman Empire and how the Great Powers might absorb what remained of it, or in the British case, how to prevent its dismemberment. The Russian long-term goal was clear: free access to the Mediterranean. The Russians had been making steady inroads into Turkey since 1783, when Catherine the Great seized the Crimea, and in two wars in 1806 and 1828 they conquered more Ottoman territory. However, once war broke out in 1853 and the British and French joined forces with the Turks in 1854, the Russians were placed on the defensive. The Suez Canal had not yet been built, and the British felt Russian expansion would threaten important land routes through the Levant to India. They were therefore committed to maintaining the integrity of the Ottoman Empire as a bulwark against the Russian southward push. In July 1853 a Russian army occupied the Danubian principalities of Moldavia and Wallachia (which correspond roughly to Rumania before its expansion after World War I). These provinces were not strictly speaking Ottoman territory, but rather protectorates

Introduction

of the empire. The Russians claimed they were occupying them temporarily to put pressure on the Sultan to settle the religious issues. In fact the Tsar would have liked to appropriate the principalities as well as part of Bulgaria, and he hoped for control of Constantinople and the Turkish Straits as well. Interestingly, the occupation of the principalities was not the immediate cause of the war. However, it did make war more likely because it was at this point that the French and British put their fleets on a war footing.

After repeated fruitless attempts on the part of the other Great Powers to mediate, on 4 October 1853 the Sultan, pushed by public opinion in Constantinople and by his assumption that the British and French would support him, declared war on Russia. Five months later, in March 1854, Russian troops crossed the Danube into Bulgaria and laid siege to the Turkish fortress of Silistria. Because Bulgaria was real Ottoman territory, not an Ottoman protectorate, on 27 and 28 March 1854 the British and French officially declared war on Russia. The new allies expected the principal scene of action to be the lower Danube and therefore sent troops to Bulgaria to support the Turkish army. But on 22 June 1854, just as British and French troops were landing in Bulgaria, diplomatic pressure forced the Russians to lift the siege of Silistria and evacuate the principalities. The allies were left in Bulgaria with no enemy to fight. With an army and fleet so close to Sevastopol, the British cabinet decided to use this opportunity to destroy Russian naval power in the Black Sea—a political, not a military decision.

The war aims of the Russians and British after April 1854 were clear: both governments were protecting their empires. The French goals were somewhat diffuse. Napoleon III thought an alliance with the British could bring France out of the diplomatic isolation which the 1815 Congress of Vienna settlement had imposed and could re-establish her as a major European diplomatic power. Furthermore, if war did occur, he did not want to lose his share of the spoils as a result of not having participated. He was not interested in power politics in the Black Sea but went along with the British plan of attacking Sevastopol in the hope of winning a glorious military victory which would restore the reputation of the French army in Europe, and might make his much more limited Second Empire look more like Napoleon I's First Empire. Military victory might

Introduction

also help shore up his not entirely secure throne. The fact that the aims of the two traditional enemies who were now allies were not aligned would make their conduct of the war more difficult. This was compounded by the fact that there was never a unified command: the British and French generals consulted, but the two armies always acted independently.

As well as the Danubian campaign, the Sultan was also fighting the Russians in the Caucasus, the traditional second front in all the Russo-Turkish wars – the Russians had been fighting the mountaineers almost continuously since the time of Peter the Great. A skillful leader of the Caucasian Muslim tribes, an imam named Shamil, emerged in the 1820s and would cause the Russians considerable trouble in 1853 and 1854. Both the British and French governments sent arms and ammunition to the mountaineers. Contemporaries called the Crimean War the Eastern or Russian War – these are really better names, because the Crimean campaign was only one of many. As well as the fighting in the Caucasus, Crimea, Black Sea, and along the Danube as mentioned above, the war was fought in the White Sea, Barents Sea, North Pacific, Baltic Sea, and Sea of Azov. However, it was in the Crimea that the heaviest fighting took place and where nursing came to the forefront. Therefore this book deals primarily with the Crimean campaign.

What do these political, diplomatic, and military events have to do with nursing in the Crimea? A very great deal, and it is the aim of this book to show why and how military affairs, cultural assumptions, and the political and economic structure of each of the five countries involved shaped the beginning of female military nursing and, in the English-speaking world, female nursing in general. There are many excellent histories of the Crimean War and multiple studies of Florence Nightingale, but there is no book on Crimean War nursing as such, and no adequate international investigation of nursing in the five armies. Yet the Crimean War saw the birth of modern nursing in four of those five armies, a significant event in both nursing and military history. The great Russian military surgeon Nikolai Pirogov described the introduction of trained female nurses into his army's medical department as a revolution. He and his surgeons became highly dependent on these women and attributed much of their success to them.

Introduction

The imperialist aims of four imperial governments and a fifth minor expansionist power were certainly the cause of the war, but imperialism had no impact on the military nurses. Scholars of imperialism, colonialism, and post-colonialism have criticized the 'white man's burden' of the British or the *'mission civilisatrice'* of the French as a rationalization for exploitation and racism in the pursuit of self-interest. This is justified in many instances, and is precisely what the Russian armies fighting contemporaneously in the Caucasus were doing. Aggrandizement and Russification were primary goals there. By contrast, in the case of the nurses in the Crimea, there is nothing to support these historians' interpretation of nurses as agents of empire, imposing economic policies and Western medicine and values on foreign peoples.

Susan Armstrong-Reid has pointed out that recent post-colonial scholars have persuasively contested this binary framework because it fits so poorly with the complex, cross-cultural, humanitarian challenges transnational nurses faced and the way they had to constantly negotiate and contest their professional space.[2] In her most recent work, Armstrong-Reid studied Western nurses who worked side-by-side with Chinese nurses, but in the case of the Crimean War, even if they had wanted to, neither the allied nor the Russian nurses had any opportunity to work with or impose their values on the other armies or Russian civilians. They remained isolated in their own camps and none of the nurses in any of the sources used here ever expressed or even mentioned imperialist aims in any context. Florence Nightingale was disappointed that the allies did not pursue the war further and in later years became rather a jingoist. However, in her enormous correspondence during the war she never expressed any imperial hopes or goals, or any wish to foist British nursing practices or values on the other armies' medical departments. At the same time, like Armstrong-Reid's nurses in China, the Crimean nurses were indeed constantly contesting and negotiating their professional space in terms of class, gender, and nursing knowledge. British nurses struggled against a rigid sense of class which demeaned working-class women and an ideology of separate spheres which dictated an unrealistic role for women; the French army found it difficult to recruit male soldier nurses because nursing was considered a feminine pursuit; Piedmontese nurses had their letters censored because of the Prime

Introduction

Minister's difficult political situation; a corrupt Ottoman government failed to give Turkish orderlies either the training or the resources they needed to nurse effectively; and, when the war ended, a corrupt medical department stripped the Russian nurses of the powerful position they had succeeded in gaining in military hospitals.

Beyond Nightingale treats medicine and nursing as international disciplines, which shared many commonalities in the five armies but followed rather different courses in each. In the following chapters, the book will examine the various historiographical debates regarding the Crimean nurses and the value the armies placed on their contributions. The historiographical arguments are complex, and easier to understand when the reader has some grasp of the events which caused the controversies. Because it takes a transnational perspective, comparing the medical and nursing services of the five armies, this book is divided into three parts. The first studies British nursing, a politically driven nursing service that the government forced on a medical department which did not want female nurses. The second part looks at the religious nursing Sisters in the British, French, and Piedmont-Sardinian armies. The third part is devoted to nursing services which doctors directed in the British navy and in the British and Russian armies. At the end of the war each army's nursing service had developed differently, reflecting its own national culture and political and economic structure. However, whether badly or well organized, smoothly functioning or damaged by political and sectarian infighting, well funded or severely underfunded, or working under almost impossible conditions, in every case – even that of the Turks, who had the least effective medical department – the nurses relieved some of the suffering of the sick and wounded.

Notes

1 Figes, *Crimean War*, pp. 122, 147–50, 159–60; Baumgart, *Crimean War 1853–1856*, pp. 13–16.
2 Armstrong-Reid, *China Gadabouts*, pp. 268–9.

1

The wider context of military nursing in the Crimean War

Introduction

In many ways the Crimean War was the first of the new industrial wars, but it also retained many characteristics of the old 'gentlemanly war.' Diplomacy played a major role and prevented it from becoming a more generalized European war. 'In contrast to the wars of the twentieth century, but in common with most European wars in modern history up to the nineteenth century,' diplomatic historian Winfried Baumgart wrote, 'the outbreak of the Crimean War did not stop the frantic and continuous diplomatic activities of the belligerent powers.' The concept of unconditional surrender demanded in World War II, which leaves little room for compromise and makes diplomacy irrelevant, did not exist in the 1850s. Diplomats continued trying to find a means of making peace throughout the war. Moreover, all of the armies involved respected some of the old rules of warfare, and a certain sense of chivalry still remained.

There are numerous examples of this kind of gentlemanly war. Truces to clear the wounded and dead from the field were frequent. Count Osten-Sacken, latterly the commanding general in Sevastopol, expressed in the most flattering terms his great admiration for the courage of the French troops. He had French prisoners buried with all the honors which he said were owed to their exemplary bravery. The Baron de Bazancourt, the official French historian of the war, deemed Osten-Sacken 'a true and knightly gentleman.'[1] The Russians treated prisoners well. A British colonel taken prisoner lived comfortably in a Russian general's home,[2] and from time to time a British aide-de-camp went into Sevastopol under a flag of truce taking letters from Russian officers who were British prisoners and bringing money,

The wider context of military nursing in the Crimean War

letters, and baggage to British officers who were Russian prisoners.[3] The French also took a chivalrous attitude toward the enemy. Major Jean François Herbé, a ten-year veteran and St. Cyr trained officer, admired the courage and valor of the Russian officers who led sorties into the French trenches. They fought 'with a vigour and intrepidity to which we must render homage,' he said. Two days after a major sortie, when an armistice was declared to collect the dead and those wounded who were still alive, French and Russian soldiers, subalterns, and officers all shook hands, congratulated each other on their fighting prowess, and exchanged tobacco and cigars. Herbé thought that no one would ever have guessed that these men, only a few minutes earlier, had been trying to kill each other.[4]

But if the Crimean War had elements of the old warfare, it also presaged twentieth-century total war. The siege of Sevastopol involved the trench warfare which characterized the western front of World War I. Many features of the Crimean War demonstrate the power of industrialization: global attacks on Russian naval bases, newspaper correspondents, photographers, the telegraph, the new Russian land and sea mines, massive bombardments of civilian homes and civilian participation in the building and constant maintenance of Sevastopol's formidable defenses, and for our purposes, the introduction of secular female nurses, some of whom were trained. In the American Civil War a few years later, the Union's technological and economic superiority led to its victory over the Confederacy. Similarly, despite the brilliant and innovative Russian defense, the far greater industrial capacities of the British and French were the decisive factors in achieving allied victory.

An agrarian society at war with industrialized countries

The Russian and Ottoman economies were essentially agrarian and pre-industrial. The Ottoman army played a small part in the siege of Sevastopol and the Piedmont-Sardinian army was actively involved for only a few months. However, unlike Turkey, Piedmont-Sardinia was an industrialized country. By contrast, Russian society was based on serf labor; significant industrialization would not begin until after the war. Captain Edouard Ivanovich Totleben, the brilliant young army engineer who designed the awesome defenses of Sevastopol,

The wider context of military nursing in the Crimean War

identified two major consequences of Russia's backward economy: first, the allies had overwhelmingly greater sea power, and second, allied gunnery was much superior. In both allied navies about one third of the ships were steam powered, a much larger proportion than in the Russian navy. In the naval campaign in the Baltic in 1855–56 the British used only steamships as well as the new iron-clad ships that were then called 'floating batteries.' The French navy was somewhat smaller than the British – 300 warships as opposed to 385 – but equally modern. Anglo-French fleets burnt and pillaged Russian towns in the Black Sea and Sea of Azov, in the Baltic and White Seas, and in the northern Pacific.[5] After the fall of Sevastopol the French used their new iron-clad ships with great success during the bombardment of Kinburn. The Russians put up a gallant resistance, much admired by the enemy, but in the face of such devastating fire, overwhelming force, and the invulnerability of the iron ships to Russian shells, had to surrender.[6] Recent historians have pointed out that the British expected their war effort to be primarily a war at sea. Anticipating that the French would be mainly responsible for the land war, they originally sent a small army of only 26,000 men to the Crimea. Very early on, beginning with the fierce fight the Russians put up in the face of overwhelming odds at the Battle of the Alma on 20 September 1854 and the failure of the allies' First Bombardment of Sevastopol in October, it became clear that Sevastopol was not going to fall in three weeks as the allies had hoped. The French therefore doubled the size of their army during the fall of 1854. The British enlarged their army but could not keep it up to strength.[7]

Totleben identified the superior firepower, accuracy, and range of the allies' new Minié rifles and bullets as the second element that placed the Russians at a catastrophic disadvantage. Almost all the British foot soldiers were armed with these new rifles, and in 1855 the British issued the Enfield rifle, which was lighter and even more lethal than the Minié.[8] The Zouaves, the French elite troops, all had Minié rifles; the rest of the French infantry carried smooth-bore muskets but shot Minié bullets, which had a longer range than the old musket balls.[9] The Minié's range was 1,200 or more paces, while the Russian muskets had a range of no more than 300. Russian soldiers were therefore helpless until they were at close range, and even then were at a disadvantage because Russian muskets were old, top-heavy,

The wider context of military nursing in the Crimean War

and poorly made with stocks of light softwood that broke easily. The British soldiers could twist and break them with their hands.[10] The Russian armourers were perfectly competent to make good arms, but because of the pervasive graft in the army, many colonels bought the cheapest possible weapons and kept the money the government gave them for supplying their men for themselves.[11]

What do Enfield rifles and Minié bullets have to do with medical and nursing care? A very great deal: because they had longer range, greater accuracy, and far more intense power of penetration than the old musket ball, the Russian surgeons and their nurses had to deal with an exponentially increased number of more severe wounds.[12] One cannot speak too highly of the Minié rifle, Dr John Morton declared. Morton was an American doctor from Nashville, Tennessee who was working with the Russians. He pointed out that, with its greater power of penetration, when a Minié bullet struck a bone, a comminuted fracture necessitating amputation resulted.[13] The Russians did have a few Minié-type rifles which they gave to their sharpshooters. They used a heavier bullet than those of the allies, which produced immense comminuted fractures.[14] Although their artillerists were excellent,[15] the Russian guns were also inferior to those of the allies. At the Alma, because the French guns were of heavier caliber and longer range, the French kept the Russian gunners at a distance where Russian shells could not reach them. Some of the Zouaves taunted the Russians by dancing a polka in front of their guns. The French made it a policy to avoid close combat where the Russians could give as good as they got; when the Russian battalions charged they retired beyond the reach of the Russian muskets and then poured a murderous fusillade into them. Furthermore, Russian troops were trained to rely on their bayonets, and marched and attacked in the old-fashioned oblong column. Therefore, only the men in the first two ranks could use their muskets, while the columns made an easy target for the allies with their Minié bullets – which at short range could go through two men and lodge in a third. The allies also used different tactics, fighting in lines only two deep, which made the most of their infinitely superior firepower.[16]

The Russians realized immediately that they had to get more rifles and, because they could not manufacture them themselves, they would have to buy them abroad. The Belgians produced excellent

The wider context of military nursing in the Crimean War

rifles but they were selling them to the British and agreed to sell only 13,900 to the Russians, and then at a very high price. Since the allied navies controlled the Baltic Sea, only about 3,000 of those 13,900 rifles reached Russia before the fighting ended. Of the 102½ battalions that the Russians put into action at the Battle of the Tchernaya in August 1855 only three were rifle battalions. There was only a small munitions industry in Russia and the army soon began to suffer from a shortage of gunpowder and projectiles. The Minister of War sent people all over Russia searching for gunpowder but the Russian powder factories had a limited output and their delivery was slow, with the result that by January 1855 the Russians were firing only half as many rounds as the allies.[17] It speaks to their accuracy that Herbé, who was an experienced observer, thought the Russian cannonades were always stronger and more violent than those of the allies.[18] The allies' mortars and explosive shells devastated civilian buildings and hospitals as well as military objectives. As a result many women and children were among the wounded,[19] an additional burden on the Russian doctors and nurses which the allies did not face.

Totleben pinpointed the vast extent of the Russian frontiers as another severe major military disadvantage. For the Russians the Crimean campaign was only a small part of a much larger war. They worried about a naval attack on Cronstadt, the great naval base that defended St. Petersburg, and feared possible attacks all along their long western frontier.[20] At the same time as they were defending Sevastopol, as mentioned earlier, the Russians were also fighting fierce mountaineers under Shamil in the Caucasus. The enormous extent of the Russian frontiers made it almost impossible to concentrate troops. In all of Russia there was only one rail line, which ran from St. Petersburg to Moscow. Russian soldiers had to march on foot from various distant points across the empire to the Crimea, where they arrived utterly exhausted and having lost many men on the way. It took Captain Hodasevich (who will appear again in a later chapter) and his regiment six months to march from their home base in Ninji Novgorod to Sevastopol. He described the march as a long, dreary, and fatiguing journey.[21] With railroads to their home ports and steamships to the Crimea, the British and French could send troops to Russia, although 3,000 miles away, far more quickly than the Russians could bring troops from the provinces. Also communications were poor in Russia; there was no telegraph system in the Crimea. By contrast, in April 1855 the allies completed a telegraph system that connected London and Paris with the Crimea and they also had telegraph wires connecting the principal points of their siege works in front of Sevastopol. In January 1855 the British shipped navvies with their horses to Balaclava to build a railroad which carried provisions and ordnance up to the camp from Balaclava. The navvies completed the railroad at the end of March.[22] Land transport was a terrible problem for both the allies and the Russians, but the railroad solved it for the British.

Sevastopol was designed as a small peacetime garrison and did not have the land transport and magazines required for a major campaign such as it now faced. Before the allied landing in September 1854 the Russians had increased the number of troops in the Crimea to 50,000. Six months later they had 300,000 men and 100,000 animals in the city, all of whom had to be fed. The Crimea produced mainly grapes and cattle, but had always depended on importing grain and forage from the Don basin. Food for the newly enlarged army had to be brought by ox-cart over hundreds of miles of dirt roads which in winter became tracks of deep mud. By contrast, the British had only seven or eight miles of such roads from the Balaclava harbor up to the camp on the heights and after March 1855 they had their railroad. The French had even fewer miles because their harbor and base in Kamiesch were closer to the camp. Shortage of hay was a critical problem throughout the siege for both sides. Russian wagons could not hold enough hay for both the horses and oxen pulling them and a supply for the animals in Sevastopol. As a result, the draft animals were poorly fed and horribly overworked, resulting in two-thirds of the animals dying.[23] At times the shortage of hay was so great that the Russian cavalry was feeding brush, or chopped oak leaves mixed with flour, which resulted in the death of the horses and the demise of the cavalry.[24] The British cavalry did not even have oak leaves and flour so their horses ate each other's tails as they starved to death.[25]

Russian and Ottoman society had changed little since the end of the Napoleonic Wars; by contrast industrialization had changed British, French, and Piedmont-Sardinian society very considerably. It developed later in France and Piedmont-Sardinia than in Britain, but by 1854 they both had decidedly industrial economies. The

The wider context of military nursing in the Crimean War

accompanying better standard of living and education in the industrialized nations produced significant cultural shifts, one of which was a humanitarian movement. For example, in Britain the campaign for the reform of criminal law began at the end of the Napoleonic Wars, the Society for the Prevention of Cruelty to Animals was founded in 1824, and in 1833 laws abolishing slavery in the colonies were passed. The educated public began taking an interest in the welfare of the working classes. A more literate public was horrified when it read about the lack of care for the wounded and sick after the Alma. We are fortunate in having the diary of a humane and perceptive professional British soldier, Sir George Bell (1794–1877), who entered the Crimean War as a 60 year old veteran of the Napoleonic Wars. In the Napoleonic Wars, the ordinary soldiers 'were not looked upon as parts of humanity,' Bell wrote, but now the public included the private soldiers as well as the officers in their demand for better medical care for the army.[26] The terrible mortality and destruction of the British army at Sevastopol was not any worse than in many earlier wars, most recently the first years of the Peninsular War,[27] but then there were no newspaper correspondents and photographers or soldiers who were adequately literate to write home about the horrible conditions. In 1854 the newspapers had correspondents and photographers actually in the war zone delivering eye-witness accounts and pictures to the home front. When the new telegraph connections were completed in April 1855, war news could reach Britain within a few hours and the public read it eagerly.[28] 'That terror of all tyrants, the press,' Bell wrote:

> had not the power, nor the pen, nor the freedom, nor the courage to speak out for the army as they have in the present day. So all heroic deeds were forgotten or held in abeyance, and clouds of darkness overshadowed the lives of hundreds of brave men who died in obscurity.[29]

In April 1855 Brevet-Major Henry Clifford, a much younger veteran British officer than Bell, commented, '"The Times" is certainly a most wonderful Commanding Officer. What Raglan doesn't think of or doesn't get done this all powerful paper brings about in no time.' Only a week after *The Times* wrote that there was no general on duty in the trenches Lord Raglan, the commander of the British army in the Crimea, had a general visiting the trenches by day and remaining

The wider context of military nursing in the Crimean War

in them at night. Clifford himself had always visited the trenches at all hours of the night as well as the day, but he had been almost the only member of the general staff who did.[30]

Beginning in the 1820s the British public started demanding abolition of flogging. In Wellington's army men were flogged every day for drunkenness. Bell saw men 'suffer 500 to 700 lashes before being taken down, the blood running down into their shoes, and their backs flayed like raw red-chopped sausages.'[31] Many army officers resisted abolition because they thought they would be unable to maintain discipline without it. Nevertheless, public pressure forced the army to make it less vicious. By 1850 the maximum number of lashes which could be awarded was reduced to fifty, and twenty-five was the average number, while flogging was supposed to be seldom used and only in aggravated cases.[32] The French were surprised that flogging continued at all. 'The sight of these corporal punishments disgusted us,' one French soldier wrote, 'reminding us that the Revolution of 89 abolished flogging in the [French] army when it established universal conscription.'[33] When he reached the Crimea in 1854, 22 year old Dr David Greig, an assistant surgeon, was also surprised to learn that flogging was still in use in the British army, but he surmised that the army could not manage without it. The surgeon in his dress uniform stood by, so that if the man became ill or fainted, he could stop the punishment. In Grieg's unit there were floggings every three to four days; he had just witnessed one when he wrote to his family. Three men who had all been drunk and disorderly were punished. The first man got twenty-five lashes, the second fifteen, and the third ten.[34] The flogging ceremonies were supposed to show the soldiers the rewards of disobedience but their efficacy was questionable. Clifford noted in January 1855 that about fifteen or twenty men in his regiment, 'all bad characters,' had deserted to the Russians in the preceding fortnight. Most of these men had just undergone corporal punishment. Flogging in the British army would not be abolished until 1881.[35]

A veteran soldier in the Crimean War

Military patients were very different from civilian patients: they were accustomed to horrors which civilians rarely see and used to suffering with little or no medical or nursing support. Bell illustrates this well.

The wider context of military nursing in the Crimean War

He joined the army as a 17 year old ensign in 1811 and was shipped to Lisbon to join Wellington's forces in the Peninsular War. He was billeted in a small room with a cot in the corner in an ugly part of the town. He soon learned that soldiers had to take a different approach to sickness. Two days after landing in Lisbon he became violently ill, unable to leave his bed for many days. No one in his unit knew where he was: some thought he had been kidnapped, others thought he had deserted, while his commanding officer never gave Bell's absence even a thought. The only person he saw while he lay sick on his cot was the maid who brought him rice-water every day.[36] Bell recovered, rejoined his regiment, and fought through the rest of the campaign. He and his fellow soldiers would be sick many times, some almost constantly. On the retreat from Madrid large numbers of soldiers, including Bell, fell ill with ague and fever. Bell was fortunate to be billeted with a peasant family who were very kind to him. Exceedingly poor and dressed in sheepskins, the father herded goats all day on the hills, returning at night to make the family meal himself. It was always the same: a loaf of brown bread cut up and mixed with olive oil and hot water. Despite their poverty the family was extremely courteous, never sitting down to eat without first inviting Bell to join them. He could not remember how long he lay prostrate on his cot in a corner of their kitchen, but he did remember that the regimental surgeon came every day. The surgeon's equipment consisted of only 'his carving tools [amputation kit], blue pill and salts,[37] and his good name which carried him through an honourable life with success.' All he had to offer Bell was a kind and encouraging word. The sick soldiers who had less kindly billets or none at all died by the score for lack of medical care and food. Uncertain whether he would recover, Bell yearned for his home during his long illness but as his health gradually came back his homesickness resolved.

As in Bell's case in the Napoleonic Wars, in 1854 army doctors certainly dealt with wounded men, but by far the greatest number of their patients suffered and died from diseases that we now tend to associate with the tropics. Malaria, cholera, typhoid fever, and typhus were prevalent in all parts of Europe in the first part of the nineteenth century. Bell's 'ague' was malaria, for it recurred every two days and would some years later be treated successfully with quinine. Although he would sometimes have to take the day off and lie prostrate under

The wider context of military nursing in the Crimean War

a tree, somehow Bell always managed to catch up with the regiment the next day.[38] During the Peninsular campaign Bell also suffered from severe rheumatism; at one point it doubled him up for three weeks. In July 1814, as the victorious army fought its way through the Pyrenees into France, Bell was lying under an apple tree having one of his very worst ague days when the drums beat to arms and the bugles sounded. It was a point of honor with the officers and men never to be absent when there was a chance for a brush with the enemy so Bell joined his company, dragging himself along with difficulty, faint and weary with pain and debility. The following day, although he was still quite shaky, he and an assistant surgeon were ordered to take a number of the wounded to the hospital in Alizando, a distance of a two days' trek.[39]

In the Crimea Bell and his colleagues would again frequently be ill but the same point of honor of always participating in a fight with the enemy prevailed in all the armies. For example, when the French troops were preparing to leave Bulgaria for the Crimea Lt. Masquelez had been suffering from diarrhoea for two months. He was barely able to eat and utterly exhausted, so on 25 August he went to see the regimental doctor, Dr Gerrier. He had complete confidence in Gerrier but when he told him he should not even think of going to the Crimea Masquelez insisted he had to go. Gerrier then gave him some laudanum, which did not help at all so he went back two days later, at which point Gerrier gave him an enormous dose which did help. His 'infernal indisposition' came back violently twice on shipboard and he had to take even more enormous doses of laudanum. At the Battle of the Alma Masquelez and his men were among those Zouaves who turned the tide by clambering up the dirt track to the top of the escarpment on the allies' right flank. The Russians, who had not thought anyone could attack up such a steep hill, were astonished. They sent their reserve artillery at the gallop to confront them, followed by two regiments of infantry. The Zouaves remained under severe fire while their colleagues in the artillery struggled to ford the river and drag their guns up the mountainous path. There were thirty-two Russian cannons firing at Masquelez and his company when the first gun arrived and forty before all the others reached the top. Masquelez was hit by a shell in the side and hand, and severely wounded in the foot.[40]

The wider context of military nursing in the Crimean War

The allied armies were already very sick armies – Masquelez is one example – before they reached the Crimea. The war coincided with one of the worst nineteenth-century cholera epidemics, and by the end of July diarrhea and cholera were wreaking havoc among the soldiers in Bulgaria. Tormented by a plague of locusts which swarmed by the thousands on the soldiers' faces, hands, and eyes, many officers and men died. Cholera struck the French even harder than the British and soon spread to both fleets. In August, as the British army prepared to leave Bulgaria for the Crimea it was losing so many men every day that morale sank. Nevertheless, the allied fleet crossed the Black Sea and anchored in the bay at Eupatoria on 12 September 1854. The day after disembarking, Bell became very ill with fever but, in traditional military fashion, managed to soldier on to the banks of the Alma River where the allies defeated a smaller but well entrenched Russian army. Bell and his regiment were in the thick of the fight.[41] The night before the battle cholera attacked some 150 men. There were not enough surgeons to care for them but they were eventually collected and put on piles of hay. Those who were in their death throes were quiet but the moans, cries, and hollow plaintive pleas of those in the crisis of the disease as they begged the passers-by to rub their cramped limbs were pitiful.[42] Bell, who had been feeling unwell in Bulgaria, was now severely smitten with cholera.[43]

The Battle of the Alma ended around 4 o'clock in the afternoon; the French had all their wounded off the field before nightfall and had set up tented field hospitals equipped with operating theaters. By contrast, the British wounded lay on the ground, begging the men who were pursuing the retreating Russians not to ride over them. There were no ambulance wagons and there were no orderlies. Fifteen or twenty bandsmen from each regiment were assigned to carry the wounded off the field, but at the start of the battle they were at least a mile away from the fighting. Each regiment had only eight stretchers on which they were supposed to carry all their wounded, and they were completely untrained for this work. The navy sent a thousand sailors who worked for two days collecting the wounded and sick and burying the dead. The sailors carried the men in hammocks slung on oars two and a half miles to the beach to be loaded onto the ships for Constantinople. Many died on the way and many more would perish once on board for lack of medical aid. The surgeons worked

The wider context of military nursing in the Crimean War

indefatigably but there were far too few. It took nearly three days before the army was ready to move on. When the British ships sailed for Scutari with their wounded they left one doctor behind, together with an orderly, to look after 630 Russian wounded.[44] The absence of proper transport and medical equipment occurred through no fault of the army medical department. When the army embarked for the Crimea, to save space for more fighting men on the ships, Lord Raglan ordered that no regimental hospital equipment of any kind was to be allowed on board. The medical department was a civilian department, and as civilians the doctors protested in vain.[45]

When the allied armies reached Sevastopol a few days later they pitched camp on the heights in front of the south side of Sevastopol. The British established their base hospital, which they called the General or Balaclava General Hospital, in what had been a school. The wounded and sick continued to suffer horribly. On the one night of 2 October a regimental surgeon and forty-six men died in the Balaclava Hospital. When nine tents for Bell's regiment arrived in the camp they were assigned to the officers and regimental hospitals, but they made very poor hospitals because they had been lying in store for forty years and were almost in rags. In addition, the doctors had no medical comforts to offer.[46] Usually the daily ration for a full hospital diet was a pound of meat, a pound of potatoes, two pints of tea, and a half pint of porter. 'Medical comforts' consisted entirely of edible items such as wine, mutton chops, milk, eggs, rice pudding, or jellies which the doctors ordered for individual patients and which the orderlies or later the nurses, not the army kitchen, prepared.[47] In October Bell became quite crippled again with rheumatism. When he felt well enough to eat, one of his mess chums, who was a doctor and who took good care of him otherwise, had only the standard salt pork to feed him. As in the Peninsular War, amputation tools were his only equipment. The whole medical department was 'shamefully and cruelly neglected,' Bell declared, while the positive reports which (later Sir) John Hall, the chief doctor in the Crimean army, was sending to the newspapers were completely untrue.[48] In the Peninsular War Bell had considered the miserable field hospitals and the surgeons' lack of equipment simply a fact of life. It is a reflection of the great strides civilian hospitals had made that he now had much greater expectations of the medical department.

On 14 October the Russians opened a massive bombardment and the next day the allies began what they called their First Bombardment. The allied bombardment was a failure: the Russians suffered very little and were enormously encouraged.[49] The allies had won the Battle of the Alma but the Battle of Balaclava on 25 October, when the Russians attacked the British lines, was a different story. It is usually represented as a British victory, or at the very least as a kind of draw, but from the Russian point of view it was a great Russian victory. Many roads north of Sevastopol had remained open so that supplies and reinforcements poured rapidly into the city, but now the Russians had gained control of the Vorontzov Road, the only metalled road in the Crimea; the British were confined to their inner defense lines where there were only dirt tracks on which to convey their supplies up from the harbor to their camps. The Russians celebrated their Balaclava victory, parading through the town with trophies from the battlefield – British horses, overcoats, swords, and most importantly the British guns they had captured.[50]

The Battle of Inkerman on 5 November more than counterbalanced the Russian victory at Balaclava, for it was a major defeat of a daring Russian attack on the right wing of the British camp. The Russians took the British by surprise early in the morning and appeared to be winning in the early afternoon when Raglan called in French aid, which saved the day. Bell and his regiment were again in the thick of the fight. The next day the British began collecting the Russian wounded. The doctors used an old garden enclosure as a kind of holding pen for them.

> They were ranged round the walls, as thick as they could lie, for the convenience of the army surgeons to use their carving-knives, who were amputating for three days. The unfortunate disabled were day and night exposed to the cold without any covering, nothing to lie on but the wet sod, groaning, yelling, agonised, and dying.

The whole countryside was covered with wounded, and as the dead were removed from the holding pen new Russians were brought in to take their places. It took three days for fatigue parties from every corps to collect them. After lying out in the cold and rain for two nights the soldiers' wounds opened afresh when they were lifted from the ground, and many died before they reached the holding pen. It made Bell's

The wider context of military nursing in the Crimean War

heart bleed to see these Russian soldiers who had fought so bravely suffering so horribly.[51] He thought that in all his forty-three years of soldiering he had never seen such a frightful scene of human misery, and Bell had seen the aftermaths of thirteen great battles as well as many smaller ones and heard the groans and cries of the wounded who were trampled on, both by their own men and the enemy. They were left to the mercy of the French, a ferocious enemy, and the camp followers who rushed out and stripped the wounded and dying, not only of valuables but of their clothes, sometimes leaving them completely naked.[52] One of the English nurses said the men who were wounded at Inkerman often told her how in the long wait to be collected after the battle they lay on the ground listening to the soldiers' piteous cries for water while scavengers passed and repassed them searching for plunder. The officers were a particular target because they went into battle in full dress uniform wearing their decorations and jewellery, and were often killed for the sake of their watches and rings.[53]

As the bitter Crimean winter closed in, the siege continued more or less at a stalemate until April. When the army's baggage finally reached the camp at the end of October the British soldiers' clothing was all in tatters. They were cutting up dead Russians' knapsacks to bind round their legs. Many had no shoes and were barefoot, while others cut up Russian coats to make sandals out of them.[54] Then on 14 November the worst storm in local living memory, referred to in contemporary accounts as a hurricane, struck Sevastopol. It blew down the tents, whirled the weaker men off their feet, and blew horses from their picket posts. The new British screw steamer, the *Prince*, went down with medical supplies and 40,000 warm winter uniforms plus all but six of its 150-man crew. The *Resolute* sank with its cargo of ten million Minié bullets. In Kamiesch the *Henri Quatre*, a battleship, and the steamer *Pluton* sank, while the merchant navy lost two ships with all their crews and supplies.[55] The French army also suffered from the harsh weather, but being better prepared, not as severely. However, its condition worsened as the winter progressed. The commissariat provided inadequate amounts of conserved vegetables, potatoes, and onions, and in the bitter January weather frostbite became a major problem.[56] Like the British, the French artillery was relatively inactive because it was so difficult to transport ammunition from the harbor up to the camp.[57] The British camp was left a sea of

The wider context of military nursing in the Crimean War

mud, with officers and men dragging out their miserable existence in the mud wearing rags with short rations and no fuel. The draft animals were so underfed, weak, and exhausted that they no longer had the strength to pull supplies up to the camp. 'Continued heavy rains,' Bell wrote in late November,

> constant alarms, rations falling short, no rum today, a terrible damper to the poor men. They consider this their greatest privation. They go down to the trenches wet, come back wet, go into the hospital tents wet, die the same night, and are buried in their wet blankets the next morning![58]

Bell asked the regimental surgeon if there wasn't anything that could be done to save the sick. He replied that the men were too far gone when they entered the hospital tents, and since he had no medical restoratives they simply died. Bell thought the surgeons did all they could but their continual demands for necessary supplies were completely ignored.[59] And the reinforcements the army was sending out consisted of what Bell called young inexperienced lads, who quickly succumbed to the harsh living conditions and disease. 'The young lads cannot endure the fatigue,' Bell wrote, 'they lie down wet on the wet sod, helpless, unattended and shiver away their young lives in silent sorrow.'[60] As early as 2 October Clifford had made the same complaint. The replacements had very little training and could not withstand the hardships of the campaign.[61]

By December all the trees and shrubs within walking distance of the camp had been cut down for fuel. The men grubbed up roots to use for cooking their rations. In January some pickaxes were issued for digging the roots out from under the deep snow but soon there was not even a root left within reach of the camp. The French had to help the British bring shot and shell up from Balaclava. At the same time the British government was shipping all kinds of provisions and goods into Balaclava but the commissariat had no way to get the goods up to the camp. The draft animals died from overwork, starvation, and the cold; Bell saw nine cavalry horses die in one night. One morning Bell found five men in his own regiment frozen to death in their tents. 'The early cry is "Bring out your dead!" – something like the London Plague in 1666,' he wrote. Many of his men were badly frostbitten, their hands, fingers, and feet dropping off from gangrene.[62] Ravens swooped overhead while in the rush to get the

The wider context of military nursing in the Crimean War

men buried quickly some dying men were shovelled under while still breathing.[63] The regimental hospitals had little to offer. 'What is an hospital?' Bell asked. 'Any old tent where sick and disabled are huddled together unfit for duty and under the care of a medical officer.'[64] The men lay on wet ground and were so badly cared for that few went into the hospital voluntarily. Their officers had to order them to go.[65] On 19 February Bell found seven of his regiment outside their tent, sewn up in their blankets waiting to be buried. Meanwhile in Balaclava there were thousands of bales of goods with no transport system to deliver them.[66]

At the end of February 1855 Bell himself became very unwell with general debility, failing eyesight, and incapacity for work. A medical board ordered him home. He left Balaclava on 16 March, just when the huge amounts of money the British government was pouring into the war effort began to yield results. Better administration and transport arrangements enabled the army to feed and clothe its men generously. Bell missed the Second Bombardment, the failed assault on Sevastopol on 18 June 1855, the Russians' last desperate attempt to break the siege at the Battle of the Tchernaya on 16 August, and finally on 8 September 1855, after a horrifically bloody fight, the fall of the south side of Sevastopol.

Military medicine in 1854

Although germ theory and aseptic technique would not come until later in the century, medicine had made enormous strides in the seventy years which preceded the Crimean War. It became increasingly based on anatomy and physiology, with doctors aspiring to be considered scientific professionals.[67] Rather than the traditional depleting methods – bleeding, purging, and vomiting – the new medicine emphasized supportive treatments: generous diet, a great deal of alcohol (because at that time it was thought to be a stimulant) as well as cleanliness, rest, and fresh air.[68] Well before anesthesia came in, surgeons were perfecting new and complicated operations, many of which required a good length of time on the operating table for the fully conscious patient. Surgeons aimed to preserve limbs for which previously the only option had been amputation. They called this new approach 'conservative surgery' because they were conserving rather

The wider context of military nursing in the Crimean War

than amputating limbs.[69] Then came the great discovery of anesthesia which gave the surgeons so much more scope for lengthy, complex, and delicate operations. First used in Europe in London in 1846, there was some opposition to it but that died quickly. By the mid-1850s it was in common use and would be widely used in the Crimea.

Military surgery was rather different from civilian surgery because it dealt with problems rarely encountered in civilian life: wounded men. From a surgical point of view, however, as Thomas Longmore (who served in the Crimean War and was later Surgeon-General) pointed out, the advent of the new rifles and bullets meant that gunshot wounds totally outnumbered all other kinds of wounds and were far more severe than those inflicted by the old musket balls. Men with gunshot wounds suffered from pain and especially horribly from thirst as a result of loss of blood, while complications from these wounds could be lethal. Bell was wounded three times during the Peninsular War but never suffered any broken bones. However, he remembered the terrible thirst and drinking more water at that time than he normally did in a whole month.[70] Tissue which died in the track of a bullet sloughed off but could also become gangrenous. Tetanus was considered the worst complication of a gunshot wound because there was nothing the surgeon could do to alleviate it, much less cure it. Gunshot wounds were also especially prone to erysipelas, which was also much dreaded for it could spread and attack deeper structures. Furthermore, it was very difficult to eradicate.[71] A large number of men died from pyemia, which was characterized by high temperature, fever, chills, and painfully swollen joints.[72] Hospital gangrene was a dreadful problem in the Peninsular War, but not a major issue in the Crimean War hospitals, with the exception of the earlier part of the war when many men, who were sent to Scutari by ship with no attendants, suffered from it. Another less lethal but very irritating complication of gunshot wounds was maggots. What appeared to be the common housefly appeared in swarms in the warmer weather in the Crimea and invaded the wounds and settled on the faces and exposed parts of the men. There seemed no way to keep them in check. The best the hospital staff could do was to lay cotton gauze net over wounds which were exposed to the air and they also covered the patients' faces to enable them to get some rest and sleep.[73]

Treatment for all of these complications was typically very labor-intensive. What was known as distant or distal gangrene meant gangrene starting, for example, in the toes or fingers as opposed to beginning in a wound. It was treated with warmth, proper posturing, and wrapping the limb in cotton wool. If the gangrene continued up the limb, amputation was required. Local gangrene was treated by trying to increase the patient's strength. Patients were given easily digested food and stimulants in small quantities, ideally at frequent intervals, and opium for pain. Soldiers with erysipelas were placed in an airy atmosphere, preferably in tents, and, if they were reasonably strong, given purgatives plus diaphoretics and tonics. Wine, alcohol, beef tea, milk, and other light foods were urged if the patient was able to take them. These treatments could only be administered by what Longmore called 'careful and judicious nursing.' Treatment of local inflamed areas varied from surgeon to surgeon. Some surgeons preferred fomentations and linseed poultices; others used leeches, cupping, and repeated punctures. Longmore used the puncture system, which consisted of repeated longitudinal incisions through the integuments about 1½" in length and 2–4" apart, followed by fomentations to promote the escape of blood and serum to ease the patient.[74]

But wounds, however important, accounted for only a small part of the army doctors' work. A far larger proportion of the military doctors' work was with diseases that are also suffered in civilian life. Bowel disease was always the primary medical problem in field armies. At that time doctors recognized three kinds of bowel disease: cholera, dysentery, and diarrhea. There were five different kinds of diarrhea, each requiring a different treatment.[75] All of these different treatments required experienced, knowledgeable nurses. Fevers were the second commonest type of illness. Their treatment was extremely labor-intensive too, because in the days before intravenous fluids these patients had to be spoon-fed fluids frequently, sometimes as often as every five minutes although every half hour was more standard. Frostbite was also common, and the problem all the nurses thought more painful and difficult to treat than gunshot wounds. For a frostbitten foot the standard treatment was to cover the whole foot and ankle with a large linseed poultice. When removed, as well as decayed flesh, the nurses would sometimes find toes in them.[76]

The wider context of military nursing in the Crimean War

There were severe epidemics of typhus leading to extensive bedsores and rapidly spreading hospital gangrene,[77] the worst occurring in the French and Russian armies in the second winter of the war. Scurvy was an almost universal affliction in the British and French armies because the standard field diet consisted of just salt pork and biscuit. In the winter of 1854–55 it affected almost every officer and man in the British army to a greater or lesser extent. It was an underlying disease in almost all the other ailments and radically slowed their recovery.[78] The treatment was purely dietetic, but the necessary lime or lemon juice and vegetables were often unattainable.[79]

All of these treatments, both medical and surgical, placed heavy responsibility on the nurses and required a higher level of competence than most nurses had at the time. Careful and judicious nursing could only be achieved by prior training or by long clinical experience. The French and Piedmontese did have trained nurses in their armies from the beginning and the Russians introduced them in the winter of 1854–55. The Ottoman army had untrained orderlies but appears to have had no nurses as such. The British relied mainly on untrained orderlies as well, but when Florence Nightingale introduced female nurses there were a considerable number of trained religious nurses and many experienced and competent hospital nurses among them. They would make a very big difference in the nursing care.

Notes

1 Bazancourt, *Cinq Mois*, pp. 14–15, 73.
2 Gordon, *Letters*, p. 28.
3 Calthorpe, *Letters from Headquarters*, pp. 276, 281–2.
4 Herbé, *Français & Russes*, pp. 220–1, 226–7; Bazancourt, *Cinq Mois*, pp. 140–5.
5 Totleben, *Défense*, vol. 1, pp. 201–5.
6 Duckers, *War at Sea*, pp. 135–40.
7 Lambert, *Grand Strategy*, pp. 12, 213–14.
8 Longmore, *Gunshot Injuries*, pp. 31–3.
9 Curtiss, *Russian Army*, pp. 126–7.
10 Woods, *Past Campaign*, vol. 1, pp. 363–5; Peard, *Campaign in the Crimea*, pp. 67–8.
11 Curtiss, *Russian Army*, pp. 212–17.
12 Longmore, *Gunshot Injuries*, pp. 43–5.
13 Margrave, 'Dr John W. Morton,' p. 23.

The wider context of military nursing in the Crimean War

14 Macleod, *Surgery in the Crimea*, pp. 98–9.
15 Clifford, *Letters*, p. 50; Small, *From the Ranks*, p. 111; Calthorpe, *Letters from Headquarters*, pp. 107–9.
16 Figes, *Crimean War*, pp. 209–10, 214–15; Curtiss, *Crimean War*, p. 309; Goodlake, *Sharpshooter*, p. 50; Macleod, *Surgery in the Crimea*, p. 115.
17 Curtiss, *Russian Army*, pp. 126–8, 130.
18 Herbé, *Français & Russes*, p. 181.
19 Figes, *Crimean War*, pp. 357–8.
20 Totleben, *Défense*, vol. 1, pp. 41, 45; Curtiss, *Crimean War*, pp. 188–9; Lambert, *Grand Strategy*, pp. 302–3.
21 Hodasevich, *Within Sebastopol*, p. 14.
22 Lambert, *Grand Strategy*, pp. 349–50, Figes, *Crimean War*, pp. 305, 355–6.
23 Draft animals consisted of oxen, horses, ponies, mules, and occasionally camels. Later in the first winter, out of desperation, some of the cavalry horses were used as draft animals.
24 Lambert, *Grand Strategy*, pp. 171–2; Curtiss, *Crimean War*, pp. 337–8.
25 Clifford, *Letters*, p. 106.
26 Bell, *Rough Notes*, p. 96.
27 The Peninsular War consisted of Wellington's campaign pushing the French out of the Iberian peninsula into France from 1808 to 1814.
28 Fortescue, *British Army*, vol. 12, pp. 158–9; Figes, *Crimean War*, pp. 304–11.
29 Bell, *Rough Notes*, p. 127; Figes, *Crimean War*, p. 305.
30 Clifford, *Letters*, p. 197.
31 Bell, *Rough Notes*, pp. 44, 96–7, 30–1.
32 Strachan, *Wellington's Legacy*, pp. 79–82.
33 Figes, *Crimean War*, pp. 177–8.
34 Greig, *Letters from the Crimea*, p. 84.
35 Clifford, *Letters*, p. 144.
36 Bell, *Rough Notes*, pp. 5–6.
37 Blue pill and salts were both essentially cathartics.
38 Bell, *Rough Notes*, pp. 61–2, 64–5, 80–1.
39 Ibid, pp. 80–1, 95.
40 Masquelez, *Journal d'un Officier*, pp. 84–6, 89, 110–15.
41 Bell, *Rough Notes*, pp. 201–3, 205–8, 212–17.
42 Woods, *Past Campaign*, vol. 1, pp. 315–16.
43 Bell, *Rough Notes*, pp. 220–1.
44 Ibid, p. 217; Heath, *Letters*, pp. 63–4, 67; Woods, *Past Campaign*, vol. 1, pp. 371–3.
45 Cantlie, *Medical Department*, vol. 2, pp. 47–8.
46 Bell, *Rough Notes*, pp. 228–9, 231.
47 Taylor, *Eastern Hospitals*, vol. 1, pp. 74, 78.
48 Bell, *Rough Notes*, pp. 231–2.
49 Figes, *Crimean War*, pp. 240–1; Lambert, *Grand Strategy*, pp. 158–63.

The wider context of military nursing in the Crimean War

50 Lambert, *Grand Strategy*, p. 164; Figes, *Crimean War*, pp. 253–4.
51 Bell, *Rough Notes*, p. 247.
52 Ibid, pp. 27, 100, 137.
53 Goodman, *English Sister of Mercy*, pp. 72–3.
54 Bell, *Rough Notes*, p. 241.
55 Ibid, pp. 252–4; Figes, *Crimean War*, pp. 278–80.
56 Scrive, *Relation*, pp. 286–7.
57 Herbé, *Français & Russes*, p. 181.
58 Bell, *Rough Notes*, p. 255.
59 Ibid.
60 Ibid, p. 263.
61 Clifford, *Letters*, pp. 57, 154–5.
62 Bell, *Rough Notes*, pp. 261–7, 273, 275.
63 Ibid, p. 254.
64 Ibid, pp. 261–7.
65 Goodlake, *Sharpshooter*, p. 82.
66 Bell, *Rough Notes*, pp. 277, 279–80.
67 Bynum, *Practice of Medicine*, pp. 94–5, 112–44.
68 Helmstadter and Godden, *Before Nightingale*, pp. 4–8.
69 Lawrence, 'Historiography of Surgery,' pp. 24–5.
70 Longmore, *Gunshot Injuries*, pp. v, 43–4, 55, 57, 155; Bell, *Rough Notes*, p. 81.
71 Longmore, *Gunshot Injuries*, pp. 198–9, 253–4.
72 Ibid, pp. 230, 233, 237.
73 Ibid, pp. 212–17, 399.
74 Ibid, pp. 394–6, 417–20.
75 Cantlie, *Medical Department*, vol. 2, pp. 186–7.
76 Longmore, *Gunshot Injuries*, p. 418; Doyle, 'Memories,' p. 23; Nicol, *Ismeer*, pp. 33–5; Goodman, *English Sister of Mercy*, p. 90.
77 Longmore, *Gunshot Injuries*, pp. 216–17.
78 *Parliamentary Papers* (hereafter *PP*), 1854–55, vol. 20, pp. 8, 11–12; Longmore, *Gunshot Injuries*, p. 202.
79 Cantlie, *Medical Department*, vol. 2, pp. 188–9.

Part I
Government-imposed nursing

2

British nursing at the beginning of the Crimean War

Introduction

There was little nursing in the British army before the Crimean War, and what little there was, was done by doctors. The introduction of female nurses in 1854 would be a major innovation fraught with many difficulties. Perhaps the greatest difficulty was the fact that the government forced female nurses on an unwilling army medical department, placing Florence Nightingale in a complex and highly politicized position. The terrible reputation of hospital nurses, which in many cases was deserved, was not the least of her many challenges. Hospital nurses belonged to the lowest rank of domestic service, and while there were certainly some very able and sober old-style nurses, drink was a dreadful problem among them. From the doctors' point of view, their most egregious shortcoming was failure to carry out medical orders. Young Dr Benjamin Golding was one of the new breed of so-called 'scientific doctors,' the men who based their practice on anatomy and physiology. In 1819 he pointed out that doctors lost many important cases because nurses frequently did not implement doctors' orders, and this was especially true of the night nurses, who were the least competent members of the old nursing staffs. But at the same time, Golding said, many patients whom the doctors had given up as lost had been cured by the kind attentions of a good nurse.[1] Generally speaking, however, at the beginning of the nineteenth century it was only doctors in leading-edge teaching hospitals, such as St. Thomas's where Golding practiced, who appreciated the importance of nursing care. The Charity Commissioners described the hospital nurses in 1837 as performing all the usual duties of servants: they waited on and cleaned the patients, beds, furniture, wards, and stairs.[2]

Government-imposed nursing

Placing patients in the same category as the furniture and stairs was characteristic of the way the upper classes viewed the lower classes. Almost two generations ago Leonore Davidoff delineated this scornful attitude.[3] Gertrude Himmelfarb argued that the upper classes identified the working classes with the effluvia of their polluted cities.[4] Himmelfarb's conclusion seems rather extreme, but the fact was that hospital nurses actually worked with the effluvia of their patients. Traditionally the first duty of the head nurse was to see that the ward was always neat and clean and that all filth and stools were carried out twice a day. As late as 1864 the Charity Commissioner reported on inspecting St. Thomas's Hospital that although the windows were always wide open twenty-four hours a day, the wards had 'an almost intolerable stench,'[5] and this was at a time when bad smells were believed to cause disease. The nurses, on their hands and knees, scoured and cleaned the beds, other furniture, floors of the wards and the halls, stairs, and garrets. In addition, they cleaned incontinent patients and their bedding, attended the surgeons while they dressed the patients, taking away all the foul materials and providing clean dressings. They also attended the working of all enemas and vomits.[6]

At mid-century the term 'servant' would more accurately have described the assistant nurses. In the 1850s 'assistant nurse' meant what we might now call a floor nurse (or staff nurse in the UK), the regular nurse as opposed to head nurses, or sisters as they were called in the medieval hospitals and Guy's Hospital. Because today an assistant nurse usually refers to a practical nurse who has a much shorter training than a Registered Nurse, I will refer to the earlier nineteenth-century assistant nurses simply as nurses to prevent them from being confused with the modern, less well-trained assistant nurses. British hospital nurses in 1854 were actually charwomen who also attended to the wants of bedridden patients, and in less important cases made and applied poultices. Some of the sisters, although by no means all, were what we would now call real nurses. If they were interested in their patients and worked in a ward where the doctor was willing to teach them, sisters could become very effective nurses.[7] Two of Nightingale's best working-class nurses, Eliza Roberts and Susan Cator, were head nurses with many years of experience. Dr Steele, the highly competent and very observant professional administrator at Guy's Hospital, thought the trend to increase the number of nurses per patient and to separate nursing work from that of ordinary domestic service had only started in the late 1850s, in other words after the Crimean War. Steele was referring to the nursing sisterhood of St. John's House, who took over the nursing at King's College Hospital in 1856 and began the systematic reform of nursing. Their reforms were based on treating the nurses with respect, heavier staffing, and removing all the cleaning duties from the nurses. From the point of view of most hospital administrators in 1854, however, nurses were essentially maids and not an important part of patient care. It would be many years before this attitude changed.

The British army medical department in 1854: a civilian department in a decentralized and antiquated army

Introducing female nurses into the British army was made doubly difficult because the army medical department was hobbled by an outdated administration. The French medical department suffered from the same structural problem of an administration which had not kept up with advances in warfare and military medicine. There had been significant improvements in the qualifications required of British army surgeons since the Napoleonic Wars but the position of regimental surgeon remained in the gift of the colonel and was still often openly bought and sold. For example, Sir James McGrigor, Director General of the Army Medical Department from 1815–51, bought his position in the Connaught Rangers for £150.[8] There was an insurmountable divide between the regular army officers and the army surgeons, whom the officers very much looked down upon. Because the medical service was a civilian department, doctors had no authority over their orderlies or patients. Making its administration even more difficult, there were two distinct branches of medical staff, the regimental surgeons and the medical officers. Each regiment had its own surgeon, who did not report to Dr Andrew Smith, the Director General of the Army Medical Department, but rather to the regiment's colonel, giving the Director little control of regimental doctors. As well as having no authority over his orderlies and patients, the regimental surgeon had no resources, supplies, or transport services except what his colonel was willing to give him. That was often very little, as Bell learned when he was ill, because

Government-imposed nursing

the needs of the fighting men were considered more important than those of the wounded and sick. The second branch of the department consisted of the medical staff officers who served at headquarters, in the few peacetime hospitals, and in the base hospitals that were established for expeditionary forces. The Director General did have control over these doctors.[9]

At the beginning of the Crimean War the medical department suffered grievously from belonging to an antiquated army. The officer corps tended to be aristocrats, men who had 'influence,' or very wealthy men who bought their commissions and whose military education tended to be poor.[10] Placing social status above military competency, as the purchase of commissions did, caused what Geoffrey Best called gerontocracy, snobbishness, and inflexibility in the officer corps. It would be a central problem in the army until the Cardwell reforms in 1871.[11] Bell is an illustration of the gerontocracy. He was 60 years old when he landed in Turkey in 1854, admittedly younger than Raglan who was 65 and Sir John Burgoyne, the army's chief engineer who was 72,[12] but nevertheless an older man. Although Bell had a great deal of talent he had progressed very slowly through the upper ranks because he had neither money nor influence. For the private soldiers there was no draft as in continental armies. Men volunteered but the pay was so low and their term of service so long – twenty-one years – that the army as a career had little appeal to anyone except those who were desperately poor. During the war, in an effort to attract more recruits, the army introduced two new classes: a term of two years and a term of ten.[13] In the early 1850s the British economy was booming and able young men could easily find much better jobs. Efforts to attract more volunteers only resulted in the young, untrained lads whom Bell described as unable to endure the fatigue of trench warfare and lying down helplessly on the wet ground and dying. When these new drafts arrived they were hardly trained at all: they were young campaigners who did not know their trade.[14]

Inkerman was a disaster for the Russian army, which lost 11,959 men. The official figure for allied losses was 4,338, which was probably too low because the French always under-reported their losses. The British army did not recover until the following spring and the Russian army never really recovered. But it was a pyrrhic victory for the allies, and as the bad weather set in and desertions from the allied camps increased, Raglan desperately needed more soldiers. Unable to recruit men at home, the British government was forced to hire mercenary soldiers. By the 1850s international law deemed recruiting foreign soldiers a breach of neutrality, which made this process difficult. In the summer of 1854 the British army in the East was roughly 21,500 men, about a third the size of the French army. It was not until it was planning the unrealized 1856 campaign that the army reached equality with the French and somewhat outnumbered them. Then the French had 96,000 men in the field and the British 107,000, but only 61,000 of the 107,000 were British – the rest were foreign troops.[15] To add to the difficulties of this conglomerate army, it was a parliamentary army and Parliament had constantly curbed army expenditure during the peace years between 1815 and 1854.[16] In addition, the army's administration, like much of the British government in the earlier nineteenth century, was highly decentralized. The Crown exercised nominal control of the army but executive control lay with three Secretaries of State: Home, Foreign Affairs, and War and the Colonies. The control of the Home and Foreign Affairs offices was rather tenuous. The Foreign Office had some responsibility for troops used abroad in places outside the colonies and the Home Office was in charge of forces in the United Kingdom, leaving the Secretary of State for War and the Colonies as the primary political director of the army.

The Treasury played a major part in army administration. The Secretary *at* War, basically a financial officer, was a member of this department; he did not report to the Secretary *of* War and the Colonies. However, in order to function properly there had to be collaboration between the various departments. The Commander-in-Chief of the Army in 1854, Viscount Henry Hardinge, did better than most because he was a close friend of Sidney Herbert, then Secretary at War, and they worked well together.[17] The Secretary at War was also responsible to the Master-General of Ordnance. The commissariat, like the medical department, was a wholly civilian department so the army officers had no control over it. It reported to the Treasury – not War and the Colonies – and supplied food, non-military stores, fuel, forage, and light. It also supplied its own transport, which it failed to provide in the first winter of the war. Smith commented in 1855 that

Government-imposed nursing

he could have done all his work twice as fast if he had been reporting to a single person.[18] Lord Palmerston, who had been Secretary at War for many years, made somewhat of an understatement when he wrote in 1836, 'The present subdivision of the administration of the affairs of the Army into several departments is inconvenient.'[19]

The 'regular forms,' or bureaucratic red tape, presented another horrible problem. In addition to all of the duplications of responsibilities, the army was hamstrung with narrow bureaucratic regulations and forms, making quick action almost impossible and denying any kind of initiative to individuals. When the Roebuck Commission, one of several parliamentary commissions established to investigate the conduct of the war, questioned Smith, the commissioners were quite incredulous when he described the uncertainty of authority and conflicts between the various departments that the medical department had to deal with. Surely the purveyor did not have the authority to countermand the superior medical authority in the hospital?, one commissioner asked. Smith replied that he did not think he did, but the purveyor thought differently. In his lengthy evidence of over eighty printed pages Smith explained that, after being expected to save money for forty years, when Herbert gave him a much bigger budget he could not believe he had the power to spend money without going through the regular forms.[20]

The 64 year old James Filder, who had been recalled from retirement to become head of the commissariat, would later defend the actions of his department by saying that he had not distributed lime juice and vegetables or provided fuel for the soldiers – all of which were actually right in Balaclava, in ships in the harbor – because he had not been given specific orders to do so.[21] When the British Ambassador to Turkey sent a whole ship of cabbages and vegetables to Balaclava, no one was willing to take the responsibility of signing for them because they had not been issued by the commissariat and the clerks were afraid they would be held personally financially responsible. As a result the vegetables rotted and in the end were all thrown overboard. When supplies came in, the shot and shell were usually packed on top of other items such as medical supplies and clothing. Because the commissariat officers at Balaclava had specific orders to unpack the ammunition but no specific orders to unload anything else, the ships often left with the warm clothing still on board.[22] Smith said that some of the supplies he sent to the Scutari hospitals 'knocked about' for a month or two before being delivered.[23]

When Nightingale dealt directly with Purveyor-General Matthew Wreford, whom she called 'that vain, silly, swearing old man,' she fared no better. Wreford refused to supply carpenters with knives and forks although he had 7,500 in his store, and would not give them rations 'unless the officer of engineers wrote "urgent" on the form and asked it as "as a favour."'[24] Worse still, by November 1854 the army's transport system for provisions and ordnance, as well as transport for the wounded and sick, was almost non-existent. The standard practice had been to contract with local civilians for wagons and draft animals but the army was operating on a small strip of land in enemy territory (see Map 4) and quickly exhausted local supplies.[25] In the Peninsular War the army recruited Spanish muleteers whom Bell considered 'the very life and sustenance of the army.' They formed the land transport corps, then called the Royal Waggon (*sic*) Train, a part of the army which Wellington considered absolutely essential, but it was disbanded in 1833 to save money. Raglan asked to have it re-established but this did not happen until March 1855.[26]

The declaration of war at the end of March 1854 did force a number of major improvements in army administration. Lord Aberdeen launched a good deal of centralization before his government fell at the end of January 1855. The decision to transfer the commissariat from the Treasury to the War Department, making it a military department, was made in May 1854 and completed by December 1854. However, more responsibility was not transferred to army officers in the field.[27] Within a week of assuming office as Secretary of War in the new Palmerston government in February 1855, Lord Panmure merged the office of Secretary at War with that of Secretary for War. He then insisted that a chief of staff be appointed to supervise Raglan's staff officers and ensure that Raglan's orders were enforced. Panmure was both an experienced army officer and an experienced politician. He spent twelve years, from 1819 to 1831, in the army before entering politics in 1835. He served as Secretary at War in Lord John Russell's government, which took power in 1846. Moreover he had a personal interest in the dreadful conditions under which the Crimean army was laboring because his brother, Colonel Lauderdale Maule of the Highland Brigade, died of cholera in

Bulgaria in August 1854. Panmure was known as the 'Bison' because of his shaggy head of hair and hot temper but he was a real army reformer. Previously four independent army forces worked side by side: the Royal Engineers planned and laid out batteries and parallels; the infantry built and defended them; the Royal Artillery and the Naval Brigade mounted and fought the guns. By June 1855 Panmure had placed the military branch of the Ordnance, the artillery and engineers, under the Commander-in-Chief and the civilian branches under his own direction. The War Department took charge of the soldiers' clothing, the commissariat, and medical departments. Only the office of Commander-in-Chief maintained a separate existence. The Duke of Newcastle, then Secretary for War and the Colonies, sent the civilian navvies to build a railroad from the port in Balaclava up to the camp on the heights, but it was Panmure who sent a commission to investigate the supply system and who re-established the Royal Waggon Train with the new name of Land Transport Corps.[28]

The question of female nurses for the army: social conventions versus nursing efficiency

Before war was declared Smith placed orders with the Admiralty for invalid foods, palliasses, hospital beds, blankets, sheets, hospital canteens, and other medical supplies. Due to the lack of coordination between the various departments that provided and transported these supplies, none had left England when the expeditionary force sailed at the end of March.[29] Smith did not see providing nurses as his most pressing job, but at the beginning of the war the War Department did ask the army doctors to consider the French practice of using female nurses in their military hospitals. The army doctors were opposed to the idea because, they explained, they had tried hospital nurses (who in Britain at this time were all women) on a number of occasions and they were 'very much addicted to drink, and often more callous to the sufferings of the soldiers than those male attendants [orderlies] who had been employed more recently.'[30] The government was forced to take a different approach to female military nurses when on 12 October 1854 Thomas Chenery set off a public outcry with his famous article in *The Times* describing the lack of care for the soldiers following the Alma. The army did not have enough surgeons, Chenery

British nursing at the beginning of the Crimean War

reported, and had no dressers or nurses. The next day he described the French medical corps and its well-equipped base hospitals in Constantinople run by the Daughters of Charity. On 14 October *The Times* published a letter asking:

> Why have we no Sisters of Charity? There are numbers of able-bodied and tender-hearted English women who would joyfully and with alacrity go out to devote themselves to nursing the sick and wounded, if they could be associated for that purpose, and placed under proper protection.[31]

This letter expressed both the public's distress about the poor care of the soldiers and the widespread belief that nursing was an inborn talent of women, who were widely believed to be naturally more kindly than men. Their biological role as mothers made them innately good nurses so they needed no special education or experience in hospital nursing. They had only to be able-bodied, tender-hearted and, as supposedly vulnerable and innocent persons, needed proper protection. The terrible uproar in the press created a severe public relations problem for the government, forcing it to reconsider the issue of female nurses.

Despite the disapproval of the military doctors, Newcastle was open to women nurses. But, he explained, 'The difficulty was to find any lady who was competent to undertake so great a task as the organisation of such a body; and I confess I despaired, having seen one or two [of the ladies who volunteered] of making the attempt …'[32] This was indeed a major obstacle because although hospital matrons, who would be the obvious choice today, were responsible for all the female servants including the nurses, in the earlier nineteenth century matrons were not nurses, nor were they responsible for the nursing care of the patients. It was the more conscientious doctors and their medical students who took on the nursing of the acutely ill.[33] The matron's job was to see that the hospital was in good order and clean, the linen supply and furniture well maintained, meals properly prepared and served on time, and – what Golding considered the most important part of her work – she presided over the morals of the female staff, seeing that they carried out their duties in a respectable manner. The matron also, Golding explained, 'superintends those departments which could not be so well regulated by a person of the other sex.'[34] Victorian society was ideologically divided into two separate spheres, a male or public arena, and for upper-class ladies, a domestic or female arena. In the class-bound society of mid-Victorian England the term 'lady' usually meant a middle- or upper-class woman who did not support herself, which differentiated her from working-class women, women who worked for a wage. Women were thought intellectually and physically inferior to men, and if the woman was a lady she had a special mission – she should be high-minded, more religious, and if married, totally dedicated to motherhood and submissive to her husband. Women also had to be directed by women, as Golding indicated, and it was inappropriate for ladies to interact with men in the public sphere of which hospitals, and especially the all male military hospitals, were a part. A later chapter will demonstrate that this British convention did not obtain in Russia: there it was not a problem when a man directed female nurses.

The concept of woman's mission, and the relegation of ladies to an entirely domestic sphere seems alien, if not silly, to us today, but it is important to keep in mind that it was widely accepted by both sexes in the earlier nineteenth century. Anna Jameson, a leader of the woman's movement, wrote in the 1850s that despite their celebrated surgeons and physicians, hospitals lacked the 'tender, human, sympathizing love' which only 'thoughtful and kindly women of higher classes' could provide. Hospitals needed the 'presence of feminine nature to *minister* through love as well as the masculine intellect to rule through power.'[35] In other words, it was only upper-class women who were thoughtful and kindly, while women in general lacked intellect and could not rule through power. Men, on the other hand, lacked tender love and the ability to nurture. In the following chapters this idea will appear again and again, although far more often in the British setting. One must remember that while this belief appears to be class and gender bias to us today, women, even a leader of the women's movement, believed it to be a fact of life in the Crimean War era.

When Herbert suggested Florence Nightingale as a possible director for female nurses, Newcastle took heart because he knew her personally. 'We felt,' he said, 'that anything she undertook would be successful.'[36] And indeed Nightingale was uniquely qualified for the position. She was not an aristocrat but she moved easily in aristocratic circles. Her father had given her the education of a man: her Greek and Latin were better than that of most men she would work with, she spoke and wrote excellent French, knew Italian and German, and had a good grasp of constitutional history and mathematics.[37] She had trained for three months at the Deaconess' Institute of Kaiserswerth, and gained considerable clinical nursing knowledge and administrative experience running a small London hospital for gentlewomen in Harley Street, London. Equally importantly, she was well prepared for this politically driven appointment because she came from a very political family. Her grandfather, William Smith, an MP for forty-six years, was a leader in the movements to reform Parliament, abolish the slave trade, and repeal the Test and Corporations Act. Smith was very fond of his grandchildren, visiting them frequently, and Nightingale was 15 when he died so she knew him well. Her father, W. E. Nightingale, served as a county administrator. In 1832 he and her uncle, MP John Bonham-Carter, helped organize Lord Palmerston's campaign for re-election. In 1834, W. E. Nightingale stood for Parliament himself but was not elected.[38] Florence was also very charming and socially accomplished. After meeting her in 1844 Julia Ward Howe described her as 'rather elegant than beautiful; she was tall and graceful of figure, her countenance mobile and expressive, her conversation most interesting.'[39] She was deeply religious although not conventionally so, and a mystic. For Nightingale, Crimean War nursing was a sacred mission. On 20 October 1854, the day before leaving for the East, she wrote a prayer of self-dedication in her copy of Thomas à Kempis. She prayed:

> I adore your eternal designs; I submit myself to them with all my heart, for the love of You. I will everything, I accept everything, I offer you everything and I make my sacrifice one with that of Jesus Christ my Saviour.[40]

On 14 October 1854 she wrote to her friend Elizabeth (Lizzie) Herbert that she was about to lead a small private expedition to Scutari. She planned to go privately with several nurses.[41] She and her nurses would be no cost to the government. Smith and Lord Palmerston, then Home Secretary in the Aberdeen government and a Nightingale family friend, had already approved the plan. Nightingale was anxious to know what Lizzie's husband Sidney, as Secretary at War, thought of the scheme. Did Mr Herbert think the

Government-imposed nursing

authorities would object, and would he give any advice or letters of recommendation? Although Dr Smith said nothing was needed, did Mr Herbert think they should take any supplies for the hospital? Lord Palmerston had asked Lord Clarendon, the Foreign Secretary, to write to the ambassador in Constantinople for his support of the venture. She wondered if she should apply to the Duke of Newcastle for his approval. While she appreciated that she needed government authorization, Nightingale did not seek official government status. 'Perhaps it is better,' she told Lizzie, 'to keep it quite a private thing and not apply to government qua government.'

Nightingale was well aware of the latent opposition to female nurses. She thought the fate of the expedition lay entirely in Smith's hands. Irritated by *The Times*' unfavorable accounts of the army medical department, he was prepared to support Nightingale and her small party if they went quietly and privately. But, she wrote, 'if we went with a great body of nurses to take possession of the hospital he would decidedly oppose us.' Smith was actually not opposed to female nurses as such: he suggested that Nightingale start with a few nurses and then, if they were well accepted, have another group follow in ten days.[42] Nightingale thought it would be 'infinitely easier to pioneer the way with three or four women than to march in (even supposing it possible) with a great batch of undisciplined women not knowing what places to assign them, in so new a position as a military hospital.'[43] She hoped to start the following Tuesday '*if* we go,' she told Lizzie Herbert. On reaching Constantinople she planned on leaving her nurses there,

> thinking the Medical Staff at Scutari will be more frightened than amused at being bombarded by a parcel of women, & I cross over to Scutari with someone from the Embassy to present my credentials from Dr Smith, & put ourselves at the disposal of the Drs. My uncle went down this morning to ask my father & mother's consent.[44]

It is indicative of the restraints Victorian society placed on unmarried women that Nightingale, who was then 34 years old and had been running a hospital in London for a year, required her parents' permission to go to the East. When Herbert appealed to her to organize the nursing team, he asked, 'There is one point which I have hardly a right to touch upon, but I know you will pardon me. If you were inclined to undertake this great work, would Mr and Mrs Nightingale give their consent?' In fact, Nightingale's parents had already partly agreed to her projected private expedition and were enthusiastic about the government project.[45] In the same way Nightingale could not go to Scutari without a chaperone. Her old friends Charles and Selena Bracebridge agreed to go with her. Like everyone else, they were expecting the war to be over quickly and hoped to be home within two months.[46]

On receiving Herbert's letter, dated 15 October, Nightingale immediately dropped her plan for the private expedition. Like Newcastle, Herbert did not think the ladies who had volunteered were competent to direct a nursing team. They had no conception of what a hospital was, the nature of nursing duties, or the need for strict obedience to military regulations. Nightingale was the only person in England whom he considered capable of organizing a large staff of female nurses. He thought it impossible for women to nurse in the field but Scutari was a fixed base hospital, hundreds of miles from the war zone and would therefore be safe. Thinking of Scutari as the only base hospital, Herbert officially appointed her 'Superintendent of the female nursing establishment in the English General Military Hospitals in Turkey.' Hall, as Chief Medical Officer, would later use this title to claim that Nightingale had no jurisdiction over the nurses in Russia. Herbert knew how hard it would be to find respectable nurses and how difficult it would be to introduce a system among them. Getting the new nursing team to work smoothly with the medical and military authorities was an additional difficulty, but he knew Nightingale could do it. 'Your own personal qualities,' he told her, 'your knowledge and your power of administration, and among greater things your rank and position in Society give you advantages in such a work which no other person possesses.'[47] Herbert's view that Nightingale's social status placed her at a greater advantage than did her nursing and administrative abilities was entirely correct – British society in the 1850s was hierarchical and highly deferential. While today we might resent the manifold privileges and power the upper classes enjoyed, in the first part of the nineteenth century, generally speaking, the lower classes accepted this social structure as ordained by God and a fact of life.[48] Apart from the small number of doctors who had worked with Nightingale at Harley Street, few

Government-imposed nursing

people would even have been aware of her nursing knowledge and administrative abilities, and much less respected them, whereas her many government and aristocratic connections were all widely esteemed.

The arrangements were made very quickly. Nightingale met Herbert on 16 October.[49] Two days later the Cabinet unanimously approved her appointment as superintendent of a female nursing team.[50] The next day she received her official appointment. She was given complete authority over the nurses subject to the sanction and approval of the chief medical officer under whose orders she was placed.[51] Strict obedience to doctors was essential because government-paid female nurses were a new experiment that the army doctors originally refused, and the politicians were anxious that the nurses cause as little disruption as possible. Nightingale would later summarize Herbert's instructions as first, 'Establish no separate action from the Medical Men but be their lieutenant & purveyor to carry out their intentions,' and second, she was to prevent the hospitals from becoming a 'polemical arena' for all the various religious denominations among her nurses.[52] Indicating the centrality of religion and religious controversy in contemporary politics, Herbert asked Nightingale to engage nurses from all religious sects. The number of Roman Catholics in Britain was steadily increasing as Irish immigrants flooded into the workplace, intensifying the powerful tradition of anti-Catholicism in Britain, which went back to the sixteenth century. There had been no Roman Catholic bishops in England since the Reformation, but in 1850 the Pope re-established the standard ecclesiastical hierarchy of bishops. This came to be called the 'Papal Aggression,' and set off a virulent wave of anti-Catholicism.[53] Both Lord Aberdeen's coalition government, which sent Nightingale to the East, and Palmerston's Whig government, which came into power at the beginning of February 1855, were dependent on the Irish vote in Parliament and therefore tried to avoid alienating Roman Catholics.[54]

Herbert therefore instructed Nightingale not to show favoritism to any one religious confession: he definitely wanted Catholics in the nursing team, but only a limited number. He ordered Nightingale to maintain a ratio of one Catholic nurse to every three Protestants in any given hospital.[55] In his written instructions on 19 October 1854 he told Nightingale:

> I rely on your discretion and vigilance carefully to guard against any attempt being made among those under your authority, selected as they are with a view to fitness and without any reference to religious creed, to make use of their position in the Hospitals to tamper with or disturb the religious opinions of the patients of any denomination whatever, and at once to check any such tendency and to take, if necessary, severe measures to prevent its repetition.[56]

Herbert's instructions are another illustration of the very political nature of Nightingale's mission. She fully understood this aspect of her mission and, with one major exception, strictly obeyed Herbert's orders throughout her stay in the East. The exception was that she almost immediately started using a higher ratio of Roman Catholic to Protestant nurses. Her reason for this was that Catholic nuns were eminently respectable and many were accomplished nurses. However, she insisted that the nurses care only for the bodily needs of the patients and leave spiritual care to the chaplains.

Recruiting the first party of nurses: clinical experience and political considerations

Between the afternoon of 16 October when she met with Herbert and 21 October when she left London for Paris, there were four days to find forty nurses. For political reasons Herbert was anxious to send a good number, and Nightingale appreciated Herbert's political position and agreed to take a party of forty. 'I sacrificed my own judgment and went out with forty females,' she later told him,

> well knowing that half that number would be both more efficient and less trouble – and that the difficulty of inducing forty untrained women, in so extraordinary a position as this (turned loose among 3000 men) to observe any order or even any of the directions of the medical men, would be Herculean.[57]

Her most difficult job at Harley Street had been building a trustworthy nursing staff, a problem shared by all London hospitals, including the prestigious and wealthy teaching institutions such as St. Bartholomew's and St. Thomas's. At Harley Street Nightingale had only one nurse, Theresa Foster, with whom she was completely satisfied.[58] She described her other nurses as slovenly, unhandsome, and unpunctual.[59] The nurses' lack of punctuality was by no means their fault for clocks were a rarity in hospitals in the 1850s. When Nightingale made this comment she was actually writing to her mother to thank her for donating a clock to the hospital. Her comments about the nurses' appearance can sound unkind to the modern ear but they were an accurate description. The nurses' unattractive appearance was a result of their living and working conditions. Nursing was usually a job of last resort which attracted older unskilled women. As well as their dreadful workload, as described earlier, the nurses' living conditions exacerbated their inability to acquire a neat, tidy appearance. In the first half of the century they worked sixteen-hour days with one day off a month at best; they lived in the often rat-infested hospitals' attics and cellars, which were cold in winter and hot in summer. At St. Bartholomew's Hospital, the wealthiest of the London hospitals, about half the nurses lived in tiny rooms carved out of the space under the staircases in the hall. The rooms had no windows and only two beds for three nurses. Each nurse had to work every third night after her day shift and then work the next day's day shift, making a thirty-six-hour shift, but it did free up a bed for the third nurse. There was usually a bathroom for the patients in the basement of the hospital where they were to be bathed before being admitted to the wards, but no water closets or bathrooms for the nurses, who usually did their laundry in the scullery when working nights.[60] It is probable that most nurses never had a bath in their lives; water was a scarce commodity for the poor. At the Westminster Hospital Dr Roe hesitated to prescribe warm baths for his patients because it meant the nurses had to carry so many pails of hot water from the basement along the passages and up the stairs to the moveable bath tubs on the wards.[61] It is unlikely that after finishing her sixteen-hour shift a nurse would be prepared to go to so much trouble in order to have a bath. With the best will in the world, these nurses could not help appearing untidy and unattractive. Nightingale was describing a reality, not being unkind when she called her nurses slovenly and unhandsome.

Furthermore, these working conditions led the working classes to what the wealthy young Friedrich Engels called 'the maddest excess.' Engels was a very sympathetic observer who knew the working classes intimately, in part because he lived monogamously with an Irish

British nursing at the beginning of the Crimean War

mill girl for twenty years, until she died. They never married because Engels considered marriage, and especially church-ordained marriage, oppression. 'All conceivable evils,' he wrote in 1844, 'are heaped upon the heads of the poor,' especially in big cities. 'They are deprived of all enjoyments except that of sexual indulgence and drunkenness, and are worked every day to the point of complete exhaustion of their mental and physical energies, and are thus constantly spurred on to the maddest excess in the only two enjoyments at their command.'[62] Drunkenness was one of the major failings of nurses and orderlies, as the next chapters will show. The working classes also showed the lack of restraint – or what we would call lack of the self-discipline which was so important to the Victorian middle classes – in squabbling, bickering, and failure to control their tempers. Like drunkenness, the new lady superintendents would have to deal constantly with squabbling and displays of temper.

These common characteristics of many hospital nurses made it very difficult to recruit an efficient team of clinically experienced women for the new venture of female nurses in military hospitals. Nightingale felt under severe pressure to find nurses she could rely on to maintain respectability, which the Victorians usually referred to as 'propriety'. She took only one nurse from Harley Street, her matron Mrs Clarke whom she considered invaluable, 'an army in herself.'[63] Clarke was not what we would now call a nurse but, as Dr Steele pointed out, people did not distinguish between nursing and domestic service at that time. But where to find another thirty-nine experienced and respectable nurses? Nightingale went first to women's organizations. There were two that were devoted entirely to nursing: Mrs Fry's Devonshire Square Sisters and St. John's House. Founded in 1840 by Elizabeth Fry, the Quaker philanthropist and prison reformer, the Devonshire Sisters of Mercy were not, as their name would suggest, a religious sisterhood, but rather secular nurses who had a little hospital experience.[64] The Sisters' board of governors, at this point, was not willing to send nurses to the East unless they remained under their own control. Nightingale, who already had to report to three authorities – the army doctors, the military officers, and the War Department – did not want a fourth, so no Fry nurses went in the original party. Nightingale was disappointed because it was a very Protestant institution and would have demonstrated her effort to avoid sectarianism.[65] Later the Devonshire Square Sisters sent three nurses to the army hospitals and three to the naval hospital at Therapia.[66]

Next, Nightingale went to St. John's House. Like Mrs Fry's Sisters, St. John's House was devoted entirely to nursing, but unlike them it was a real sisterhood, albeit a lay sisterhood: the Sisters did not take lifelong vows. Founded in 1848, this sisterhood was quite revolutionary in that it trained both lady and working-class nurses together. A lady could do charitable work part-time, but to work for a salary meant a loss of social status – it made her a working-class woman. St. John's House got around this problem by paying their working-class nurses but not the lady nurses. Their full-time unpaid work qualified as traditional Christian charity so they maintained their social status as ladies. Still, to most people it was unthinkable for ladies to work side by side with working-class women, doing what was considered menial work. Nightingale knew St. John's House personally. She had had many discussions with Miss Elizabeth Frere, their first Lady Superintendent, when she was preparing to take over the Harley Street hospital, and Frere had taken her to visit the sisterhood's home. At the end of May 1853 Nightingale sent Theresa Foster there for three months' training.[67] Since St. John's House nurses did only nursing care and no cleaning, at Harley Street Foster refused to do any housework. Nightingale and Clarke found this problematic, but Nightingale still considered Foster her most satisfactory nurse.[68] On 19 October Herbert, Army Chaplain-General George Gleig, Charles Bracebridge, Nightingale's father, and Nightingale herself met with the St. John's House Council. Six working-class nurses volunteered. The Council agreed to suspend its rules and accepted the government contract. Nightingale would have sole control of the nurses and the government would give the nurses a generous wage and pay for their uniforms, board, and round trip to Scutari. It would not pay their return fare if they were fired. In the contract Nightingale named as causes for dismissal what she considered the three worst failings of hospital nurses: neglect of duty, immoral conduct, and intoxication.[69]

Nightingale went to two more Anglican sisterhoods. These sisterhoods were High Church, which St. John's House was not, and they differed from St. John's House also in that they did social work as well as nursing. The first was the Order of the Holy Cross, more commonly known as the Park Village sisterhood because it was situated near Regent's Park. Mother Superior Emma Langston, Sister Etheldreda Pillans, and the Honorable Harriet Erskine, who was visiting the sisterhood but not yet a member, all volunteered. The second sisterhood, the Devonport Sisters of Mercy, was founded by Priscilla Lydia Sellon in 1848. Nightingale had followed these Sisters' work during the cholera epidemic of 1849 when they established and ran a temporary hospital, and they nursed again in the cholera outbreak of 1853. Sellon sent five Sisters: Sarah Anne Terrot, Clara Sharpe, Bertha Turnbull, Margaret Goodman, and Elizabeth Wheeler. On the night before the eight Sisters left London, Mother Emma was formally made Superior of the small group; Erskine was made a novice, and she and Goodman, who was an aspirant, received Sisters' habits.[70] In an effort to disassociate herself from the much maligned High Church practices of the Devonport and Park Village sisterhoods, Nightingale always referred to these Sisters as Sellonites, but no one else used this term. Finally, the Roman Catholic Bishop of Southwark, Dr Thomas Grant, sent five nuns from the Convent of Mercy at Bermondsey. Grant wanted to make up his full quota of ten of the forty nurses and tried to recruit five Sisters from the Irish Sisters of Mercy but, although later they would send a contingent of fifteen nuns, they did not send any in October 1854. Grant then recruited five nuns from the Convent of Our Lady of the Orphans in Norwood.[71]

Because they had clinical experience, Nightingale was anxious to enlist hospital nurses, and asked her friends Elizabeth Herbert, Mary Stanley, and Selena Bracebridge to advertise publicly for them, stipulating that applicants must have clinical experience and be at least 24 years old. The three ladies interviewed applicants in the Herberts' Belgrave Square home. Many women applied – there are letters and testimonials from 617 women in the National Archives and many more women, who either could not write or did not have references, appeared in person. Stanley reported that they scoured London, sending emissaries in every direction, but found very few nurses who seemed suitable. In the end they hired sixteen hospital nurses so that with the ten Roman Catholic nuns, eight Anglican Sisters, and six St. John's House nurses they met Herbert's desired number of thirty Protestants and ten Catholics. However, while in Paris Nightingale

Government-imposed nursing

tried to recruit more Catholic Sisters from the Daughters of Charity but was unsuccessful.

When the nursing party reached Constantinople there were only thirty-eight women in addition to Nightingale. Before leaving London Nightingale decided that Nurse Dorothy Travers was unsuitable, and Nurse Larscher became ill in Marseilles and had to return home.[72] Hence only fourteen working-class nurses – or hospital nurses as the ladies called them, although not all had hospital experience – arrived in the East on 4 November 1854. Then, before the party disembarked in Constantinople, Nightingale fired another nurse, Nurse Wilson, sending her home immediately. Wilson had arrived at the railway station in London so drunk that the station master turned her away. She then went to Nightingale's parents who gave her money to go to Marseilles where, having travelled first class, she joined the other nurses. On the voyage to the East she announced that she had not come for the paltry ten shillings a week which the government was to pay her, but planned to desert at the first opportunity.[73]

The principal British nurses: the untrained orderlies

Nightingale could not take care of all the thousands of sick and wounded in Scutari with thirty-seven nurses; she had to rely heavily on hospital orderlies for most of the basic nursing care. The traditional method of recruiting these men consisted of the military commandant of the hospital asking the various regiments to send him men who could be used as orderlies, stewards, shopkeepers, and cooks. Doctors also used convalescent soldiers as orderlies. As a general rule the regimental officers sent their worst soldiers, men they were glad to be rid of. These men were given no training whatsoever for the various jobs they were assigned,[74] while the convalescent orderlies were sent back to the front as soon as they were well enough so they had no opportunity to learn from experience.[75] Private Edward Jennings was in the latter group. He had arrived sick at the Scutari General Hospital on 22 September 1854 and was made an orderly on 29 September, the day the wounded began pouring in from the Alma. 'I did not like to go as orderly,' he explained later, 'but the adjutant picked me out of the ranks with others as the strongest men.'[76] The regimental hospitals used the same system as the base hospitals for

50

British nursing at the beginning of the Crimean War

supplying orderlies: officers sent the men who were usually the least good soldiers; but many regimental hospital tents in Balaclava did not have orderlies.

The orderly's job was impossible. His day began at 6:30 a.m. when he went to the purveyor's office to get the bread for his ward. Since there were nearly 200 orderlies at the Barrack Hospital it took an hour and a half to serve it out. At 9 a.m. he got in line for the raw meat and salt for the dinners. It could take up to four hours of standing in line before receiving his portion. Next he had to take the meat to the kitchen and wait while it was cooked.[77] Alexis Soyer, the famous chef from the Reform Club, visited the Crimea in 1855 and found the army's cooking system very inefficient. He made many suggestions for better organizing the kitchens and improving the cooking. He thought the copper boilers, in which soup, meat, and potatoes were cooked, were excellent but needed retinning. Joints of meat were tied together very tightly and placed on a wooden board before being put in the boiler, with the result that the meat in the middle was usually barely cooked. The orderlies labeled their respective pieces of meat with pieces of cloth cut from an old jacket, or buttons tied together, or old knives, forks, and scissors. One orderly tied an old pair of snuffers to his portion. When Soyer pointed out to him that the snuffers were quite dirty the man replied, 'How can it be dirty, sir? Sure they have been boiling this last month.' Soyer was also distressed to see the cooks throwing out the rich broth that was left when the meat had been served out. Furthermore, the kitchen at dinner time was in a state of utter confusion. Each orderly was given two cans for his patients' soup; they ran about crashing into each other trying to get as much as they could, with the result that some got more soup than others and some got none.[78] Nightingale thought the system of drawing raw rations seemed to have been invented deliberately to waste as much of the orderlies' time as possible. 'The scene of confusion, delay, and disappointment, where all these raw diets are being weighed out, by twos and threes and fours, is impossible to conceive unless one has seen it,' she wrote. It was impossible to imagine the abuses the system led to – for example raw meat drawn too late to be cooked had to stand all night in the wards.[79]

After the orderly received his cooked meat he had to carry it up to the wards, which could be quite a distance because the hospital had three stories, each nearly a mile long. He then had to cut up the meat and serve the food to the men. Most orderlies just left the food next to the patients' beds, sometimes out of their reach. They fed only those patients who had both arms disabled, and even those few orderlies who were kind and did try to feed the men, did not know how to give food to an invalid and just crammed it down their throats.[80] After the dinner was served the orderlies then had to cook the extra diets. This required considerable ingenuity for, unlike the civilian hospitals in London which had sculleries attached to each ward, the military hospitals did not have extra kitchens. Some orderlies cooked their extras on the ward stoves (which of course were designed for heating, not cooking), some finagled the army kitchen cooks into cooking it, while others made a fire in some outhouse and cooked it in their own mess tins. Jennings used the outhouse system. He did not boil the extras in the kitchen coppers because if he had, he would have had to wait until the next day. Rather, he boiled them in a shed in an old tin belonging to a man in his ward. Like the other orderlies he cooked the extras all at once so that the patients had to eat them all at one time if they wanted them hot, and then they went hungry for the rest of the day. The same thing was true of fluids. Nightingale cited the case of a man who was given his daily allowance of 20 ounces of wine, immediately drank all of it, becoming quite drunk, and then had to go without liquids for the rest of the day.[81] Not surprisingly Dr Duncan Menzies, who was in charge of the Scutari hospitals when Nightingale arrived, thought that as well as an inadequate number of orderlies, the kitchen for the Barrack Hospital was not large enough. The meals were never cooked on time, he said, and the food was poor.[82] For these reasons, shortly after arriving in Scutari Nightingale established her own extra diet kitchens.[83]

Orderlies clearly had little time left for nursing care and few were interested in it, often finding it distasteful. 'I have seen men I thought well of as patients,' one of the Anglican Sisters wrote, 'who on recovering and being made orderlies, show[ed] a negligence, hardness and indifference that surprised me, and I scarcely knew an orderly who could get leave to go out and come in sober.' The orderlies suffered from the same failings as many of the hospital nurses: they often drank the men's wine and brandy themselves, did not carry out doctors' orders, and stole articles and money from dying and dead patients. The orderlies' working conditions intensified these problems. They had to eat and sleep in what was believed to be the malignant, infectious air of their wards; the only fresh air they got was when they took the corpses out to be buried. Every third night they were expected to sit up with the patients, but usually they lay down and slept so soundly they did not hear the cries of men asking for help.[84] The number of patients rapidly increased as the fall wore on and their condition grew worse and worse; they were indescribably filthy, with death written on their discolored faces. On admission to the hospital, stretcher-bearers carried the men from ward to ward searching for an empty bed. 'We have no room, be off,' an orderly would tell the stretcher-bearers. 'We don't want any more of his sort here, we have more already than we can look to.' The bearers would carry the man off saying, 'What are we to do with him? We cannot keep walking around the hospital all day.' Usually the only bed they would find was one from which a corpse had just been removed.[85]

Orderlies require intelligence, respectable character, and previous training in large hospitals, declared one of the many sets of commissioners whom Parliament sent out to investigate the military hospitals. The commissioners thought the orderlies the most radical defect in the British hospitals,[86] and as one army doctor pointed out, without a trained hospital corps doctors could accomplish little.[87] With encouragement from some of the religious Sisters a few orderlies became excellent nurses, but generally speaking, in the wards where there were no female nurses the patients were very much neglected.[88] In London, Smith was well aware of the failings of the orderly system and tried to create a hospital corps of at least 600 men who would be ambulance drivers and hospital orderlies. However, so few young men volunteered that Smith had to accept pensioners who, he knew, would be unsatisfactory. But even taking these older, less promising men he was only able to raise 370,[89] and they proved to be a disaster. They arrived in Bulgaria at the end of July 1854 and drunkenness, disease, and a complete lack of discipline soon decimated them. The drivers were so incompetent that sometimes the sick soldiers had to drive the ambulances themselves. Most of this corps died or disappeared before the army embarked for the Crimea.[90] Yet until Nightingale arrived these untrained, temporary and often unwilling orderlies were the only nurses, and would remain so in many wards throughout the war. This was because Nightingale had no authority in the military hospitals except that over her nurses. She could not assign nurses to the wards; she had to wait for a doctor to ask for a nurse, and many doctors refused to have women in their wards.[91] Some doctors used the nurses only occasionally while others, largely the younger men, came to rely heavily on them.[92]

Nightingale identified the orderlies' lack of training and experience as well as their horrible living and working conditions as the central problem. She wrote to Lord Raglan at the beginning of January 1855 asking if it would not be possible to make some of the orderlies permanent. 'The comforts of the sick do not depend so much upon the skilful surgeon even as upon the careful orderly' she said, and the constant change of orderlies continually thwarted the surgeons' orders. Would it be possible, she asked Raglan, to issue an order that convalescents who were good orderlies should not be sent back to the ranks? Second, could Lord Raglan not issue an order that each regiment should send ten men, 'not young soldiers but men of good character,' to serve as permanent orderlies?' Similarly, she continued, good order in the ward was heavily dependent on the ward masters (non-commissioned officers who were responsible for the orderlies and their work).[93] The ward masters were supposed to visit all the wards every night, but Sister Mary Aloysius Doyle, one of the Irish nuns, reported that they frequently did not. The orderlies, she wrote, knew when the ward master was coming, and as soon as he raised the latch of the door an orderly would shout out, 'All right, your honour,' and on hearing that all was well the ward master would not come in. Many a time Doyle said to herself, 'All wrong,' but she thought one could scarcely blame him when the pestilential air of the wards could easily have killed him. In any case, she added, there was little he could have done even if he had come in.[94]

Nightingale pointed out to Raglan that, like the convalescent soldiers, the ward masters were recalled to the front as soon as they were starting to learn their duties. Perhaps three sergeants, she suggested, could be chosen from each regiment to serve as permanent ward masters. While she appreciated that her request might be impossible, hundreds of lives would be saved if it were implemented.[95] 'We have nothing but such raw corporals and sergeants as can be spared, new to their work, to place in charge [of the orderlies],' she explained to

Sidney Herbert on the same day she wrote to Raglan. There simply had to be a better caliber of ward master if there was ever to be the remotest hope of efficient orderlies. She outlined a plan for improving their working conditions. 'The Orderlies,' she said, 'ought to be well paid – well fed – well housed. They are now over-worked, ill fed & under paid. The sickness & mortality among them is extraordinary – ten took sick in one Division tonight.' They were currently given only four pence a day in addition to their standard army pay of one shilling a week. They should not have to eat and sleep in their wards. Rather there should be an orderlies' ward room in each division where they could sleep, and they should be rotated on and off nights rather than having to sit up every third night with no time to make up for the lack of sleep. They should have a mess table and a kitchen with an orderly assigned to do the cooking. Half the staff at a time should go off duty for their meals while the other half covered their wards. Two weeks later Nightingale reported back to Herbert that her system of orderlies eating and sleeping outside their wards had been successfully implemented in one division. She wished the ward masters could be placed under the command of the senior medical officer, not under the command of the army officers.[96]

The winter of 1854–55 was not a good time to remove men from the ranks. In November, with sickness on the increase, men being brought in from the trenches with frozen limbs, and cholera raging, Raglan started visiting the regimental hospitals. He did try to get the medical supplies that the surgeons so badly needed and begged for, but he also told all of his generals that, in order to make the hours the men had to spend in the trenches shorter, they must reduce the number of camp guards and orderlies.[97] Later Nightingale would be more successful in obtaining permanent orderlies, although, like the female nurses, this innovation met with resistance from some of the commanding officers, who understandably hated to give up good fighting men. Lt. Colonel Sterling, first a brigade major and later an assistant adjutant-general in the Highland Division, objected strenuously to Nightingale's presence in the army. She 'queens it with absolute power,' he wrote. He considered women useful but not as nurses. Rather, when the purveyor lacked something you could get it immediately from the ladies. Illustrating the government's new, more serious weighting of public opinion, he declared sardonically,

'The ladies would appeal to public opinion, which would back them right or wrong.' On Nightingale's first visit to Balaclava in May 1855 Sterling wrote that he was forced to take some of his finest men out of the ranks and send them to the hospitals as orderlies. He had just sent nine great big grenadiers to be permanent nurses. It was a great waste of military training and also meant the remaining soldiers had to put in longer hours in the trenches. Sterling's ideas for a better system would be to use army officers who were not in good health, and soldiers with weak constitutions, with a few medical officers to instruct them in cooking and other skills needed for the comfort of the sick. A few working-class women could be added to do the woman's work of washing and sewing. Then the army would not be weakened and 'Miss Nightingale might have had her wicked will of them without the interference of any officers except those belonging to the sick department.' The way orderlies were being provided now was absurd and made Sterling ill. 'Philanthropy is a plaything to these ladies,' he concluded.[98]

In December 1854 the War Office did accept Nightingale's suggestion to form an orderly corps but the plan was not implemented until June 1855. The first contingent of 300 men arrived only in November 1855. Called the Medical Staff Corps, it consisted of civilians recruited in England, some non-commissioned officers who were unfit for active service, and some men who transferred from the new (civilian) Land Transport Corps. The Medical Staff Corps was not devoted exclusively to orderlies but provided stewards, ward masters, cooks, washermen, issuers, and barbers. Hall took 150 for orderlies. The men were given only two weeks' instruction in drill and first aid before arriving. For those who were chosen as orderlies, instruction was supposed to continue in the hospitals. Their duties were described as attending and assisting the patients, applying fomentations, other 'simple portions of their treatment,' and cleaning the ward. The Corps was abolished later in 1856.[99]

Nightingale considered the work some of her nurses did training the orderlies one of her most important contributions to the war effort. Immediately after returning home her own goal was to work in a military hospital where she would be in charge of the linen, cooking, nursing, and teaching the orderlies.[100] When in 1858 she projected plans for introducing female nurses into military hospitals

British nursing at the beginning of the Crimean War

on a permanent basis, she suggested one female head nurse and three orderlies for a forty-bed ward as the minimum staffing. 'The introduction of Female Nurses into Military Hospitals is not intended to supply the place of Orderlies, but to perform a class of duties which never has been performed at all in the Army,' she wrote. The nurses' chief duties would be taking care of the linen and supervising the issue of extra diets. However, she hoped that feeding helpless patients – pouring nourishment down their throats drop by drop – inspecting the beds of cholera and erysipelas patients and those of patients with discharging wounds and bedsores, and doing minor dressings such as poultices would be added to the nurses' duties. Nurses should administer the medicines and see that the patients and orderlies carried out the doctors' orders.[101]

Nightingale arrived in Scutari with only thirty-seven nurses, but by the end of the war the government had sent approximately 225 women. About half of these women did not work under Nightingale's direction. The next chapter looks at the women Nightingale did direct.

Notes

1 Golding, *St. Thomas's*, pp. 214–15 and passim.
2 London Metropolitan Archives (hereafter LMA) H09/GY/A71/1, *Charity Commissioners' Report 1837*, p. 54. Also see Charing Cross Hospital, Minutes of Board of Governors (1834–45), pp. 78–9.
3 Davidoff, 'Class and Gender,' pp. 17–20.
4 Himmelfarb, 'Mayhew's Poor,' pp. 307–20.
5 LMA/H01/ST/A44/2, pp. 65–6.
6 LMA/H1/ST/A25, Duties of Sisters, Nurses, Watchers and Patients, n. d. but eighteenth century, no pagination.
7 South, *Hospital Nurses*, pp. 9–10, 12–14.
8 Ackroyd et al., *Advancing with the Army*, pp. 22–3, 37.
9 Cantlie, *Medical Department*, vol. 1, pp. 2–3.
10 Duberly, *Mrs Duberly's War*, pp. xiv–xv.
11 Best, *War and Society*, pp. 237–40.
12 Figes, *Crimean War*, p. 180.
13 British Library Additional Manuscripts (hereafter BL) 45796, FN to Pincoffs, 2 February 1857, fol. 134.
14 Bell, *Rough Notes*, pp. 229, 263.
15 Baumgart, *Crimean War*, pp. 79–84.

Government-imposed nursing

16 Sweetman, *War and Administration*, p. 35.

17 Strachan, *Wellington's Legacy*, pp. 37–43, 229–31.

18 Cantlie, *Medical Department*, vol. 2, pp. 6–9.

19 Sweetman, *War and Administration*, p. 13; Strachan, *Wellington's Legacy*, pp. 229–31.

20 *PP* 1854–55, vol. 9, Part I, pp. 409–10.

21 Sweetman, *War and Administration*, pp. 46–9, 57.

22 Steevens, *Crimean Campaign*, pp. 163–7.

23 *PP* 1854–55, vol. 9, Part I, p. 402.

24 BL 43393, Nightingale to Herbert, 19 February 1855, fol. 167.

25 Sweetman, *War and Administration*, pp. 43, 50, 54; Sweetman, 'Maule, Fox.'

26 Bell, *Rough Notes*, pp. 30–1; Goodlake, *Sharpshooter*, pp. 206–7.

27 Strachan, *Wellington's Legacy*, pp. 259–62; Sweetman, *War and Administration*, pp. 50–1; Fortescue, *British Army*, vol.12, pp. 169–70.

28 Fortescue, *British Army*, 12, pp. 169–70; Wood, *Crimea in 1854*, p. 195; Sweetman, 'Maule, Fox'; Panmure, *Panmure Papers*, vol. 1, pp. 177–8.

29 Cantlie, *Medical Department*, vol. 2, p. 221.

30 *PP* 1854–55, vol. 9, Part II, p. 132; Jameson, *Sisters of Charity*, pp. 112–13fn.

31 Cook, *Nightingale*, vol. 1, pp. 145–8.

32 *PP* 1854–55, vol. 9, Part II, p. 132.

33 Helmstadter and Godden, *Before Nightingale*, p. 45.

34 Golding, *St. Thomas's*, p. 204.

35 Jameson, *Sisters of Charity*, pp. 12–13, 173–8.

36 *PP* 1854–55, vol. 9, Part II, p. 132.

37 Cook, *Nightingale*, vol. 1, pp. 12–13.

38 Davis, *William Smith*, pp. xiii–xv, 250; Dossey, *Florence Nightingale*, pp. 24–6, 31–2.

39 Cook, *Nightingale*, vol. 1, p. 37.

40 McDonald, 'Introduction,' p. 6; Nightingale, *Spiritual Journey*, p. 388.

41 BL 43396, FN to Elizabeth Herbert, 14 October 1854, fols 10–14.

42 BL 43396, Nightingale to Elizabeth Herbert, 14 October 1854, fols 10–13.

43 WI Ms 8994, Nightingale to 'My dear friend' [Selena Bracebridge], [*c*.14–15 October 1854], Letter 113.

44 BL 43396, Nightingale to Elizabeth Herbert, 14 October 1854, fols 10–13.

45 Cook, *Nightingale*, vol. 1, pp. 154–5.

46 Boston University Nursing Archives (hereafter BU) 2/3/B1, Selena Bracebridge to Mary, 24 October 1854; Bostridge, *Florence Nightingale*, p. 280.

47 Cook, *Nightingale*, vol. 1, pp. 151–5.

48 Cannadine, *Class in Britain*, pp. 62–3, 97–8, 104.

49 Wiltshire County Record Office/2057/F4/66, Nightingale to Herbert, 16 October 1854.

50 Bostridge, *Florence Nightingale*, p. 209.

British nursing at the beginning of the Crimean War

51 Cook, *Nightingale*, vol. 1, pp. 155–7.

52 BL 43393, FN to Herbert, 15 December 1854, fols 45–6.

53 Chadwick, *Victorian Church*, vol. 1, pp. 271–309; Gilley, 'Roman Catholicism,' p. 33.

54 Chadwick, *Victorian Church*, vol. 1, pp. 271–91.

55 BL 39867, Nightingale to Sir John Hall, 15 October 1855, fols 44–6.

56 Cook, *Nightingale*, vol. 1, pp. 156–7.

57 BL 43393, FN to Herbert, 15 December 1854, fols 34–5.

58 WI Ms 8994, Nightingale to her mother, 17 November 1853, Letter 57.

59 WI MS 8994, Nightingale to her mother, 30 September [1853], Letter 44.

60 Helmstadter and Godden, *Before Nightingale*, pp. 42–3, 54–5, 59–63.

61 LMA/H02/WH/A1/28, Minutes of House Committee, 13 August 1828.

62 Engels, *Working Class in England*, pp. 108–9.

63 WI Ms 8994, Nightingale to her family, [1853], Letter 87.

64 Helmstadter and Godden, *Before Nightingale*, pp. 72–5.

65 Cook, *Nightingale*, vol. 1, p. 159.

66 LMA/H01/ST/NC8/1, Nurses Sent to Military Hospitals in the East, [1854–55] (hereafter referred to as Register of Nurses), pp. 17–18; WI/SA/QNI/W2/4, Minutes of Committee, 20 October 1854, 9 February 1855, 25 April, 29 August 1856.

67 LMA/H01/ST/SJ/A20/2, Lady Superintendent's Diary 1852–54, 4, 7, and 28 May, 18 July, 26 and 29 September 1853.

68 WI Ms 8994, Nightingale to Dearest [her mother], 17 November 1853, Letter 57.

69 LMA/H01/ST/SJ/A2/1, Council Meeting, 20 October 1854; LMA/H01/ST/NC3/SU1, Copy of nurses' contract.

70 Williams and Campbell, *Park Village*, pp. 64–7, 93, 135, 136; Williams, *Sellon*, p. 145.

71 Archives of Convent of Mercy, London, Bermondsey Annals (hereafter BA), 1854, p. 221.

72 Cook, *Nightingale*, vol. 1, pp. 158–9; Rappaport, *No Place for Ladies*, pp. 101, 107–8.

73 WI Ms 8994, Nightingale to her family, 4 November 1854, Letter 1.

74 Cantlie, *Medical Department*, vol. 2, p. 11.

75 Pincoffs, *Experiences of a Civilian*, pp. 178–9.

76 *PP* 1854–55, vol. 23, p. 315.

77 *PP* 1854–55, vol. 9, Part I, pp. 108, 113–15, 120–1, 556–60.

78 Soyer, *Culinary Campaign*, pp. 113–14.

79 BL 43393, Nightingale to Sidney Herbert, 28 January 1855, fols 114–15.

80 *PP* 1854–55, vol. 9, Part I, pp. 556–60; Terrot, *Reminiscences*, pp. 68–9.

81 Cantlie, *Medical Department*, vol. 2, pp. 87–8; *PP* 1854–55, vol. 33, pp. 314–15, 329–30.

82 *PP* 1854–55, vol. 9, Part I, pp. 556–60.

Government-imposed nursing

83 BL 43393, Nightingale to Herbert, 10 December 1854, fol. 28.

84 Doyle, 'Memories,' pp. 20–1, 38; Terrot, *Reminiscences*, pp. 38–40; *PP* 1854–55, vol. 9, Part I, p. 280.

85 Terrot, *Reminiscences*, p. 37.

86 *PP* 1854–55, vol. 9, Part I, pp. 556–60, 671; vol. 33, pp. 346–7; vol. 20, p. 40.

87 Cantlie, *Medical Department*, vol. 2, p. 22.

88 Taylor, *Eastern Hospitals*, vol. 1, pp. 203, 235–6; Terrot, *Reminiscences*, p. 39.

89 Cantlie, *Medical Department*, vol. 2, pp. 11–12.

90 Pack, *Sebastopol Trenches*, pp. 201–3.

91 Nightingale, *Health of the British Army*, p. 743.

92 Young Dr McGrigor, who was in charge of the Barrack Hospital, was Nightingale's principal supporter among the doctors. See Woodham-Smith, *Florence Nightingale*, pp. 175, 177, 201–2.

93 Leicestershire Record Office, Raglan Papers, Nightingale to Lord Raglan, 8 January 1855.

94 Doyle, 'Memories,' p. 22.

95 *PP* 1854–55, vol. 9, Part I, pp. 108, 556–60, Part II, pp. 113–15, 120–1; Leicestershire Record Office, Raglan Papers, Nightingale to Lord Raglan, 8 January 1855.

96 BL 43393, Nightingale to Herbert, 8 and 22 January 1855, fols 77–80, 103.

97 Calthorpe, *Letters from Headquarters*, pp. 189–90.

98 Sterling, *Letters*, pp. 262–3, 313–17.

99 Shepherd, *Crimean Doctors*, vol. 2, pp. 533–4; Cantlie, *Medical Department*, vol. 2, pp. 149–50, 171.

100 BL 43397, Nightingale to Col. LeFroy, 25 August 1856, fol. 240.

101 Nightingale, 'Introduction of Female Nursing,' pp. 16, 23, 60–1.

3

Nightingale's team of nurses

Introduction

Nightingale faced three central problems in the East: first, she had to win over the many army officers and doctors who resisted the project of female nurses; second, it would be a major effort to keep track of the different British military hospitals in Turkey and Russia; and third, Nightingale had to establish control of the conglomerate group of women who volunteered to be nurses. Some of the working-class nurses were very undisciplined and disorderly, while a few of the lady nurses and one group of Roman Catholic nuns would prove extremely recalcitrant.

Nightingale did not accomplish all of her enormous improvements in the Eastern hospitals with her original team of thirty-eight nurses as many people thought at the time and many still think today. In fact, she had to deal with more than a hundred women. Beginning in December 1855, the government sent eight more parties of nurses to twelve base hospitals.[1] The precise number of government nurses varies because sometimes the ladies in London who sent the nurses did not count the lady superintendents and at other times they did, and Nightingale hired two ladies in the East. The lady superintendents were asked to send reports on their nurses to the ladies who recruited them in London. Most did, although some such as Mary Stanley and Margaret Wear did not. The ladies in London then created a register with abstracts of the superintendents' reports, but with the exception of Nightingale's reports, the superintendents' reports themselves have been lost.[2] While there are vast amounts of primary sources for Nightingale, this very succinct register is the fullest primary source we have for most of the individual nurses.

61

Hospital nurses were considered so lowly and unimportant that the London teaching hospitals did not start to keep records of the nurses on their staffs until the training schools came in. Unfortunately, we have only one memoir from a working-class nurse, Elizabeth Davis; all our other sources give us the perspective of the lady nurses, patients, or doctors. Because working-class girls were so poorly educated they simply did not have the ability to write a book. A professional writer helped Davis put her book together.[3]

The military hospitals where the nurses worked opened and closed at different times throughout the war. Five were close to Constantinople. There were two in Scutari: the General Hospital was about half a mile away from the more famous Barrack Hospital. The Koulali Upper and Lower hospitals opened at the end of January 1855 and closed the following November. The Upper Hospital was originally a barrack for the Turkish army and the Lower its stable. As a result the two buildings were sometimes referred to as one, and sometimes as two hospitals. Counting the Koulali hospitals as two, the fifth hospital, Haida Pasha or the Sultan's Palace Hospital, a few miles north of Scutari, was a hospital for officers. Nightingale had nothing to do with this hospital because originally she was supposed to care only for enlisted men. It closed in December 1855, at which time the officers were transferred to the Scutari General Hospital. Five hospitals were in Russia. The Balaclava General Hospital opened as a base hospital shortly after the siege started in October 1854, the Castle Hospital opened in April 1855, and the Monastery Hospital, a convalescent hospital, opened in the summer of 1855. In March 1856 Nightingale took over the nursing in the two Land Transport Corps hospitals in Karanyi, a town close to Balaclava. In addition to these ten military hospitals, the War Office established two civilian hospitals in Turkey at Smyrna and Renkioi. Called civilian hospitals because they were staffed entirely by civilian rather than army doctors, they used the same system of government-paid female nurses. These nurses were not under Nightingale's direction – she had nothing to do with the civilian hospitals. Both hospitals closed before the war finished because they were underused. When they closed, some of the nurses transferred to the military hospitals where Nightingale was superintendent. Despite these transfers Nightingale never met or supervised most of the sixty-nine nurses whom the War Office sent to Renkioi and Smyrna.

Nightingale's team of nurses

Nightingale and her first group of nurses arrived in Scutari on 4 November 1854, the eve of the Battle of Inkerman. Revd Mother Mary Clare Moore, the Superior of the Bermondsey nuns who would become one of Nightingale's main supporters, described the major difficulties that immediately confronted her. The working-class nurses were discontented and troublesome, the purveyors were unwilling to give her supplies, the medical officers opposed her mission, and at first every single doctor refused to ask for any of her nurses. Nevertheless, by being very diplomatic, within a week Nightingale succeeded in getting a number of nurses into the Scutari General Hospital. The situation changed when, on 9 and 10 November following the Battle of Inkerman, hundreds of wounded men arrived, covered in vermin and in the worst stages of destitution. Most doctors in the Scutari hospitals were then happy to have any help they could get and began asking for Nightingale's nurses.[4] Although some doctors never used them and others used them only occasionally,[5] from this point on more and more doctors started requesting nurses.

If Nightingale gradually gained the support of most doctors, however, some were never reconciled to her presence, in part because she was violating the Victorian belief in separate spheres which prohibited ladies from acting in public institutions. Some medical men were appalled when Nightingale attended operations on naked men. For example, Assistant Surgeon Alexander Struthers wrote, 'She may be a lady, but I don't think she has the modesty of anyone deserving to be a woman.'[6] The soldiers, however, all loved the kind, efficient care that Nightingale and her nurses provided, and within a few months she had become a legend. But while she gained the backing of most doctors and the love of the soldiers and the public at home, Nightingale never succeeded in gaining full cooperation from the purveyors, and she failed to win the support of two very important persons, Mother Francis Bridgeman (who will be studied in detail in the next chapter), and Sir John Hall. Hall was obviously the one doctor whose support she most needed but unfortunately he took the presence of the female nurses as an insult; he thought the government sent them because it considered his staff incompetent. Furthermore, he bitterly resented Nightingale's ability to deal directly with the War Office which he himself could not do, and he consistently tried to undermine her. When she was in Turkey, he was limited in his ability

Government-imposed nursing

to thwart her, but in the Crimea he became an ally of two rebellious nurses, Margaret Wear and Mother Francis Bridgeman. Nightingale made three trips to the Crimea, in May and November 1855 and March 1856. When she was there, Hall made her life as difficult as he could. She believed, and with good reason, that Hall emboldened Wear and Bridgeman to reject her authority.[7] It was not until the last two weeks of the war, in March 1856 when the fighting was finished, that Nightingale succeeded in getting a general order stating clearly that she was in charge of the nursing in all the army's base hospitals in both Turkey and Russia.[8]

Clinical experience combined with lack of respectability

It was indicative of Nightingale's overriding concern for propriety that the first nurses she assigned to the Scutari hospitals were religious Sisters. She sent two Bermondsey nuns and three Anglican Sisters with some hospital nurses to the Scutari General Hospital and assigned Moore and her other two Sisters to the Barrack Hospital. At first Nightingale placed Moore in charge of the linen and storerooms. Soon after, she put her in control of the newly opened extra diet kitchen.[9] In the first three months Nightingale and Mary Stanley, who became lady superintendent of the Koulali hospitals, dismissed a striking number of the working-class nurses. On arriving in Turkey Stanley immediately dismissed two for intoxication and a third as too old for the work. By 21 December 1854 Nightingale had dismissed eleven nurses. She sent the five nuns from the convent for orphans home because they had no hospital experience and let go three of the Anglican Sisters, one because she was ill, with a second to nurse her, and the third, Sister Elizabeth Wheeler, was dismissed because she had written a letter to a relative asking him to send supplies which were so sadly lacking in the hospitals. The relative published the letter in the newspapers,[10] which inflamed the public outcry against the medical department – precisely what the government was trying to appease. The doctors were furious because they believed they could not admit publicly that they were lacking supplies. They demanded that Nightingale dismiss Wheeler, which Nightingale was quite happy to do because she had been very demanding and troublesome.[11]

Of the fourteen original working-class nurses who arrived in

Constantinople, Nightingale had dismissed eight by mid-January. Wilson and Williams were fired for intoxication, Jones for both intoxication and misconduct, and Faulkner for drunkenness and buying and selling items for patients in the hospital. Faulkner was an experienced and good nurse otherwise,[12] and buying and selling was a fairly common practice in the London hospitals, but one that management generally disapproved of. On 15 January Nightingale dismissed four more nurses – four of the six St. John's House nurses: Emma Fagge, Mary Ann Bournett, Mary Ann Coyle, and Ann Higgins. Nightingale's negotiations for the dismissal of these four trained nurses give us an example of what she looked for in the working-class nurses. The four women also provide an excellent illustration of the position of nursing, as well as of class relationships, in mid-nineteenth-century Britain. Three of the St. John's House nurses wrote to Sister Mary Jones, their superior at home in London, describing how unhappy they were under Nightingale's direction. Elizabeth Drake, one of the two St. John's House nurses whom Nightingale did keep, wrote to Jones early in December 1854:

> We do not look for many comforts but we do feel we ought to be trusted. We are not allowed to go into the wards without one of the lady nurses. We must not speak one word of comfort to a poor dying man or read to him. We are prevented from doing what our hearts prompt us to do. We feel we are not so useful as we expected to be.

Drake only wished that 'someone from home' had come out with them to support them. The six nurses, she said, had tried in every way to conduct themselves properly but they never got a kind word.[13] Mary Ann Coyle also wished that someone from home had accompanied the nurses. She wrote:

> Wee[14] are all so very unappey Miss Nightingale have sum spite against us but for wat cawse we know not: and Mrs Brasebridg has treated us with Contempt ever since the day Mr Sheperd[15] left us: I woold not mind minde wat harde ships wee had to incaunenter with if they would be kinde to us: they treate us worse than the Coman low wimon they brate [brought] out. I was never so unappey in My life … Mrs Clarke the housekeeper Is A Complete tirant she insults us every time she sees us Maryan in particular.[16]

The third nurse, who did not sign her letter, said that Nightingale treated them with disrespect and unkindness while Clarke all but

Government-imposed nursing

starved them. 'This low woman,' as the anonymous nurse described her, also made up terrible, untrue stories about the St. John's House nurses that Nightingale completely believed.[17] Coyle believed the St. John's House nurses were the only ones who had come out with 'a good motive' and all the other nurses had volunteered because of the high pay. Still, she said, 'We will do the thing that is rite and if god be for us, will need not fear.'[18] The military nurses' pay was indeed very high, ranging from ten to fourteen shillings a week, rising to eighteen to twenty shillings after a year of good conduct. The average starting wage in the London hospitals, which paid better than those in the provinces, ranged from six to nine shillings and sixpence, usually with some food and accommodation.[19] The government paid for all the nurses' travel expenses, uniforms, and room and board.

Selena Bracebridge was very hard on the working-class nurses, while not one of the nurses – ladies, Sisters, or working class – could say anything good about Clarke. Even the generous and forgiving Mother Mary Clare Moore complained about her. Moore worked with her in the extra diet kitchens where, she said, Clarke was seldom sober and measured out the food for the nuns and nurses in scanty portions, using the 'lowest and most abusive language.'[20] Sister Sarah Anne Terrot characterized Clarke as someone who was abrupt, quick to anger, and enjoyed scolding people. Terrot always tried to get her requisitions from Moore because she was patient, calm, and attentive to every request.[21] Clarke had previously been matron of a union workhouse in Sheffield and worked for Nightingale's grandmother before Nightingale hired her as matron at the Harley Street hospital.[22] Nightingale originally had complete confidence in her, but by the spring of 1855 finally realized that Clarke was causing serious problems. 'Do you remember saying to me,' Nightingale wrote to her Aunt Mai,

> that Mrs Clarke was not to be trusted with the morals of the servants? that if any thing happened – she would prove, either that she knew it all the time or that it was quite right not to know it. Alas! what you said was quite true & Clarke either gets drunk herself, or connives at the drunkenness of others Fortunately she had wished to go before- & therefore without a quarrel of any sort, she goes – She was so utterly incapable of controlling the Nurses. that I am glad to part But I never can forget what we owe her- & therefore I am equally glad to have had no blow up[23]

Nightingale recorded the cause of her dismissal as illness and gave her an £8 gratuity, more than the standard £5 she usually gave.[24]

Mother Mary Clare Moore described the six St. John's House nurses as 'of a more respectable class' than the other hospital nurses.[25] They had not been guilty of immoral conduct, neglect of duty, or drunkenness, but they had disobeyed Nightingale's orders. They went into the wards at night without a lady accompanying them and they fed the men without medical orders.[26] Early in December Nightingale began arranging to get rid of them because she believed that, as well as not following her rules, they were not skillful nurses. She asked St. John's House to send letters of recall so that she would not have to officially fire them. It was the only diplomatic move she made during the course of the negotiations. After working with them for a month, Nightingale told St. John's House,

> I fear nothing can be made of them here, tho' I've no doubt that as private nurses in England they may be very good. Their manners are so flibberty-gibbet (though, with the exception of Mrs Higgins, I suspect no greater impropriety) that they do not command the respect imperatively necessary where forty women are turned loose among three thousand men.

Nightingale shared Golding's view that the most important part of the matron's job was maintaining the propriety of her nurses. She went on to say that the nurses' dressing of wounds was careless and slovenly, and Lawfield, the other St. John's House nurse Nightingale did keep, did not recognize a fracture when she saw one. Furthermore, they refused to take a hint except from Nightingale herself. As a result Nightingale felt obliged to use them for making stump pillows rather than for nursing. They complained, saying they had not come to the East to do needlework.[27]

Nightingale would always disdain private nursing and prize hospital experience above respectability. For example, Eliza Roberts, the nurse whom she made her head nurse, was extraordinarily competent; with 24 years of clinical experience at St. Thomas's, she was the most experienced nurse on Nightingale's team. Nightingale immediately recognized her wealth of nursing knowledge and expertise and paid her more than any of the other nurses – £65 a year as compared to a range of £26 to £46/16/- for the other nurses.[28] 'She is indeed a surgical nurse of the first order, of that race that is now almost extinct,'

Government-imposed nursing

Nightingale wrote, 'since, in Civil Hospitals, dressers now do almost all that the "Sisters" used to do.'[29] Nightingale was very impressed by Roberts's facility with dressings, and reported that the senior medical officer agreed that she dressed wounds and fractures more skillfully than any of the dressers or assistant surgeons.[30] However, while Roberts was respectable in the sense of being hard-working, sober, chaste, and devoted to Nightingale, she was barely able to read and talked incessantly in an uncouth way using bad language. She fought with the other nurses and had a terrible temper, of which she was very proud. When Nightingale tried to correct her she would respond by threatening to resign and go home. This tactic was effective because she knew how much Nightingale depended on her.[31] Nightingale's clinical experience was limited to approximately fifteen months in two small hospitals which had few acute cases.

In terms of clinical experience the St. John's House nurses did not begin to compare to Roberts and some of the other more experienced hospital nurses. After they finished their probationary period of three months in a teaching hospital the St. John's House nurses did mostly private nursing, because private patients paid better than hospitals and profits from their nursing were one of the ways the sisterhood supported its training school. Of the two nurses that Nightingale kept Rebecca Lawfield was the more experienced, having entered St. John's House in 1852. Nightingale asked Lawfield to resign in November because she thought she was impertinent for complaining about how ugly the uniform caps were. When Lawfield begged for a second chance, she allowed her to stay on. Nightingale thought she was not a clever or skilled nurse but found her kind and impeccably proper. Elizabeth Drake, whom Nightingale considered the only completely acceptable nurse of the six, was inexperienced, having started training only in January 1854. However, she was an exceptionally amiable and kind nurse whom Nightingale deemed 'a treasure.'[32] Her patients all commented on her gentle and respectful manner, her unwearying good temper, and her quiet and well-conducted behavior.[33] Of the four dismissed nurses, Emma Fagge had been at St. John's House since 1853. The distinguished surgeon (later Sir) William Bowman frequently asked for her to assist him with his operation cases.[34] Ann Higgins had been at St. John's House only since December 1853,[35] while Mary Ann Coyle and Mary Ann

Bournett had only just completed their probation in September and October 1854.[36] However, Lawfield, Higgins, Fagge, and Coyle had all worked in the cholera ward at the Westminster Hospital in September 1854.[37]

Nightingale's letter caused a furor at St. John's House. The Council delegated Bowman, a Council member, and Jones to reply. Bowman's letter is not extant, but in her response Jones supported her nurses and, after discussing it with her Council, gave Nightingale a sharp reprimand. She shared the nurses' regret that 'someone from home to whom they could have looked for kind counsel in obeying your rules and carrying out your directions' had not accompanied them. Jones was sorry that:

> in a matter of such grave import to the nurses as a complaint of their conduct . expressions should have been used which would seem to betoken a want of consideration towards women who volunteered to aid, in carrying out, under your control & guidance a good, though difficult – & arduous work on an hitherto, untried field of labour.

Jones was not quite certain what to make of 'flibberty-gibbet' behavior, and pointed out with reference to diagnosing fractures that the nurses were trained as nurses, not as surgeons. As to their refusal to take a hint from anyone other than Nightingale, Jones reminded her that 'your most express instruction to these nurses, and which you asked me to impress upon them, was that they *were to obey no one but you, nor to take orders from any one else.*' Jones feared they might have taken those directions too literally. She enclosed the four letters of recall.[38]

Nightingale replied to the Council with an even more condescending letter. She could not understand Jones's references to the nurses' lack of surgical skill so, trying to understand their accusations, she had questioned the four nurses personally. Their letters, she said, were hasty and inaccurate as might be expected from those who were 'not much accustomed to detail facts or to explain their feelings in writing.' She found their only complaint was that Mrs Clarke did not speak to them respectfully and they said they were not used to being treated with disrespect. 'Mrs Clarke,' she wrote, 'as I believe though somewhat brusque, sets them an example of incessant labour and anxiety to fulfil her duties.' The four nurses' real complaints,

Government-imposed nursing

Nightingale claimed, were against their own colleagues, Lawfield and Drake. She concluded,

> I trust that it may not be deemed offensive to say that the frivolous and really unfounded charges of these letters, which have obtained such grave consideration at your hands, confirms me in the idea that the St. John's Nurses are not well fitted for the work of this Hospital, – nor have they improved by experience ... I had hoped to find some serious devotion to the cause we are engaged in ... I cannot too strongly draw your attention to the difference between a Military & a London Hospital – to the consequent necessity of different rules & to the probability of the Nurses in question doing extremely well in private nursing at home – but not among the officers here.[39]

She had therefore given the four nurses Jones's letters of recall. It was ironic that Nightingale thought the nurses lacked devotion to the cause while they thought they were the only ones committed to it. At the same time, while Nightingale's interrogation obviously must have intimidated them, it was true that the nurses quarrelled amongst themselves although in public they conducted themselves properly.[40] It speaks well of both Jones and Nightingale that, despite these unpleasant exchanges, after the war they became very close friends and Jones was Nightingale's chief mentor when she was establishing her school at St. Thomas's.[41]

Drake, who contracted low fever in Balaclava and died in August, gives us a touching insight into the life and standard of living of a first-class, well-paid nurse in 1855. Nightingale was not surprised when she died; she thought Drake had suffered so much in life that she was not attached to it. Before leaving for the Crimea she had packed up all her belongings to be sent to St. John's House in case of her death. Her dresses all belonged to St. John's House but she bequeathed a bottle of scent to Sister Mary Jones, a pair of slippers to Miss Gipps, one of the St. John's House Sisters, a jar for flowers to Miss Bartlett, another Sister, and to the four nurses who were sent home from Scutari, a glass box, three cups, and a necklace. Anything else and her wages owing were to go to her widowed sister and her fatherless children.[42] By law the money should have gone to Drake's father, a wool gatherer, but he signed a letter with his mark (an X) agreeing that it could go to the sister.[43]

The dismissal of the St. John's House nurses demonstrates how tenuous Nightingale felt her position was when she first arrived in the East. Herbert had impressed on her the importance of strictly obeying the doctors, so it was understandable that Nightingale did her best to avoid antagonizing them and told the nurses they could only give care that doctors had specifically ordered. One of the lady nurses who sometimes accompanied Nightingale on her evening rounds found refusing feverish men who so pitifully begged for a drink the most difficult part of her job, but if there were no medical orders for fluids Nightingale would not allow the nurses to give them. It is hard to believe that doctors would have objected to giving dehydrated men fluids but in such a hostile atmosphere Nightingale feared they would use any excuse to attack her. She took Herbert's order about preventing 'a polemical arena' just as seriously as his order to obey the doctors. She forbade the nurses to read to the men because she was afraid they might read from the many widely distributed, scurrilous, sectarian pamphlets that could easily give rise to religious disputes, and she also feared it might give opportunities for improper relationships with the soldiers.[44]

From the perspective of the St. John's House nurses, however, it was impossible to understand Nightingale's draconian insistence that doctors' orders, or lack of orders, be literally followed. They were serious nurses, trained in the latest modern supportive therapies and used to being trusted. They did not complain about the horrible living conditions – the scanty food in the first months, their crowded, unheated, and flea-infested room with broken windows and a leaking roof[45] – but they did expect to be treated with respect. They were devastated by the way Nightingale and Bracebridge behaved towards them – as if they were the lowest order of domestic servant, which of course is precisely what nurses were historically. In addition, Selena Bracebridge and Margaret Wear, then superintendent of the Balaclava General Hospital, also articulated the widespread upper-class fear of the working classes. For example, Wear dismissed Mrs Disney, an experienced and highly recommended nurse from St. Thomas's, because she had been drunk and behaved towards her in what Wear deemed a 'violent and unruly manner.' Bracebridge described Disney as 'a most dangerous woman.'[46] The dismissal of the four St. John's House nurses and threatened dismissal of a fifth also illustrate upper-class expectations of deference from the working classes. It was

Government-imposed nursing

highly unusual for a lady to accept Eliza Roberts's foul mouth and ill-mannered behavior but Nightingale made an exception for her because of her nursing expertise. Be that as it may, she did not take an egalitarian view of her nurses. She assumed the hospital hierarchy should reflect the hierarchy of social class. 'In truth the only lady in a hospital should be the chief of the women, whether called Matron or Superintendent,' she wrote two years after the Crimean War.

> The efficiency of her office requires that she should rank as a lady and an officer of the hospital. At the same time, I think it is important that every Matron and Superintendent (unless during war service, when the rough-and-ready life and work required will probably be best undergone by women of a higher class) should be a person of the middle classes ... The real and faithful discharge of the duties of the wards of a General [civilian] Hospital, whether with reference to superiors, companions, or patients, is incompatible with the status, as such, of ladies.[47]

At the same time, if there were a lady superintendent, it was essential that she be clinically experienced. Nightingale deplored volunteer untrained ladies, whom she considered a real danger and 'the greatest mischief of all' in military hospitals.[48]

Head nurses should be middle class, while the regular nurses should be working-class women. Nightingale often referred to the nurses as servants, describing them as useful or not useful. She did sometimes call the lady nurses useful but never referred to them as servants and she treated them with far more consideration. Apart from Sister Elizabeth Wheeler, whom she fired on the specific order of the doctors, the only lady nurse whom Nightingale personally fired was Charlotte Salisbury. Salisbury had been governess to the family of the British consul in Patras, Greece for eleven years when Nightingale hired her in May 1855 to assist Selena Bracebridge in the Free Gift Store. The store consisted of vast numbers of gifts that the general public began sending when *The Times* published Wheeler's letter asking for food and supplies for the soldiers, and it was so large it required a full-time manager. Salisbury took charge of the Free Gifts and the housekeeping in Nightingale's house when the Bracebridges went home at the end of July. She immediately began stealing from both Nightingale personally and wholesale from the Free Gifts, which she used to distribute largesse to her friends. Nightingale soon discovered the thefts and fired her on 29 September 1855.[49] She made all kinds of special dispensations for her when she dismissed her. She paid her, out of her own pocket, six weeks' salary as compensation for the short notice of dismissal and, because the government did not pay the way home for dismissed nurses, offered to pay her passage to England herself. In addition, Salisbury had relatives in Australia so Nightingale deposited a sum of money in England to pay her fare to Australia if she wished to go there in order to start anew.[50] But Nightingale, revealing again the upper-class view of the proper relations between the upper and lower classes, was absolutely horrified when she saw a letter a corporal, a former assistant wardsman, wrote to Salisbury. The letter was couched, Nightingale said,

> in the most familiar terms – *asking her* [Salisbury] *to write to him about the Nurses thanking her for her presents* – in the most off-handed manner & the most intimate referring to change among the Nurses & Wardmasters & to her & his opinion about them & signing himself 'your affecte. friend' … this comes home to me that she is one of the lowest creatures that walks the earth, that the woman who was always for taking such great care of the nurses, who undertook their charge on the written understanding that they were to have none but the necessary intercourse with patients or orderlies, should be on terms of correspondence with a corporal about them, seems to me something so low that I really should be surprised at nothing that I could learn of her now?[51]

Salisbury's willingness to treat a working-class soldier as a friend, really an equal, seemed more shocking to Nightingale than her wholesale thievery.

Nightingale would never completely trust the working-class nurses. Ideally she would have liked to see only head nurses placed in military hospitals because 'as a body,' she believed, 'the mass of Assistant-Nurses [the regular nurses in modern parlance] are too low in moral principle, and too flighty in manner' to be of any use in military hospitals. Even most of the head nurses in the great civilian hospitals would not do. Hospital head nurses came mainly from the class of tradesmen's and servants' widows and Nightingale thought that the majority did little nursing but rather stood by while others did their work for them.[52] Like most Victorians, Nightingale worried especially about illicit sexual liaisons, and not without reason because the men often took advantage of the nurses, as was frequently the case with medical students and young doctors in the civilian hospitals.[53]

Government-imposed nursing

Both to escape this type of encounter and, equally or more important, to prevent the nurses from going out with soldiers, Nightingale locked all the nurses – Sisters, ladies, and working-class – into the nurses' quarters at 8:30 every night and slept with the key under her pillow. At first she had expected the military authorities to support her efforts to maintain propriety, but found they did the opposite. She was proud of the fact that when she was ill in the Crimea in May and June 1855,

> not one of my Nurses, thank God, but a new-made (soldier's) widow whom I had taken in as servant, left the Quarters at night & passed several successive nights in the store of a Sergeant of the 1st Class – (The consequences were soon obvious).

However, when Nightingale sought help from the commandant, Lord William Paulet, he would not even reprimand the sergeant.[54]

Nightingale, as would other British lady superintendents, made it a rule that the nurses had to be accompanied by a lady nurse when they went out walking for their exercise in the fresh air because when two or even three nurses were together alone the soldiers made appointments to meet them later.[55] The Barrack Hospital building was not all devoted to the hospital; part of it was still used as a depot for troops, so there were many soldiers about. The various parliamentary commissions that investigated the hospital arrangements all deplored soldiers and hospitals sharing the same building.[56] Two years after the war, one of Nightingale's goals in training military nurses was to 'protect and to restrain, to elevate in purifying, so far as may be permitted, a number, more or less, of poor and virtuous women.' In the 1850s the only hospital nurses who were generally considered respectable were religious Sisters or those trained by them, but Nightingale did not envisage founding a religious order. This was partly because she believed religious nurses could be prudish. They were therefore less qualified than working-class women to be hands-on nurses.[57]

Nightingale would not tolerate sexual liaisons or disgracefully drunken behavior in public but had to put up with what she called 'intemperate' women as opposed to 'case-hardened drinkers.' Nurse Tandy was one of the cleverest, handiest, most useful women she had ever known, an excellent cook, and a good nurse and servant, but she had one fault: intemperance – not intoxication.[58] Nightingale was

Nightingale's team of nurses

very fond of Elizabeth Hawkins, who was an excellent nurse, but she was only able to keep Hawkins sober by placing the brandy under lock and key and changing her from ward to ward so she would not be with friends who might lead her astray. Removing a nurse from association with other nurses that she considered likely to be a bad influence was one of Nightingale's standard methods for maintaining the much sought after Victorian respectability. Even so, Nightingale judged Tandy and Hawkins two of her best nurses.[59] Mrs Whitehead was a first rate St. Thomas's nurse who worked in Balaclava, where she was considered most valuable. However, she indulged in 'much levity of conduct' and was a heavy drinker. Having broken her leg while drunk, she was laid up for several months. Nightingale, who was then in Balaclava, sent her to Scutari from whence she was to be sent home. Nightingale ordered that she was not to be placed in the nurses' quarters because Whitehead had acquired 'habits in the relaxed discipline' in Balaclava 'which would do *essential* mischief in our untrustworthy but disciplined set of nurses in Scutari.' If the medical men thought Whitehead was not yet well enough to undertake the voyage home she was to live in Nightingale's own house in Scutari. There she should be allowed out only in the garden, not on the streets, and could be employed with needlework.[60] Nightingale's rules for the nurses, as she often boasted, were indeed stricter than those of the other lady superintendents.

After some months in the East, Nightingale started creating a division of labor – relieving the nurses who gave good patient care of some of their housekeeping duties and using women who were not competent nurses in a clinical situation entirely for the laundry, sewing, and cooking. For example, Mrs Orton, a surgical nurse from St. Bartholomew's, was in Nightingale's opinion scarcely up to the job of maid-of-all-work but she thought her such a good creature that she placed her in the linen room under direction. In September 1855 Nightingale asked the ladies who recruited nurses in London for two women to manage the linen stores, a housekeeper 'who would have nothing to do with nursing' but would maintain discipline in the nurses' quarters, two steady, elderly, healthy maids-of-all-work,' and four nurses.[61] Three nurses who gave no patient care, Nesbitt, Eskip, and Lee, illustrate this policy. They also reflect Nightingale's commitment to close surveillance of her staff. She

Government-imposed nursing

deemed Nesbitt 'active, useful, clever, equally good cook & washer-woman, but from the long established habit of intemperance & what this always brings in its train, I have never been able to trust her from out of my own supervision, without her disgracing herself.' Mrs Eskip required 'watching, like most washerwomen to see that she does not obtain drink. But, with care, she is an excellent trustworthy servant, perfectly honest & to be depended upon.'[62] Mrs Lee was also an excellent washerwoman who was, 'under strict supervision, honest, respectable and sober.'[63]

Later, when she felt her position better established, Nightingale was less high-handed with the working-class women and would treat them more kindly, and in fact became very fond of some. However, with the exception of a very few such as Eliza Roberts, she still felt she could not trust them to behave properly unless they were directly under her own eye. For example, she sent Mrs Gailey home in disgrace because she had stayed out after hours drinking. Nightingale was very sorry to dismiss her because she liked her. Gailey, who worked at the General Hospital where Miss Tebbutt was superintendent, told Nightingale it would never have happened if she had been under Nightingale's direction in the Barrack Hospital.[64] Susan Cator was another working-class nurse whom Nightingale liked very much. Like Eliza Roberts she was a highly experienced and competent practitioner but, unlike Roberts, a pleasant and deferential person. She had worked at the London Hospital for eleven years as a regular nurse, followed by eight years as a head nurse. She originally worked in the Palace Hospital for officers but when it closed, transferred to the Scutari General Hospital.[65] Nightingale found her a job as a sister at St. Thomas's after the war and wrote of her:

> an excellent Nurse a sensible woman indefatigable with her Patients perfect in propriety sobriety I have a real affection/trustworthiness for her, & cannot but point out how when, coming under stricter discipline at the General Hospital Scutari, than she had been under before, conformed to rule, instead of, like her companion, breaking the bounds of propriety.[66]

Cator's improper companion was Ruth Dawson, who will appear in a later chapter.

Notes

1 LMA/H01/ST/NC8/1 'Nurses Sent to Military Hospitals in the East,' [1856] (hereafter Register of Nurses); WI Ms 8995, 30 November 1855, Letters 78 and 79.

2 Stanley did later add comments on individual nurses to the register.

3 Beddoe, 'Jane Williams.'

4 Bermondsey Annals (hereafter BA), 1854, pp. 227–8.

5 Nightingale, *Health of the British Army*, p. 743.

6 Shepherd, *Crimean Doctors*, vol. 1, pp. 282–3.

7 WI Ms 8995, FN to Aunt Mai Smith, 16 November 1855, Letter 75.

8 Cook, *Nightingale*, vol. 1, pp. 292–3.

9 BA 1854, pp. 227–8.

10 WI Ms 8895, Nightingale's Report, 30 November 1855, Letter 78.

11 Helmstadter and Godden, *Before Nightingale*, pp. 97–8.

12 WI Ms 8995, Nightingale Report, 30 November 1855, Letter 78; LMA/H01/ ST/NC8/1, Register of Nurses, p. 4.

13 LMA/H01/ST/NC3/SU13, Elizabeth Drake to Mary Jones, 4 December 1854.

14 I have left the original misspellings.

15 C. P. Shepherd, the sisterhood's chaplain, accompanied the St. John's House nurses to Paris where they joined Nightingale's party. He then returned home.

16 LMA/H01/ST/NC3/SU16, Mary Ann Coyle to Sister Mary Jones, 5 December 1854. Unlike other hospital nurses, all the St. John's House nurses had to be able to read and write. Coyle's letter indicates that they did not do so at a very high level.

17 LMA/H01/ST/NC3/SU15, unsigned letter to Sister Mary Jones, 4 December 1854.

18 LMA/H01/ST/NC3/SU16, Mary Ann Coyle to Sister Mary Jones, 5 December 1854.

19 Abel-Smith, *Nursing Profession*, p. 6.

20 BA 1854, pp. 252–3.

21 O'Malley, *Florence Nightingale*, p. 240; Terrot, *Reminiscences*, pp. 44–5.

22 Bostridge, *Florence Nightingale*, pp. 184–5.

23 WI Ms 8995, Nightingale to Mai Smith, 16 April 1855, Letter 11.

24 WI Ms 8995, Nightingale Report, 30 November 1855, Letter 78.

25 BA 1854, p. 226.

26 LMA/H01/ST/NC3/ SU14, Nightingale to Miss Gipps, 5 December 1854; LMA/H01/ST/NC3/SU18, FN to the Council of St. John's House, 11 January 1855; LMA/H01/ST/NC3/SU24, Selena Bracebridge to Dear Sir [Rev. C. P. Shepherd], 22 January [1855].

27 LMA/H01/ST/NC3/SU14, Nightingale to Miss Gipps, 5 December 1854.

Government-imposed nursing

28 WI Ms 8995/79, Nightingale Report, 30 November 1855, Letter 79.

29 BL Ms 43402, Nightingale Report No. IV, 26 June 1856, fol. 23.

30 BL 43393, Nightingale to Herbert, 28 January 1855, fol. 124.

31 O'Malley, *Florence Nightingale*, pp. 344, 352; BL 47715, Nightingale to Bonham-Carter, 8 August 1867, fol. 23.

32 WI Ms 8994, Nightingale to William Bowman, 14 November 1854, Letter 117.

33 LMA/H01/ST/SJ/C3/1, Register of Nurses 1849–55, p. 123.

34 Ibid, pp. 97, 113.

35 Ibid, pp. 104, 122.

36 LMA/H01/ST/SJ/A20/2, Lady Superintendent's Diary, 1852–54, 8 and 12 September 1854; LMA/H01/ST/SJ/C3/1, Register of Nurses 1849–55, p. 125.

37 LMA/H01/ST/SJ/C3/1, Register of Nurses 1849–55, pp. 81, 95, 97, 113; LMA/H01/ST/SJ/A20/2, Lady Superintendent's Diary, 4–12 September 1854.

38 LMA/H01/ST/SJ/SU17, Mary Jones to Nightingale, 22 December 1854.

39 LMA/H01/ST/SJ/NC3/SU18, Nightingale to the St. John's House Council, 11 January 1855.

40 LMA/H01/ST/NC3/SU30, W. A. Halpin to C. P. Shepherd, 3 April 1855.

41 Helmstadter and Godden, *Before Nightingale*, pp. 146–7, 162–3.

42 LMA/H01/ST/NC3/SU/35-38, Nightingale to C. P. Shepherd, 16, 21, 27, and 28 August 1855.

43 LMA/H01/ST/NC3/SU/40, John Drake to Nightingale, 10 September 1855.

44 Nightingale to Miss Gipps, 5 December 1854. LMA/H01/ST/NC3/SU14; Nightingale to the Council of St. John's House, 11 January 1855, ST/NC3/SU18; Doyle, 'Memories,' p. 28.

45 Taylor, *Eastern Hospitals*, vol. 1, p. 93; BA 1854, pp. 226–7.

46 LMA/H01/NC8/1, Register of Nurses, p. 11.

47 Nightingale, 'Introduction of Female Nursing,' pp. 8–9. This article was originally written by Jane Shaw Stewart. Nightingale edited it, deleting some portions, but left the rest in Stewart's handwriting when she sent it to the publisher.

48 BL 45818, Nightingale Note, [c.1866], fol. 33.

49 WI Ms 8895, Nightingale Report, 30 November 1855, Letter 78; O'Malley, *Florence Nightingale*, pp. 299–301, 321–7.

50 BL RP 988, Nightingale to Dear sir [Salisbury's former employer], 3 September and 17 October 1855; Nightingale, *Crimean War*, p. 291.

51 WI Ms 8995, Nightingale letter, no addressee, [c.October 1855], Letter 42.

52 Nightingale, 'Introduction of Female Nursing,' pp. 33–4.

53 See, for example, Archives of London School of Economics, Booth Collection/B/153, Cane interview, March 1896, pp. 26–8.

54 LMA/H01/ST/H01/ST/NC18/15, Nightingale to Bonham-Carter, 1 October 1869, fol. 44.

Nightingale's team of nurses

55 Leeds District Archives, Nightingale to Lady Canning, 9 September 1855, HAR/LdC/177/2/2.

56 *PP*, 1854–55, vol. 9, Part I, p. 280, Part II, p. 680.

57 Nightingale, 'Introduction of Female Nursing,' pp. 5–7.

58 BL 43402, Nightingale Report No. IV, 26 June 1856, fol. 24.

59 WI Ms 8995, Nightingale to Dear friends [Selena and Charles Bracebridge], 7 August 1855, Letter 26, [10]; BL 43402, Nightingale Report No. I, [May 1856], fols 3, 6.

60 WI Ms 8995, Nightingale note [to Aunt Mai Smith], 19 October 1855, Letter 46; Davis, *Autobiography*, vol. 2, p. 187.

61 Leeds Record Office, Nightingale to Lady Canning, 9 September 1855, HAR/LdC 177/2/2.

62 BL 43402, Nightingale Report No. III, 18 June 1856, fols 12, 17.

63 BL 43402, Nightingale Report No. II, 16 June 1856, fol. 16.

64 64 Nightingale to her mother, 12 April 1855, WI Ms 8995, Letter 10.

65 LMA/H01/ST/NC8/1, Register of Nurses, p. 31; London Hospital archives, LH/F11/4, Register of Salaries 1853, p. 38; LMA/H01/ST/ST/C2, Matron's Ward Register 1848–60, no pagination; LMA/H01/ST/NC/V48/56, Cator to Nightingale, 19 October 1856.

66 BL 43402, Nightingale Report No. III, 18 June 1856, fol. 16.

4

Lady nurses: myth and reality

Introduction: nursing and woman's mission

The religious and secular lady nurses presented Nightingale with very different problems from those of the working-class nurses. With the arrival of Mary Stanley and her forty-seven women in December 1854 secular ladies with no clinical nursing experience were introduced into Nightingale's nursing corps. As with the hospital nurses and the religious Sisters, the government paid all the volunteer lady nurses' expenses but the ten ladies in Stanley's group – eleven if we count Stanley herself – were not paid salaries, in line with the convention that ladies should not work for money. These eleven lady volunteers, and thirty-seven more ladies who were sent later, would become the substance of a myth that is still with us today. 'There went out angel women from England, determined to confront that world of horror and misery,' Alexander Kinglake wrote in his history of the Crimean War. They effected a revolution in the Barrack Hospital by doing 'no more than nurse – simply "nurse" the poor sufferers.'[1] Kinglake found it hard to believe that ladies would be willing to do the menial work of nursing, and nursing common soldiers at that. Like most people of his generation, he believed they were fulfilling woman's mission, 'the natural aptitude of their sex for ministering to those who lie prostrate from sickness or wounds.' This natural aptitude made ladies highly effective nurses and it was to these lady nurses that he attributed Nightingale's success. 'Using that tender word which likened the helplessness of the down-stricken soldier to the helplessness of infancy, the alleviation of misery when a gracious lady approached the soldier's pallet to assuage his suffering and to rule him like a sick child' enabled lady nurses to produce a complete transformation of military nursing.[2] Earlier historians of nursing perpetuated this myth of gracious ladies transforming military nursing and applied it to civilian hospitals as well. 'The whole existing system of nursing in civil hospitals was revolutionized by the introduction into them of educated, trained, and refined women,' two early American historians of nursing, Lavinia Dock and Isabel Stewart, proclaimed.[3] Nightingale differed radically in her estimation of untrained lady nurses. Accepting the class structure of English society and its belief in the superiority of the upper classes, she believed higher social status was essential for those in authority, but at the same time she believed clinical experience essential: there were no secular ladies in the first group of nurses when she controlled the selection.

Secular lady nurses: gendered constructions and nursing efficiency

After a year of working in the military hospitals, on 30 November 1855, Nightingale sent a report to the War Office describing the performance of the nurses who had worked in the hospitals she supervised. She indicated who had left and why, and who remained. Her figures include a few arithmetical mistakes: for example, she reported 108 nurses had worked under her direction but listed only 106. Nevertheless, the report gives us an excellent picture of her view of the performance of the three different categories of nurses – working-class, religious Sisters, and secular ladies. In April 1855 Nightingale had resigned all responsibility for the Koulali hospitals. They were about five miles away from Scutari, her hands were full with the two Scutari hospitals, and Mary Stanley had just left and Nightingale could not find a suitable replacement for her. She did not trust Mother Francis Bridgeman who was unofficially superintendent. She wished, she told the War Office, to be 'in no way responsible for the conduct and expenditure of those [Roman Catholic] Sisters,' whom she considered very extravagant.[4] The following October, Hall placed Bridgeman and her nuns in charge of the Balaclava General Hospital so that in November 1855 Nightingale was superintending only four hospitals: in Scutari the General and Barrack hospitals, and in the Crimea, the Castle Hospital and officially, but not in fact as will be shown later, the Monastery Hospital. Some of Nightingale's 106

Government-imposed nursing

Table 4.1 Summary of reasons for nurses leaving

Bridgeman and her 11 Sisters seceded	12
Died	6
Invalided	18
Dismissed for drunkenness	12
Dismissed for incompetence	12
Dismissed for impropriety	4
Chose to go home from Koulali when it closed	4
Other reasons	4
Total	**72**

Source: WI Ms 8895, 30 November 1855, Letter 78

nurses had previously worked in the three hospitals she was no longer superintending, and because Mary Stanley did not send Nightingale reports of the nurses at Koulali, a good deal of the information about the Koulali nurses is missing.

The nurses came out at different times in different groups; some went to the civilian hospitals, many transferred from one hospital to another, others went home sick, and a great many were dismissed. As a result, from November 1854 to July 1856 there were never more than fifty nurses, the number the doctors specified as the maximum number of female nurses they would accept, at work at the same time.[5] One of Bridgeman's original fourteen nuns, Sister Mary Bernard Dixon, went home ill in July 1855 together with a second Sister to nurse her, and a third nun died on 20 October so Bridgeman had only eleven Sisters left at the Balaclava General Hospital in November. Sickness and death accounted for the largest number who left, twenty-four nurses. There were sixteen dismissals for drunkenness and impropriety. With the exception of Charlotte Salisbury, all of these were working-class women. Of the twelve dismissed for incompetence, five were the nuns from Norwood and seven were working-class nurses. Drink was obviously the major problem of the hospital nurses. Twelve were dismissed for intoxication, of whom five were sent home immediately because it was so apparent that they would not be able to work effectively. After some months Nightingale dismissed five more who were not constantly drunk but drunk often enough to threaten the respectability of the nursing team. She gave one of these nurses a gratuity for her good work despite the drunken

Lady nurses: myth and reality

episodes.[6] It was not surprising that there were so many nurses crippled by drink, for alcohol was a horrible problem not only among the working classes but among all classes in the earlier nineteenth century; it was considered the national vice.[7] It was not normally a problem among upper-class ladies, but of the fifty ladies the government sent to the East there were two who were suspected of being heavy drinkers. Charlotte Salisbury, who helped look after sick nurses in Nightingale's house when she was the housekeeper, reported that Matron Walford ate enormous quantities of food and drank even larger amounts of wine when she was dying of fever. Mrs Roberts and another nurse later told Nightingale that Salisbury was drinking the larger half of the wine, stout, and cordials the doctor ordered for Walford. Still, at the time Nightingale seems never to have seen Salisbury drunk and did not suspect her of drinking Walford's prescriptions.[8] The second lady was Martha Clough, who was seen taking three nurses out drinking in a spirit shop when she arrived in Turkey. Later, in Balaclava, Emma Langston asked Nightingale to dismiss her because she encouraged drinking and insubordination among the working-class nurses. However, Clough left Nightingale's team to nurse at Sir Colin Campbell's Highland Brigade hospital before Nightingale could take any action. Clough may well have been fond of drink, but Sir Colin and the doctors were very pleased with her work, which would suggest that she did not overindulge.[9] For all that she dismissed so many of the working-class women, Nightingale declared that paid working-class hospital nurses were always the most useful.[10] Nevertheless, despite their usefulness, she felt only three of the twenty-two hospital nurses remaining at the end of the war were ideally suitable for work in a military hospital; the other nineteen lacked the requisite propriety. 'Give me [hospital] *Nurses*, with a very small admixture of *experienced* Ladies,' Nightingale wrote at the end of the war, '& a larger one of *English* [Moore's nuns as opposed to Bridgeman's] Nuns for the Army Hospitals.'[11]

In her list of nurses who were no longer employed Nightingale did not mention Mary Stanley, the most difficult of the secular ladies. A personal friend of Nightingale, she was one of the ladies who helped to interview and recruit the hospital nurses in London in October 1854. Nightingale first met Stanley during the winter of 1847–48 which she spent in Rome with the Herberts and Bracebridges.

Stanley's father was the Bishop of Norwich and her brother Arthur, later Dean of Westminster, was a close friend of Henry Edward Manning, another member of the Herberts' circle in Rome. At that time Manning was still an Anglican; he would convert to Catholicism in 1851. Eight years older than Nightingale, Mary Stanley became one of her ardent admirers. She had wanted to convert to Catholicism for some years, and in 1854 Nightingale was fully aware of this because Arthur had asked her to use her influence to stop Mary from following Manning into the Catholic Church.[12] In fact, Father Ronan, one of the Catholic chaplains, received her into the church while she was in Koulali.[13] Stanley had arrived in Turkey with forty-seven women, fifteen of whom were Roman Catholic nuns, on 17 December 1854. Nightingale had no positions for them in the two Scutari hospitals and sent the whole group to Therapia until she could make other arrangements. Although Herbert would affirm that the Stanley party, and Bridgeman's group in particular, were under the same rules as the first team of nurses who went out in October, Stanley insisted that he had told her to report to Dr Cumming.[14] Stanley's mother stated quite the contrary. She said that when Herbert had addressed the nuns before they left London he told them they were to obey Nightingale and referred to Stanley as Nightingale's representative until they reached Scutari.[15] Stanley, however, stubbornly refused to accept Nightingale's direction. At the same time she expected her to find the housing for her group and to pay the costs of the nursing at Koulali.[16]

Sue Goldie described Nightingale's initial refusal to accept Stanley and her party as a tactical blunder on Nightingale's part, made because she was so jealous of her position.[17] Mark Bostridge thought that what made matters even worse was that Stanley was challenging Nightingale's authority when, since meeting her in Rome in 1846, she had always been her admirer and loyal disciple.[18] Yet one can hardly blame Nightingale for being so upset when Stanley insisted that Herbert placed her under Dr Cumming's direction. Nightingale sent Herbert one of her most famous and most furious letters expressing her outrage. When she agreed to accept forty nurses rather than the smaller number she would have preferred, she reminded Herbert, he had promised her that he would send no more unless she specifically asked him to do so, and he would not send more nurses unless the doctors had given prior approval. Nightingale had no reason to disbelieve Stanley when she claimed she had been placed under Cumming's direction rather than under hers, and it is entirely understandable that she felt betrayed when she thought Herbert had sent a rival team of nurses. She submitted her resignation.[19] Herbert was a man of good faith who certainly had no intention of betraying Nightingale; there was obviously some major misunderstanding involved in his decision to send this large second party. Fanny Taylor, one of the lady nurses in Stanley's group, believed that Mr Bracebridge had written to Herbert asking for more nurses.[20] It seems possible that Herbert did misinterpret a comment in one of Bracebridge's letters, to the effect that more nurses would be welcome, to mean that Nightingale was asking for additional nurses. Herbert replied to Nightingale's angry letter informing her she was free to send Stanley's party home. He insisted that Bridgeman had come out under the same terms as Moore, and he refused to accept Nightingale's resignation.[21]

Nightingale was extremely concerned by Stanley's financial irresponsibility. When she and her forty-seven nurses arrived they had spent all of the £1,500 that the government had given them. F. B. Smith reported that she spent the money on the best hotels and travel arrangements. Neither Dr Cumming nor Nightingale felt they could give Stanley money from government funds but Nightingale lent her £90 from her own pocket and would later give her a £300 note of credit, also from her own funds.[22] Stanley had intended to chaperone her nurses to Scutari and then immediately return home, but when Nightingale had no positions for them in December she stayed on until they were in work, remaining through the beginning of April 1855. Despite all this, Nightingale felt that Stanley was better qualified to be superintendent than any of the other ladies who were available,[23] another illustration of the importance of social standing in mid-nineteenth-century England. With the exception of Jane Shaw Stewart, Stanley's social status was higher than that of all the other ladies in her party. Similarly, when Nightingale thought she was dying in 1857, even though she knew Jane Shaw Stewart was mentally unbalanced, she told Herbert, 'Mrs Shaw Stewart is the only woman I know who will do for Supt. of Army Nurses.'[24] As she would later write, 'I have always held that Female Nursing in Military Hospitals was impossible unless there were a "real lady" at the head *and* a [lay,

Government-imposed nursing

male] Governor.'[25] As lady superintendent, Stanley was well liked by the nurses who worked under her[26] but she found the actual nursing care too hard for her physically. She took on a standard nursing workload for the first two days in Koulali, after which she decided it was best if she just supervised. She lamented her inability to carry a coal-scuttle or lift a pail of water. 'I *could* not go through the nursing,' she wrote to her family. 'I cannot stand the fatigue, and therefore I gave it up at once.' In any case she felt she had learned all she needed to know in those two days.[27]

The strong Catholic representation in Stanley's group made the experiment of female military nurses even more tenuous. There had been an outcry over the ten Catholic nuns in Nightingale's original party and articles appeared in the press accusing Nightingale of Romanist and/or High Church sympathies. In the same month of December 1854, Wheeler's letter was causing more adverse publicity around the issue of whether women should be in military hospitals at all. The Bracebridges feared that the whole project of female nursing was about to collapse. *The Times* published an article on 9 January 1855 reporting that unless religious dissensions could be reconciled this was a strong possibility.[28] Nightingale's difficulties with Stanley would get worse when it became obvious that she saw nursing as a kind of pastoral calling. She wanted to use ten lady nurses as assistants to the Protestant chaplains and the ten Catholic nuns as assistants to their priests, and she also told Nightingale she wanted only lady nurses.[29] Stanley was an impressionable person who aligned herself with the redoubtable Bridgeman, helping to set up what Nightingale called an opposition party in Koulali.[30] After Stanley left Koulali in April 1855 she kept up a correspondence with Bridgeman, and it was said that Bridgeman grieved her death in 1879.[31] Stanley's request for no working-class nurses and her wish to use the nurses as assistants to the chaplains were all in line with Bridgeman's thinking. One cannot help wondering if the aggressive Bridgeman, under whose influence Stanley had fallen, might not have suggested to her that she should report to Cumming rather than Nightingale.

With the fall of the Aberdeen government Herbert went out of office, and Nightingale had to do business with Benjamin Hawes, the Deputy Secretary at War, who was often quite inimical.[32] He would later refuse to dismiss a purveyor's scurrilous 'Confidential Report'

Lady nurses: myth and reality

which denigrated Nightingale and her nurses. In March she tried to clarify her position to Lord Panmure. 'As Miss Stanley's party was not consigned to me,' she wrote,

> I can only take Miss Stanley's accounts and vouchers, as she gives them to me for expences at Therapia and Koulali, where such of the party have resided who have not joined me at Scutari or been sent by me to Balaclava. I have advanced her money since she came. Until your despatch referring to her, I have had no authority to ask for her accounts nor have I received any from her. Miss Stanley informs me that she had not the contracts with the nurses and that these were left in London, that she knows nothing precisely of their claims nor did she arrange any plan for paying those who went back. I can only refer to those who made the contracts with them.
>
> ... I beg to be distinctly instructed what authority I am deemed to have over the Scutari hospitals, as regards the Sisters and nurses generally as well as over the hospital at Balaclava, and those at Koulali. And in what way I am to be provided with means to meet their expences current and extras – and whether I am deemed to have the same authority over the whole and each individual as over those who came out with me – always, of course, under the restriction of subordination to the inspector general [Sir John Hall] and chief medical authorities as pointed out in my original instructions.[33]

Well might Nightingale tell Sidney Herbert that she found the ladies as unsatisfactory as the hospital nurses, and more ignorant of professional matters.'[34]

Charlotte Salisbury did not go to Australia but returned to London in October 1855. Stanley, who had been home since the preceding April, again demonstrated her general inconsistency and manipulability by helping Salisbury lodge a libel suit against Nightingale. It was a vicious and fraudulent attack, circulating lithographed false statements to diplomatic offices and military officers as well as launching the law suit, which was eventually dismissed. At least one lady nurse, Mrs Burton (the former Miss Innis), and several hospital nurses (Mrs Wheatstone whom Nightingale had dismissed, Mrs Davis who had never liked Nightingale, and Mrs Sansom who was sent home sick and whom Nightingale considered a mischief-maker) agreed to give evidence against Nightingale.[35] At the very same time Stanley sent Nightingale a series of nine lengthy, confused letters in December 1855 and early January 1856. Nightingale consistently strictly followed military regulations and only distributed food and goods to the soldiers if there was a requisition. Stanley admitted

Government-imposed nursing

that Salisbury should not have disobeyed Nightingale in giving out Free Gifts without requisitions, but told Nightingale she would have done the same thing herself. 'The system of requisitions you know is one which I never would adopt beyond a certain point,' she wrote to Nightingale. In this letter, she said she wanted to come back to the East to work under Nightingale but she must be able to do so openly as a Catholic. She did not understand Nightingale's nursing system although she was happy to have recently heard that Nightingale was now turning her attention to the moral diseases rather than the bodily. You know how it grieved me, Stanley continued, when you told me the War Office did not recognize the moral issues as your province. She ended her first letter saying that if Nightingale would accept her honestly as a Catholic, and recognize that she did not understand Nightingale's nursing system, 'I would come and you can scarcely tell what it would be to me if we could end this labour together.' The implication was that she did understand Bridgeman's system of nursing (which is explored in the next chapter), and would use that system rather than Nightingale's. Nightingale replied to Stanley on 19 December 1855, telling her she would have nothing more to do with her. She had tried to be supportive of Stanley, and at first thought her behavior inexplicable, but now she had decided Stanley was temporarily insane.[36]

Eight ladies who came with Stanley, or nine if we include Stanley herself, were gone by 30 November. Four ladies, Innis, Jones, Polidori, and Emily Anderson, went home sick; two, Smythe and Clough, died of fever; and two, Kate Anderson and Fanny Taylor, decided to return to England when Koulali closed rather than work under Nightingale in Scutari. Declaring herself subject only to Hall's authority, Martha Clough withdrew from Nightingale's supervision to become matron of Sir Colin Campbell's Highlanders' regimental hospital. There she became very ill and was sent to Scutari but died of fever on shipboard.[37] By 10 December 1855 when Mrs McLeod and her daughter Abigail left Koulali and came to Scutari, there were nine ladies working in Nightingale's hospitals. She described the two McLeods as 'gentle workers.' The mother had been in charge of the nurses' home in Koulali and was most amiable, but because of her age and delicate health was unable to do any serious work. Nightingale could not understand why she had been sent in the first place. The daughter,

88

Lady nurses: myth and reality

Abigail, was full of courage and energy but not at all useful.[38] The reports unfortunately give no hint of why the ladies decided she was not useful.

Nightingale made three ladies hospital superintendents. She deemed two of those three, Margaret Wear and Miss Tebbutt, unsatisfactory; in both cases she appointed them only because she had no better candidates. Their only real qualification was that they were ladies and, in the rigidly defined class structure of Victorian England, superintendents had to be ladies. As superintendent of the Balaclava General Hospital Wear was conscientious and enjoyed giving personal care to individual soldiers, but Nightingale judged her unable to manage her staff as well as completely unbusinesslike – she did not keep any accounts. After a few months in Balaclava, like Stanley and Clough, Wear rejected Nightingale's authority and transferred her allegiance to Dr Hall. When, in October 1855, Hall demoted Wear and made Bridgeman superintendent, Wear pronounced herself happy to work under her.[39] In fact, Bridgeman considered Wear as poor a superintendent as did Nightingale, saying she was kind to her patients but a consummate gossip and intensely jealous of her Sisters' superior nursing, a jealousy she vented in a very dangerous manner.[40] In mid-December Hall sent Wear to the Monastery Hospital as matron. Nightingale decided to ignore Wear's desertion and acted as if she were still working for her. Nightingale considered Tebbutt even less competent, 'entirely unfitted to be a superintendent and even less fitted to be a nurse.' But, like Wear, she was a lady and, in Nightingale's view, she did have one saving grace: she was very concerned with her nurses' morals.[41]

Nightingale believed Jane Shaw Stewart, the third lady superintendent, an unqualified success. Of the seventeen months she was in the East, she spent fifteen as superintendent of three Crimean hospitals: first the Balaclava General, then the Castle Hospital when it opened in April 1855, and finally the left wing of the Land Transport hospitals in March 1856.[42] She was well qualified to be a lady superintendent for two reasons. First, after she had been turned down when she volunteered in October 1854, at Nightingale's suggestion she then worked as a nurse at the Westminster Hospital until she left London with the second party of nurses on 2 December 1854.[43] She therefore had some real clinical experience. Second, she came from the upper

89

ranks of society. Her sister was the Duchess of Somerset, so Shaw Stewart automatically commanded respect from the lower classes.[44] At the same time Nightingale and others considered her more than half mad[45] – 'Good old mad Shaw,'[46] Nightingale called her when writing to her sister Parthenope. But she also considered her 'good and sterling.' 'Unwise, provoking, & mad as she is,' she wrote to her family, 'it is such a relief to come to something which is above, entirely above, all that is mean & petty & selfish & frivolous & low.'[47]

Nightingale was not the only one to question Shaw Stewart's mental stability. George Lawson, a young surgeon, thought she was perfectly mad. She worked twenty-four hours a day nursing the worst fever cases, seldom removing her clothes, and taking snatches of rest wrapped in a cloak lying on the ground. 'She has already had an attack of erysipelas,' Lawson wrote, 'and if she continues in her foolish ways, will probably get an attack of fever.'[48] Temple Godman, a young cavalry officer, reported her '*quite* cracked, she seems very odd.'[49] Elizabeth Davis, who worked under her in Balaclava, called her 'just and firm, though arbitrary and odd now and then.'[50] After the war, on Nightingale's recommendation, she was made lady superintendent of the army hospital at Netley. There she behaved very erratically, flying into passions, stamping her feet, slamming doors, physically beating her nurses, snapping her fingers in the doctors' faces, and sending them lengthy, unreasonable letters and memoranda. The medical staff complained vociferously and she was eventually dismissed.[51] Nevertheless, Shaw Stewart was very loyal to Nightingale and she had the virtues that Nightingale most esteemed in a nurse: devotion to the cause, untiring zeal, watchful care of the nurses, and accuracy in keeping accounts.[52]

The four remaining ladies, Clarke, Morton, Tattersall, and Écuyer, were good workers but not at what we would now call nursing. Miss Clarke was hired especially for the position of housekeeper at the Barrack Hospital. She is not to be confused with the Mrs Clarke, who had been Nightingale's matron at Harley Street and whom she fired in Scutari. Miss Clarke was in no way related to her. She was a lady who had trained at several hospitals and Nightingale described her as 'good, true, kind, faithful & well meaning.' Miss Mary Tattersall, at her own request, was the cook and housekeeper for the female staff at the Scutari General Hospital. She had spent some weeks at the Westminster Hospital working as a nurse before coming to Scutari, but thought she would do better in charge of the cooking and housekeeping rather than as a clinical nurse. Her truthfulness, good judgment, willingness to do any job no matter how menial, and her trustworthiness made her an invaluable worker.[53] Miss Écuyer, who originally worked at Smyrna but transferred to Scutari after Sevastopol fell, was matron of the Scutari General Hospital. She was 'excellent, useful, laborious, active, devoted to nursing, but, 'from a peculiarity of temper,' could only work alone.[54] Miss Anne Ward Morton was very willing to do anything assigned to her but lacked the physical strength to do a great deal of the necessary work. Nightingale made her the matron of the Barrack Hospital. In that position she took tender care of the nurses, exercising an excellent moral influence on them. She taught them reading and writing and raised their characters with moral instruction.[55] Nightingale had decided that most of her ladies were better suited to elevating the characters of the working-class nurses than tending the patients. She regretted having no position for a lady, Miss Spottiswoode, who volunteered her services, because she 'so thoroughly comprehends the work before her (which is the only true beauty).' She hoped she would have a position for her in the future because 'She seems to understand that the work of the Ladies here lies with the Nurses more than with men – which scarcely anyone has done.'[56]

Of the above four ladies, three – Clarke, Écuyer, and Tattersall – were paid, as were the two McLeods. Because they were ladies, Nightingale paid them at the top level of the government fee schedule, eighteen shillings a week. The McLeods really needed the money. Abigail wrote to Nightingale in August 1856 saying she and her mother had not been fully reimbursed for travel expenses and asked that this be rectified. She was defensive about having worked for a salary. On the voyage home Miss Tebbutt had reproached her for being paid and 'being consequently bound to do what she did not think fit to do.' To go to the Eastern hospitals was the first wish of her heart, McLeod explained, and she 'accepted a *Salary for the sake of the work*, not the work for the sake of a *Salary*. With no source of income but my mother's small pension (£40 per annum) how could I go out to the East without a salary?'[57] The silliness of the argument that she could not have gone to the East unless she was paid a salary is obvious.

It cost the volunteer ladies, paid ladies, and working-class nurses absolutely nothing to travel to the East because as well as paying all their costs in the military hospitals the government paid their travel expenses from their home town, Edinburgh in the McLeods' case, to the seaport. The only group that lost money sending nurses to the East was St. John's House. They supported their training school with private donations and the profits from the private nursing their trained nurses brought in, so they lost valuable income when they sent six nurses to Scutari.

Mlle. Écuyer, as the Smyrna ladies called her, and Mary Tattersall, who arrived in the spring of 1855, were the first paid ladies to join the nursing team. They took a less traditional approach to being paid than did Abigail McLeod and Miss Tebbutt. They are illustrations of what Frank Prochaska called the shifts in the nineteenth-century view of woman's mission.[58] We do not know what Écuyer's circumstances were, but she seems to have needed the money, for on returning to England she looked for a paid job as a matron.[59] Mary Tattersall, who was thought to be between 30 and 40 years old, appears to have come from relatively comfortable circumstances. Her father was a brewer in Leeds and she had done the traditional lady's district visiting before going to the Westminster Hospital for three weeks of training.[60] Tattersall seemed quite thrilled to be receiving a wage. She asked Nightingale to send the Westminster Hospital £5 saved from her salary, being 'the first money she ever earned, that she earnestly wishes to devote to the place where she received so much kindness when learning there.'[61] Unlike many of the other nurses and Écuyer, she never wrote to Nightingale after the war asking for her help in finding a job.

In summary, the government sent a total of forty-eight lady volunteers to the different hospitals and Nightingale hired two more ladies, Charlotte Salisbury and Mrs Walford, in the East, making a total of fifty. Of these fifty, twelve were paid and seven worked under Nightingale. The two McLeods were rather useless and Nightingale fired Salisbury, but four of the seven did excellent work in non-clinical nursing positions. Nightingale listed thirty-two nurses remaining on 30 November 1855 but she actually named thirty-six women: twenty-two hospital nurses, two Anglican and five Catholic Sisters, and seven ladies.[62] Counting the McLeods, who

Lady nurses: myth and reality

arrived on 10 December, of the nine ladies who remained only one, Jane Shaw Stewart, was competent to superintend and actually nurse in the sense of clinical work. Sister Mary Aloysius Doyle, who was considered the best nurse among Bridgeman's nuns, pointed out that the lady nurses came from luxurious homes and did not have the experience to deal with the kind of acute care nursing which confronted them in the military hospitals. They admitted, Doyle said, that they knew nothing about nursing and often regretted that they had to lean so heavily on the Sisters. By contrast, Doyle thought the Sisters' four and a half year novitiate gave them both the physical stamina and the clinical experience to withstand the shock under which the health of many ladies collapsed.[63] However, when the large group of forty-seven nurses arrived and the government sent dressers to do the dressings on the surgical wards in December 1854, the lady nurses' work became much lighter.[64] Nightingale then asked them to stop nursing individual patients and instead supervise the hospital nurses and orderlies. But '*How could they superintend without some knowledge of the work?*' Doyle asked.[65] She was absolutely right where patient care was concerned, but the ladies were of real assistance because they could see that the working-class nurses stayed at work rather than visiting the canteens to buy liquor, and they could insist that nurses carried out doctors' orders and did so promptly and accurately. While in law ladies were subordinate to their male relatives, as Anne Summers has pointed out, in their own homes and in their charitable activities they were more used to giving orders than to taking them,[66] so they tended to be good managers. Furthermore, ladies were familiar with housekeeping which the orderlies were not, and the doctors and patients very much appreciated their housekeeping and cooking.[67]

Nightingale considered thirty-six nurses an adequate number to staff the four hospitals. It would be necessary in the future, she thought, to renew the staff of female nurses every two years. She was not distressed by this high rate of turnover, attributing it to four unavoidable causes. First, many succumbed to the difficult climate and local fevers and had to go home sick, and second, the high incidence of drunkenness among the hospital nurses meant many had to be dismissed. Nightingale believed drunkenness was considered tolerable in civilian hospitals but she could not condone it in military

Government-imposed nursing

hospitals. Third, when recruiting nurses, until they were actually at work, it was very challenging to identify incompetents, adventurers, or women who were attracted solely by the exceptionally high pay that the government offered. Finally, some nurses left because they became homesick. Still, she concluded,

> taking all these draw-backs into consideration which apply (not more but perhaps) less to the female than to any other branch of the service, it is obvious that the experiment of sending Nurses to the East has been eminently successful – & that the supplying of trained instruments to the hands of the Medical Officers has saved much valuable life & remedied many deficiencies …[68]

Nightingale's best nurses

Whom did Nightingale consider her best nurses and what made them superior in her view? Nightingale wrote reports or 'characters' for the forty-six nurses who were working when the war ended in 1856. At that point she was in charge of the nursing in seven hospitals: the two in Scutari; the Monastery and Castle hospitals in Balaclava; in March 1856 she took over the nursing in the two Land Transport Corps hospitals; and the following month when Bridgeman left, the Balaclava General. She herself, together with her Aunt Mai, did not go home until August 1856 when the last patient left the hospitals, but she dispatched her nurses home in four groups in May, June, and July. With the exception of the three Bermondsey nuns who arrived in January 1856, Nightingale sent the weakest nurses home first and those she considered her very best last. The three latterly arrived Bermondsey nuns were equally as good as the three Sisters who went home in the last group; they went home earlier because they worked in the Crimean hospitals, which closed before those in Turkey.

The last party to leave for home, those whom Nightingale considered her very best nurses, consisted of two secular ladies, Jane Shaw Stewart and Anne Ward Morton, three Bermondsey Sisters, two Anglican Sisters, and five hospital nurses. The two ladies were excellent but there were problems with both. Shaw Stewart was a committed and outstanding nurse but everyone agreed that she was quite mad. Morton lacked the physical strength to do any clinical

Lady nurses: myth and reality

nursing and had to spend most of her time teaching and elevating the characters of the working-class nurses. The five religious Sisters were superlative nurses and also had the most staying power – all five came out with Nightingale in October 1854. Of the original five Bermondsey Sisters, three worked through the whole campaign; the other two stayed through all but the last two months, when Moore went home sick accompanied by Barrie to nurse her. Shaw Stewart came in December 1854 and Morton in August 1855. Of the five working-class nurses, Eliza Roberts was the only one who came in the first group. Robbins came in December 1854 and Logan, Tandy, and Taunton in April 1855. Only two of the five hospital nurses, Robbins and Logan, met Nightingale's unreasonably high standards. Robbins was a sober, respectable, kind, and excellent nurse as well as a good cook. Logan was sober, respectable, kind as well as clever, industrious, thoroughly trustworthy, and a good washerwoman. The three remaining nurses each had some failing. Nightingale herself never complained about Roberts, but she was a very difficult person who was ill-mannered and enjoyed fighting with the other nurses. Certainly Nightingale's Aunt Mai found her an unpleasant person to work with. Tandy was intemperate and Taunton did not meet Nightingale's standard of complete dedication to nursing. She was 'much given to thoughts of marriage,' which Nightingale considered very inconvenient for a nurse in the field.[69]

Still, Nightingale remained convinced that the best mix for any nursing team was a large number of working-class nurses with a few religious Sisters and ladies added 'to elevate and leaven the mass.' She said that 'under circumstances of peculiar temptation' a larger proportion of paid nurses than of ladies did well during the war.[70] In fact on 30 November 1855 out of seventy-three working-class nurses only thirty-two, or 44 percent, were still working, a figure that compares badly to that of the Catholic Sisters – twelve out of fifteen in Bridgeman's party and six out of eight in Moore's. In terms of the nurses who had given her the most support Nightingale listed five. Without them, she said, she could not have pulled through, opposed as she had been 'by all the officials here [in Scutari] & in the Crimea, thwarted & harassed on every side, with traps set for me – & *not* supported at home, at least, not with a consistent & efficient support.' The nurses were Mother Mary Clare Moore and Sister Bertha Turnbull who were both ladies and religious Sisters, Jane Shaw Stewart, Anne Ward Morton, and Mrs Roberts.

Raising character

It seems contradictory that Nightingale was committed to working-class women as the base for any nursing team when she listed four ladies out of five as her mainstays. However, there were many reasons why she considered working-class women the most useful. They had real hospital experience, were physically stronger than secular ladies, and were used to doing the heavy nursing work. Nightingale did assign the less able hospital nurses to purely housekeeping duties, but unlike the more progressive St. John's House, she never completely removed all of the housekeeping duties from the more able nurses. She retained the standard upper-class view of working-class nurses as servants and appreciated the flexibility of being able to use them as washerwomen, seamstresses, and so on as well as for patient care. Furthermore, working-class nurses were more amenable to direction than ladies. The hospital nurses could certainly be rebellious and cause trouble, but they did not have the social status to organize what Nightingale called rebellion and secession, which one paid lady nurse, Charlotte Salisbury, three secular unpaid ladies, Martha Clough, Margaret Wear, and Mary Stanley, and one religious Sister, Mother Francis Bridgeman, did.

Nightingale certainly valued clinical experience highly, but raising the characters of nurses had always been her 'principal & dearest object' in working with them.[71] Elevating working-class character was not an esoteric pursuit of Nightingale and Morton but, as Martin Wiener has demonstrated, permeated nineteenth-century culture and public policy.[72] Michael Roberts has a whole book, *Making English Morals*, arguing that moral reform was a major force in English society from the 1780s until the 1880s. Furthermore, for Nightingale nursing was more than a profession. A profession such as medicine or midwifery, she believed, required only technical knowledge, but nursing was a calling that required in addition a mystical religious commitment. Without the elevated character religious dedication conveyed, the technical knowledge of nursing was comparatively useless.[73] 'When very many years ago I planned a future,' she told her

Lady nurses: myth and reality

close friend Benjamin Jowett, Regius Professor of Greek at Oxford, 'my one idea was not organizing a Hospital, but organizing a religion.' Quoting the Magnificat, she thought a nurse should ideally be a 'handmaiden of the Lord.'[74] In 1845 she had thought of organizing 'something like a Protestant Sisterhood, without vows, for women of educated feelings,'[75] but she gave this up when she saw the hostilities that sisterhoods, both Anglican and Catholic, aroused in the Crimea. She also realized that it would be difficult to attract enough women to a nursing sisterhood.[76] Working-class nurses were the most useful for her particular plans.

Before returning to England in August 1856 Nightingale summarized the work of her nursing mission. 'A great work has been done,' she wrote. There had been problems with 'our masters, the army surgeons,' the mission had attracted women 'desirous of notoriety rather than of work,' and it had incited the restless, envious enmity of some nurses and some people in the public. 'Nor can we deny,' Nightingale continued:

> that things to be deeply regretted have happened among us. Rebellion among some ladies & some nurses, and drunkenness among some nurses have unhappily disgraced our body. Still what we came to do has been done. The suffering to be relieved has been relieved.

As she and her team prepared to return home to England she hoped that the nurses would say as little as possible about their work in the East 'since not only we are the last appointed, the fewest, & the lowest in official rank of the Queen's war-servants, but we are the first women who have been suffered in the war-service'.[77]

Notes

1 Kinglake, *Invasion of the Crimea*, vol. 4, pp. 280–1.
2 Ibid, vol. 7, pp. 359–60, 363.
3 Dock and Stewart, *Short History of Nursing*, pp. 126–7.
4 National Archives, Nightingale to Benjamin Hawes, 2 April 1855, Kew/ WO/43/963.
5 WI Ms 8895, Nightingale Report, 30 November 1855, Letter 78.
6 Ibid.
7 Webb, *Modern England*, p. 130; Harrison, *Drink and the Victorians*, pp. 37–41, 306–9.

Government-imposed nursing

8 O'Malley, *Florence Nightingale*, pp. 322, 325.

9 Roxburgh, 'Miss Clough,' pp. 87–8.

10 Nightingale, 'Introduction of Female Nursing,' p. 29.

11 BL 43402, Nightingale Report No. I, May 1856, fol. 6.

12 O'Malley, *Florence Nightingale*, pp. 135, 197–8, 251.

13 Nightingale, *Crimean War*, p. 336fn; Smith, *Reputation and Power*, p. 31.

14 Dr Alexander Cumming was a member of the three-man Parliamentary Commission sent to inquire into the state of the hospitals and was senior to Dr Duncan Menzies who was originally the Principal Medical Officer at Scutari.

15 Goldie, '*I Have Done my Duty*,' p. 50.

16 BL 43393, Nightingale to Herbert, 15 February 1855, fols 155–8.

17 Goldie, '*I Have Done my Duty*,' p. 54.

18 Bostridge, *Florence Nightingale*, pp. 240–1.

19 BL 43393, Nightingale to Herbert, 15 December 1854, fols 34–5.

20 Taylor, *English Hospitals*, vol. 1, pp. 10–11.

21 Stanmore, *Sidney Herbert*, vol. 1, pp. 370–2.

22 Smith, *Reputation and Power*, p. 46; BL 43393, Nightingale to Herbert, 12 February 1855, fols 142–5.

23 WI Ms 9020, Nightingale to Herbert, 22 January 1855, Letter 11.

24 BL 43394, Nightingale to Herbert, 26 November 1857, fol. 193.

25 BL 45754, Nightingale to Sutherland, 1 October [1869], fol. 3.

26 Taylor, *Eastern Hospitals*, vol. 1, pp. 142–3.

27 Stanmore, *Sidney Herbert*, vol. 1, pp. 377, 408.

28 Bostridge, *Florence Nightingale*, pp. 238–9, 241.

29 BL 43393, Nightingale to Herbert, 25 December 1854, fols 45–6.

30 WI Ms 8995, Nightingale to her mother, 1 February 1855, Letter 3.

31 Doyle, 'Memories,' p. 50; Bolster, *Sisters of Mercy*, p. 145.

32 Goldie, '*I Have Done my Duty*,' pp. 110–11.

33 National Archives, Nightingale to Lord Panmure, 5 March 1855, WO/43963.

34 Nightingale to Herbert, 18 March 1855 in Nightingale, *Crimean War*, p. 167.

35 BL 43397, Nightingale to Lady Cranworth, 31 January and 10 February 1856, fols 79–80, 87–9; BL 43401, Nightingale to Lord Murray, 29 September 1856, fols 252–3; WI Ms 8995, Nightingale to the Bracebridges, 7 August 1855, Letter 26; WI Ms 8996, Nightingale to Parthenope, 17 March 1856, Letter 28; Davis, *Autobiography*, vol. 2, pp. 114–17, 163–6.

36 O'Malley, *Florence Nightingale*, pp. 327–8, 355; WI Ms 8995, FN [to her family], 4 March [1855], Letter 6; WI Ms 8996, FN to 'My dearest' [Parthenope], 17 March 1856, Letter 28.

37 Roxburgh, 'Miss Clough,' pp. 71–2, 87–8,

38 BL 43402, Nightingale Report No. II, 16 June 1856, fol. 10.

39 BL 39867, Wear to Hall, 9 November 1855 and 21 December, fols 63, 73–4.

40 Bridgeman, 'Account,' pp. 200–1.

Lady nurses: myth and reality

41 Helmstadter and Godden, *Before Nightingale*, pp. 91–3; BL 42402, Nightingale Report No. II, 16 June 1856, fol. 10; LMA/H0/ST/NC8/1, Register of Nurses, p. 16.

42 BL 43402, FN Report No. IV, 26 June 1856, fol. 19.

43 LMA/H02/WH/A1/37, Minutes of House Committee, 24 October, 5 December 1854.

44 Bostridge, *Florence Nightingale*, p. 431; Lawson, *Surgeon in the Crimea*, p. 164.

45 BL 45793 FN [to family member], 19 October 1855, fol.106; Lawson, *Surgeon in the Crimea*, p. 164.

46 WI Ms 8995, Nightingale to Parthenope, 9 July 1855, Letter 22.

47 WI Ms 8995, Nightingale to her family, 28 October 1855, Letter 56.

48 Lawson, *Surgeon in the Crimea*, p. 164.

49 Godman, *Fields of War*, pp. 139–40.

50 Davis, *Autobiography*, vol. 2, p. 136.

51 Helmstadter and Godden, *Before Nightingale*, p. 94.

52 BL 43402, Nightingale Report No. I, May 1856, fol. 19.

53 Ibid, May 1856, fols 3, 16.

54 BL 43402, Nightingale Report No. IV, 26 June 1856, fol. 10.

55 Ibid, fol. 25; LMA/H01/ST/NC8/1, Register of Nurses, p. 31.

56 WI Ms 8996, Nightingale [to Aunt Mai Smith], 24 January 1856, Letter 5.

57 LMA/H01/ST/NC1/V25/56, A. McLeod to Nightingale, 28 August 1856.

58 Prochaska, *Women and Philanthropy*, pp. 1–2.

59 LMA/H01/ST/NC2/V3/56, R. M. Écuyer to Nightingale, 25 August 1856.

60 LMA/H01/ST/NC8/1, Register of Nurses, p. 23.

61 Nightingale to the Westminster Hospital, 13 August 1855, reproduced in Humble and Hansell, *Westminster Hospital*, p. 81.

62 Bridgeman picked up on this arithmetical error although she said Nightingale listed thirty-five. Bridgeman, 'Account,' p. 218.

63 Doyle, 'Memories,' pp. 27–8.

64 BL 43393, Nightingale to Herbert, 4 January 1855, fol. 64.

65 Doyle, 'Memories,' p. 28.

66 Summers, *Angels and Citizens*, p. 3.

67 Calthorpe, *Letters from Headquarters*, p. 35.

68 WI Ms 8895, Nightingale Report, 30 November 1855, Letter 78.

69 BL 43402, Nightingale Report IV, 26 June 1856, fol. 24; O'Malley, *Florence Nightingale*, pp. 344, 352.

70 Nightingale, 'Introduction of Female Nursing,' pp. 5–6, 29.

71 BL 43397, Nightingale to Lady Cranworth, 14 January 1856, fols 75–6.

72 Wiener, *Reconstructing the Criminal*, pp. 44–5.

73 Bonham-Carter, 'General Register,' p. 3. In line with her efforts to avoid public exposure, Nightingale had her views published under Bonham-Carter's name.

Government-imposed nursing

74 Luke 1:48, 'For he hath regarded the low estate of his handmaiden,' King James translation.

75 Cook, *Florence Nightingale*, vol.1, pp. 44, 366–7.

76 LMA/H01/ST/NC1/66/25, Nightingale to Sister Mary Jones, 20 December 1866.

77 BL 43402, Nightingale Note, [July to August 1856], fol. 160.

Part II

Religious nursing

5

Mother Francis Bridgeman and her Sisters of Mercy

Introduction

Of the three systems of nursing used in the Crimean War, government-imposed, nursing sisterhoods, and doctor-directed nursing, religious Sisters were obviously the most successful as a group. However, British Roman Catholic Sisters had a particularly difficult time because of the long-standing anti-Catholic tradition in Britain. Anti-Catholicism also impacted the new Anglican Sisters because they were often mistakenly identified with Catholic nuns. The French and Piedmont-Sardinian Daughters of Charity, on the other hand, had a long and distinguished tradition of military nursing and were welcomed. We are fortunate in having Mother Francis Bridgeman's own account of her mission to the East as well as those of two of her Sisters, Sister Mary Aloysius Doyle and Sister Mary Joseph Croke. In 1897 when Doyle was awarded the Royal Red Cross,[1] her diary was published in a lightly edited version. Extracts from the Croke and Bridgeman journals appeared in articles and books, but when in the 1960s a priest wished to publish the entire Croke journal, his bishop would not give permission because parts of the diary reflected badly on Croke and Bridgeman.[2] In 2004 historian Maria Luddy edited and published all three journals in full. Doyle's diary tells us the most about the nursing. Her warm, empathetic personality and her sense of humor come through strongly. She was not as infused with the suspicion and hostility toward the English that bedeviled Bridgeman and Croke and, above all, she understood Nightingale's difficult position.[3]

Bridgeman, who came to the East with a different cultural and political viewpoint, on the other hand took a militant anti-English stand. The 'Papal Aggression' in 1850 set off a venomous wave of what contemporaries called 'No Popery.' Most English people identified Roman Catholics with England's traditional enemies, France and Spain, and the much looked-down-upon Irish immigrants who were flooding into England at this time, while Protestantism represented patriotism and the heroic English spirit of enterprise and progress. They considered popery tyranny and Protestant England a free and open society. Needless to say, the Irish did not appreciate this English view. The Irish were beginning to develop a true sense of nationalism in the modern sense of the word; the Irish Question would come to dominate British politics in the second half of the century.[4]

As an English upper-class, Protestant, secular lady, Nightingale would meet resistance from Bridgeman from the very first time they came into contact. As well as their generally hostile attitude toward the English, Bridgeman and Croke disliked Nightingale personally and were proud of the encounters in which they thought Bridgeman had bested her.[5] They were very pleased when in October 1855 Bridgeman finally cut all ties with Nightingale and established her nuns as a completely independent community working under Sir John Hall. Nightingale, Croke wrote, was then 'crest-fallen since the "Sisters of Mercy" had escaped from her fangs.'[6] Doyle was more open-minded. When she set off for the East in the winter of 1854 she thought the English bigots. 'We travel in our veils, in the face of proud, bigoted England,' she wrote. 'Will not this be a triumph for our holy religion.' But on her return to Ireland in 1856, after working with the English nurses, she asserted, 'We have now many kind friends in England, and we are now determined never again to say "the cold English."' She sent her warmest remembrances to any of the English women with whom she had worked during the war who might still be alive, assuring them she kept them in her prayers.[7]

Bridgeman in the East: recreating Irish conventual practice

Bridgeman was Mother Superior of the Convent of Mercy in Kinsale (Ireland) when Sisters of Mercy were volunteering for the second party of nurses which left England on 2 December 1854. Fifteen Sisters (fourteen if we do not include Bridgeman herself) were chosen and Bridgeman offered to take charge of them. Ten came from four

Mother Francis Bridgeman and her Sisters of Mercy

convents in Ireland and five from English convents in Liverpool and Chelsea. Two were lay Sisters who mainly looked after the domestic needs of the choir Sisters and did little nursing.[8] Bridgeman and several Sisters left Ireland for London on 3 November and spent the following month at the Convent of Mercy in Chelsea. The War Office delayed sending the second group of nurses until they felt certain that the military doctors were willingly working with Nightingale. From the time they arrived in London until they left for Scutari, Bridgeman and another Sister went every day to St. George's or another teaching hospital to study English nursing practice. When they did leave England Bridgeman was unhappy with the government's travelling arrangements. In Ireland Bridgeman was used to being treated with enormous respect and was horrified when she learned that there were only three first class berths for her party on the ship and the rest of her Sisters were to travel in second class with the working-class nurses and eat together with the other second class passengers. She was appalled that her nuns would be put 'into domestic contact with this class of people,' but, in order to keep her community together, she declined the three first class places. On the very first day on board ship what she described as a crowd of coarse men rushed into the dining room and sat down right next to the Sisters. Bridgeman instantly stood up and told her nuns to retire to their sleeping room; it was better to go without dinner than to remain in close contact with such people. She was even more shocked on arriving in Turkey when Nightingale informed her that there were no positions in the hospitals for Stanley's party and sent them to the British embassy summer houses in Therapia.

When Nightingale decided to replace the inexperienced Norwood nuns with five from Bridgeman's party she wrote to Bridgeman asking her to send five nuns to Scutari; they would be placed under Moore's spiritual direction. Bridgeman thought it best to reply in person to this request, which violated her orders to keep her community together, so she and Sister Mary Bernard Dixon went to Scutari to speak face-to-face with Nightingale. Moore met them and, presumably to show them why it had been impossible to accommodate them in the Barrack Hospital, showed them the one room in which the ten Catholic nuns were living. Bridgeman wrote that she and Dixon were 'grieved and shocked beyond expression at *all* they saw and heard.'

Religious nursing

Instead of a separate wing in a large building or a house of their own, as the contract with the War Office stipulated, there was a soiled white calico screen dividing the Norwood and Bermondsey nuns from each other, and the ten Sisters had to use this one room for every purpose – bedroom, dining room, bathroom, and living room. (The Sisters at the Scutari General Hospital had the same arrangements, with only one room.) Bridgeman thought the Sisters themselves 'soiled and neglected looking,' and she was indignant because, she said, such arrangements showed no respect for the religious life.

When Nightingale herself finally appeared she seemed sweet and gracious at first, Bridgeman reported, but then she ordered in a lunch consisting of 'a small *remnant* of musty cheese, a *scrap* of dirty butter in a bowl, some sour bread, some cold potatoes' and 'something in a bottle.' Bridgeman suggested Nightingale rent a house in Scutari where she and her nuns could live separately and come to the hospital every day, but she said Nightingale refused every proposal she made. Bridgeman thereupon took an instant dislike to Nightingale. She had hoped to find a friend in Nightingale, she wrote, but when she refused to accept all fifteen nuns at once Bridgeman decided she was an ambitious woman on whom she could not rely. Nightingale seems to have intended to treat Bridgeman as kindly as Moore at first, but could not implement her proposals. As well as having no suitable accommodation for them in the hospital and no suitable houses available in Scutari, Nightingale could not accept all fifteen nuns without violating her instructions from the War Office and the doctors. The doctors refused to have more than the ten Catholic Sisters they already had in the two hospitals and Nightingale was already stretching Herbert's ratio of one Catholic to every three Protestants. Nightingale had told Bridgeman before they met face-to-face that the doctors would only allow fifty nurses in the hospitals[9] but there is no evidence that she told her of Herbert's desired quota for Roman Catholics. Perhaps she thought it was too sensitive an issue to mention. Lord William Paulet, the military commandant, declared that the fifteen nuns should not enter the hospital.[10] Where the nurses were concerned, Paulet seems to have generally reacted less from ideological reasons than from a wish not to be bothered. Equally importantly, Bridgeman refused to understand or accept Nightingale's inability to send nurses into the wards unless the doctors requested them; she seems to have

Mother Francis Bridgeman and her Sisters of Mercy

thought Nightingale could send as many nurses as she liked into any ward. Moore understood that there were no better accommodations available in Scutari than the miserable one room the ten nuns shared, and she assured Bridgeman that Nightingale did not interfere in her Sisters' religious practices outside of the wards. But, as she pointed out, although Bridgeman had signed what was essentially the same contract as Bishop Grant signed for the Bermondsey nuns, she refused to be subordinate to Nightingale. Bridgeman had the idea 'that they might hire a house in the town of Scutari, form a regular religious community and attend the hospitals as they would have done in Ireland.'[11] But Scutari was very different from England, where there were hackney coaches and furnished houses to let. There was not a house in Scutari that was in good repair or that would have been suitable for the nuns.[12]

Nightingale's orders from the War Office stated clearly:

> Everything relating to the distribution of the nurses, the hours of their attendance, their allotment to particular duties, is placed in your hands, subject, of course, to the sanction and approval of the Chief Medical Officer [of the hospital] but the selection of the nurses in the first instance is placed solely under your controul [*sic*].'[13]

She therefore asked Bridgeman to send Dixon, who had been professed by Moore, and four others whose qualifications she would discuss with Bridgeman. They would report to Nightingale in matters relating to hospital nursing and to Moore in matters relating to religious discipline. Bridgeman then decided it would be best in the future to communicate with Nightingale in writing only. She was prepared to act under Moore but she would not divest herself of her office of superior to her own nuns, nor would she share with Nightingale the right of selection of the nuns. She herself would come to the Barrack Hospital and she would select the other four.[14] Nightingale replied that two Mothers Superior could give rise to difficulties so she could not accept her as one of the five. In the end Nightingale backed down. She sent Moore on 6 January 1855 to Therapia – in an open boat in the midst of a violent snowstorm – to negotiate with Bridgeman. Moore told Bridgeman that Nightingale would accept her, and Bridgeman agreed to bring four of her nuns to Scutari, all under Moore's direction. At first Nightingale refused

Religious nursing

to yield on her right to select the other four nuns but now she replied that she would take Bridgeman, Dixon, and three more nuns whom Bridgeman and Moore agreed on. But Dixon was not included in the four nuns Bridgeman brought with her to Scutari on 8 January 1855.[15]

Nightingale was able to absorb all of Stanley's nurses by the end of January 1855 because eight nurses went to Balaclava, the Koulali hospitals opened, and so many nurses from the first two parties had been fired or invalided home. Nightingale kept five of Bridgeman's nuns in Scutari and sent Bridgeman and her remaining nine nuns with some working-class nurses to Koulali under Stanley as lady superintendent. Stanley immediately made Bridgeman superintendent of the Lower Koulali Hospital.[16] Bridgeman made a point of visiting the five Sisters at the Scutari General Hospital at least once a month, and while there, also visited Moore, her nominal chief. She spoke with Nightingale when she thought it useful although she said that was a real penance.[17] In April 1855 the opening of the Castle Hospital in Balaclava enabled Hall to keep acute cases in the Crimea and spare the soldiers the lengthy and painful voyage to Turkey. As a result, over the summer the hospitals in Turkey became largely chronic care institutions. Early in September Bridgeman decided that she and her nuns could be better used in the Crimea. She offered her services to Hall on condition that she would work directly under his supervision and would have nothing to do with Nightingale, because her system of nursing was so different from Nightingale's. Hall was delighted to have this opportunity to undercut Nightingale. He did not reply to Bridgeman for a month because, she said, he was busy 'quietly getting Miss Nightingale out of Balaclava.' When Nightingale gave up the Koulali hospitals in April 1855 they officially came under the direction of General Storks, then commandant of the British military establishments in Turkey. On 1 October 1855 Hall, without consulting Nightingale or Storks, officially appointed Bridgeman superintendent of the Balaclava General Hospital.[18] Nor did Bridgeman discuss her plans to withdraw her nuns with either Nightingale or Storks.

Nightingale, who was clearly in charge of appointing the nurses to the various hospitals, obviously could not accept these actions. Yet there was little she could do since she was subject to Hall's orders and he had made the appointment. Croke commented that Nightingale knew Bridgeman's determination not to recognize her authority 'now that Dr Hall has exercised his faculties and absolved her [Bridgeman] from subjection.'[19] Bridgeman claimed that Nightingale 'had no shadow of authority' over the ten Sisters whom she did not accept at Scutari in December 1854, and that she had agreed that the five who worked at Scutari were free to leave whenever Bridgeman wished. Nightingale had actually written this to Bridgeman when she believed Herbert had placed Dr Cumming in charge of Stanley's group. She had no power to assign nurses who were not consigned to her, she told Bridgeman then: 'You must consult with Dr Meyer or Miss Stanley.'[20] Dr Meyer was the chaperone for Stanley's party. However, all of this changed when Herbert wrote to Nightingale telling her that she was in charge of all the nurses, including Stanley's party, whom she could send back to England if she so wished.[21] Nevertheless, Bridgeman would always claim that Nightingale dissolved the contract she signed with the War Department when in December 1854 she refused to accept all fifteen nuns at once.

When in March 1856 Nightingale finally succeeded in getting the War Office to issue a General Order stating that she was in charge of all the British hospitals in Russia as well as in Turkey, she told Bridgeman that, as long as Hall was satisfied, she would not interfere in any way in her management of the hospital. However, Bridgeman must acknowledge Nightingale's overall direction of the nursing in the Crimea. Bridgeman refused to do this. '"But Revd Mother,"' Nightingale asked, '"you came out to work under me and you even signed a written agreement to that effect. How then can you object to it now?" "Experience, Miss Nightingale, the best teacher has taught me better,"' Bridgeman replied. '"I never attempted to deny that I did come out to work under you, but you refused us. You yourself denied the connection."'[22] The problems with Mary Stanley, Margaret Wear, Martha Clough, and Charlotte Salisbury were essentially internal problems for Nightingale's management and were of little interest to the government in London, but failure to secure Bridgeman's cooperation had political overtones. Nightingale was afraid the nuns would appear to be martyrs for the faith if they went home before the military hospitals closed[23] and that could mean alienation of the Roman Catholic vote in Parliament. Bridgeman resigned in April rather than admit Nightingale's supervision but by then, fortunately for Nightingale, she was well ensconced in public opinion as a

Religious nursing

national heroine and the press took little notice of the Sisters' early departure.

Nightingale has frequently been criticized for her failure to work successfully with Bridgeman. Sue Goldie and Mark Bostridge, for example, thought the two women might have worked together successfully if Nightingale had treated Bridgeman more graciously.[24] It is difficult to imagine how Nightingale could have done so when Bridgeman believed it was wrong for Catholic nuns to be subordinate to a secular lady and almost immediately decided Nightingale could not be trusted. Furthermore, before Bridgeman started work in Scutari, she had already resolved to work independently of Nightingale. While waiting in Therapia, Stanley and the nuns prayed that they might be assigned to a hospital of their own. They undertook novenas,[25] Croke wrote, asking

> to bring about the grand object of our ambition, the charge of the Hospital …[26] Our Revd Mother has expanding confidence in novenas and in putting miraculous medals under boards. The novenas have taken the hospital by storm quite from under the wings of the Nightingale.[27]

Given the violence of anti-Catholic feeling in England, Bridgeman's ambition to take charge of a Scutari hospital shows how incredibly naive she was politically.

Bridgeman's view of Nightingale's nursing

'I would not again undertake to *work with Miss Nightingale*,' Bridgeman wrote to Sir John Hall in September 1855 when she was offering her services to him, 'as I learned while I was at the Barracks Hospital, Scutari, *how very DIFFERENT from ours*, are Miss Nightingale's views of nursing, hospital arrangements etc. etc.'[28] Why did Bridgeman consider Nightingale's nursing so different? It was partly because Bridgeman was unaware of and uninterested in the administrative, religious, and political problems that encumbered Nightingale but rather interpreted her management as illustrating her incompetence and lack of system.

Before Bridgeman and her four nuns arrived in Scutari on 8 January 1855, Moore forewarned them that they would not be assigned to nurse the sick and wounded but would be working in the stores and kitchen. Bridgeman was nevertheless appalled when she and her four nuns were not immediately sent into the wards. She thought this indicated that Nightingale believed the thousands of men in the hospitals needed no nursing, when in fact it was really because Nightingale was waiting for doctors who were willing to accept Catholic nuns to request nurses. In the meantime she assigned two of the five Sisters to work under Moore in the kitchens and one to work in a storeroom while Bridgeman and the fifth Sister had no work at all for the first few days. When Nightingale did put the last two nuns to work in the kitchen, Bridgeman was disgusted. Their job consisted of serving five to ten gallons of soup to the orderlies to take up to their wards. Nightingale allowed an hour and a half for the task, when Bridgeman thought one competent person could have completed it in a few minutes if Nightingale had had any system. All the Sisters – the Norwood and Bermondsey nuns as well as Bridgeman's team – said they had never had so much spare time. Moore and one of Bridgeman's Sisters, whom she took as her assistant a few days later, were the only two in full work.

Next Nightingale assigned Bridgeman's nuns, together with some paid nurses, to unpacking and sorting clothes that were in a dark, damp, gloomy shed full of rats that ate large parts of the woolen clothing and chased about around the nuns as they worked. The Sisters left open a door to a public street so they could escape if the rats attacked them. Bridgeman had a strong sense that nuns should lead at least a partially enclosed life and considered the public exposure in the shed as well as the job of sorting clothes beneath religious Sisters. Moore and her Sisters found it a penance to work side by side with working-class hospital nurses, who were sometimes drunk, but Bridgeman and her nuns found it personally insulting. On one occasion some of Bridgeman's Sisters returned from the store, not complaining of the rats or the exposure to the public, but crying bitterly because they had to associate with drunken working-class nurses. Father Ronan, the Jesuit chaplain who arrived in January, encouraged the feeling that the nuns were not being treated with the proper respect, and declared that the Sisters had been placed in a position which was 'injurious and disreputable to religion.'[29] Indeed, some Catholic chaplains made the situation much worse. In the fall of 1854 Moore wrote that Father Ronan's activities 'were far from promoting union between the two communities of Sisters of Mercy; rather they led to a complete misunderstanding between them.' Moore therefore refused to accept him as chaplain for her team.[30] Evelyn Bolster, herself an Irish Sister of Mercy, wrote that one of the chaplains, Father Cuffe, thought Moore's influence over Nightingale was so harmful to Roman Catholic interests that he asked Grant to recall her.[31] Later, in 1856, the Jesuit chaplains in the Crimea became even more partisan. They refused confession, and therefore Holy Communion, to the Bermondsey nuns, calling them a disgrace to their church.[32] At home the Catholic clergy were more supportive of Nightingale and Moore. Westminster Vicar General Robert Whitty expressed his regret that Bridgeman was interfering over the five nuns in Scutari: he thought they should be entirely in Moore's charge. Bridgeman's bishop, Bishop Delaney, and the Mothers Superior in Dublin and Liverpool had given permission for the other ten nuns to be subdivided if necessary. However, if more Sisters were sent out Delaney wanted them placed under Moore.[33]

The Sisters' contract stated clearly: 'The nuns are to act *principally as nurses*, and are to avoid speaking on religion to those who are not Catholic,' but gave them freedom to discuss religious matters with Catholic patients. Bridgeman appears never to have made any overt effort to do what she considered converting Protestant soldiers, but Nightingale found it difficult to distinguish between trying to convert and what Bridgeman called 'instructing.'[34] Moore made herself more unpopular with Bridgeman by suggesting that she and her nuns should not give religious instruction so openly to the Catholic patients, pointing out that Grant told Moore, who was officially in charge of Bridgeman and her nuns, 'When you reach Turkey, the chief duty of the Sisters will be to act as Hospital Nurses.'[35] Bridgeman replied that if her Sisters could not freely instruct Catholic patients they would have to go home.[36] Delaney supported this view. He told Bridgeman, 'Your calling is from God, and principally for the salvation of souls, and you could not undertake the mere task of nurse tending unaccompanied by the higher functions of your order.'[37] Grant emphasized avoiding controversy, but was no less emphatic that the Bermondsey Sisters must be able to speak to Catholics on religious matters. He told Moore, 'you should always be *Nuns* as well as *Nurses*,' and if the rumor that the nuns could not instruct Catholics were true, then 'you are reduced to mere *Nurses*,' and Nightingale has more authority over the Sisters than he was prepared to give her.[38] Certainly Bridgeman was correct in thinking that many Protestants, including Nightingale, suspected the Sisters of trying to convert the Protestant soldiers. Some of these suspicions were indeed unfounded. Bridgeman, in her usual confrontational style, met the accusations head on. 'We found the only chance we had of getting through respectably,' she said, 'was to awe those who had no scruple in calumniating us into silence or at least caution, by showing ourselves willing and able to investigate and insist on proof for *every* charge which could be traced to an author.'[39]

Bridgeman's Sisters were instructing convalescents and orderlies in the Scutari General Hospital, in wards where they did not work as well as in their own wards. They followed the standard practice of not instructing patients when they were acutely ill but rather concentrated on orderlies and convalescents. Nightingale thought it looked ridiculous for 'women and young women, be they veiled or not, to stand about corridors talking to knots of orderlies or convalescents upon religious subjects or any others.'[40] When she complained to Bridgeman about her nuns going all through the hospital instructing people, Bridgeman asserted that the nuns always placed their nursing duties first, and only gave the instruction when they had finished their nursing duties. 'Has any one had reason to complain that the Sisters neglected the common duty of nursing for the religious instruction?' she asked Nightingale. Nightingale replied that no one ever had. But there were many conversions. 'Notwithstanding our strict adherence to our engagement [not to discuss religious matters with anyone except Catholic patients],' Bridgeman wrote, many were quietly received into the church and admitted to sacraments both in Scutari and Koulali. She considered the number of conversions the Sisters' greatest achievement in the East. She claimed that at least fifty soldiers converted to Catholicism at Koulali alone. Not one conversion came to the knowledge of any Protestant authority, she thought, because the soldiers did not even tell the nuns so as not to get them into trouble.[41]

Bridgeman thoroughly disapproved of Moore because she supported Nightingale. Bolster ascribed the icy relations between the two communities of nuns to Moore having attached herself unreservedly

Religious nursing

to Nightingale and being 'so well established in her good graces that she seemed to have resented sharing the privilege with any other,' and Moore therefore tried to prevent any contact between the two communities.[42] This seems unlikely. Doyle commented that although the Bermondsey Sisters were in Scutari, they were at the Barrack Hospital while Bridgeman's nuns were in the General Hospital half a mile away, so they seldom met.[43] In her journal Bridgeman never directly attacked Moore in the personal way she did Nightingale, but she did describe her as a 'perfect drudge,' always 'trotting around owing to the utter disorder and irregularity' that no one seemed willing or able to control. Bridgeman seemed to think Nightingale approved of, or at the very least saw no need to try to correct, the disorder in the two Scutari hospitals. She described the chaotic conditions in January. The orderlies came for the extras at all hours as they pleased, or did not come at all. There seemed to be no planning of what food should be prepared. If an orderly came when all the food had been served, as often happened, he was quietly told there was none for him and he went away as happy as if he had been served. The patients in such cases were left without their meals and no one seemed to care whether they were fed or not. Bridgeman did admit that the assistant surgeons bore some of the responsibility for the failure to provide adequate food because the staff surgeons often took her nuns to task for making up what they considered overly generous diet orders.[44]

In Bridgeman's opinion, the only real nursing that Nightingale's nurses did was dressing a few sores when the surgeon permitted it. Both paid and unpaid nurses had no control over the orderlies and therefore no ability to manage the feeding of the men that was a major component of nursing care at the time. The orderlies, as we have seen, usually gave everything ordered for twenty-four hours at once, and since the men often drank down all of their stimulants immediately, doctors often found their patients drunk in bed. In order to avoid the drunkenness, the doctors ordered smaller amounts of port wine and brandy than Bridgeman thought proper nursing required. She herself was very generous with the food and drink both for patients and her nuns. Nightingale considered her extravagant, especially with the Sisters' own rations.[45] Bridgeman denied extravagance. She believed Nightingale and Bracebridge were not the least interested in the comfort of anyone. They left this up to nurses, who gave the

Sisters the scantiest and least desirable portions of the most necessary items and did that in the rudest way.[46] Moore and the St. John's House nurses indicated that Matron Clarke treated everyone, not just Bridgeman's team, in this manner[47] but Bridgeman seemed oblivious to what was happening to the other nurses. She thought Nightingale supplied her five nuns at the Scutari General Hospital 'often scantily and with the refuse of the patients, such as barley that had been boiled down for the barley water ordered in the wards, made up into a really holy poverty pudding.'[48] She claimed Nightingale stinted the food of her own nurses as well, and she disapproved of the ladies and Sisters getting the same food as the paid nurses. She believed Nightingale and the Bracebridges had a French-style dinner of several courses every day at 7 p.m. Nightingale and the Bracebridges did indeed have a better dinner than the other nurses, although perhaps not as French as Bridgeman thought.[49]

Yet, proper diet, Bridgeman believed, was 'absolutely necessary to preserve the health which was so essential to our work.' She felt, and with good reason, that one of her most important duties was sustaining the health and strength of her nuns to prevent them being sent home sick and make them better able to withstand the hardships they had to endure. Bridgeman also believed Nightingale stinted on medical comforts for the soldiers. When they were desperate for things like sweetmeats, cordials, or preserves, these very items were rotting in Nightingale's stores because she refused to give them out unless she had an order signed by the doctor in attendance and countersigned by a principal medical officer. This, of course, was because Nightingale was following Herbert's instructions of strict obedience to military regulations. There was also, Bridgeman stated, a complete lack of system in the laundry. No one seemed to be in charge of anything, and all that Nightingale seemed to care about was giving out her stores. Worst of all, she let Bridgeman and her Sisters sit for hours in the one room that they shared with the five Bermondsey nuns with nothing to do while they knew that fifty to ninety men were dying every day without any care.[50]

Bridgeman's portrayal of the state of the nursing in Scutari in January 1855 is borne out in part by Eliza Mackenzie, the lady who took over the nursing at the naval hospital in Therapia. Soon after arriving in Therapia in early January 1855 Mackenzie visited the

Religious nursing

Barrack Hospital. She was a much more impartial observer than Bridgeman, but nevertheless reported that all was in a sad state of confusion:

> Miss Nightingale in bed from overwork, and Mr Bracebridge distracted. They have quantities of stores they cannot open for lack of hands. I think nothing can be done. But it is a frightful place to manage, and it would need the Duke of Wellington to cope.[51]

Unlike Bridgeman, Mackenzie appreciated the enormity of the challenge facing Nightingale. Bridgeman seems to have had no concept of the complexity of Nightingale's situation or the strength of the doctors' resistance to the Catholic nuns. Nor did she give Nightingale any credit for starting efficient extra diet kitchens, a systematic laundry system with washing machines and a drying facility, and her major efforts to improve the orderly service, as well as all the purveying she did. The non-nursing jobs Nightingale assigned the nuns were tasks which had to be done and which were beyond the capabilities of nearly all the hospital nurses unless they were closely supervised. For the same reason, although Mother Mary Clare Moore was a superb clinical nurse – Bridgeman knew she had been one of Catherine McAuley's most efficient nurses in the Dublin cholera epidemic of 1832[52] – Nightingale used her largely in administrative positions. Bridgeman herself would later use Sister Mary Aloysius Doyle, her best nurse, in the same way – not as a nurse but as the cook in the Balaclava General Hospital.[53]

Bridgeman's system of nursing

Bridgeman's nuns found the Upper Koulali hospital, which had previously been used for convalescents, in a state of complete chaos. The wards were filthy, there was no extra diet kitchen, and the only way to get water from the immense boilers in the cookhouse was to climb up a ladder over the top. The Sisters, however, were happy, Bridgeman wrote, 'because at last they could do the work they came to do and do it *freely* and *graciously*.' On their first day in the Stable Hospital the Sisters admitted 200 severely ill, helpless patients who arrived on shipboard. After Stanley left in April, Miss Amy Hutton was made superintendent of the two hospitals but Doyle said Hutton was only too glad to hand the superintendence over to the experienced Sisters. They placed a secular lady and a Sister with one or two hospital nurses in each ward.[54] 'Indeed *we* did not experience either opposition or distrust from the medical officers,' Bridgeman declared. The doctors appreciated the Sisters' first-rate nursing and their carefully kept accounts and linen store. According to Bridgeman the excellent name the Koulali hospitals were acquiring with the nuns' totally different style of nursing, and with the full approval of the doctors, incited Nightingale's envy. The fact that the ten Sisters were working so well independently of Nightingale made her desperately jealous and even more opposed to them. Bridgeman believed everyone was jealous of her nuns and their success. She thought Anglican Sisters Bertha Turnbull and Margaret Goodman were 'gnawed with jealousy' to the point of being enraged because Bridgeman's Sisters constantly gave their patients religious instruction, which Nightingale did not allow the Anglicans to do. There is no evidence of gnawing envy in Goodman's or Nightingale's writings. The doctors in Scutari, Bridgeman believed, generally disliked Nightingale and 'her assumption of authority, surgical skill, etc., her attending unsuitable operations, etc., *disgusted them.*'[55] The Sisters' rule prevented them from assisting at operations when the men were naked but Nightingale, and sometimes the chaplains, did help at operations. In the days before hemostats, antiseptic, and aseptic technique, there was little need for nurses in the operating theater but extra people were helpful in positioning patients and applying pressure to arteries to stop the bleeding. Bridgeman considered it shockingly indecorous for a lady to do these things, and claimed that everyone who had seen Nightingale's nursing thought it a total failure. 'There seems no second opinion amongst the medical officers on this point and those who have come out to inspect, and who have made minute inquiries from proper quarters, have concurred in the opinion,' she wrote.

Bridgeman detested the hospital nurses. 'No class of people could be more disliked and despised than the paid class of nurses in the East,' she wrote. 'They were instruments of immorality; in the very hospitals they have committed the most shameful excesses.' The secular lady nurses were just as bad in a different way. They quarrelled constantly, gossiped, flirted with the chaplains, and generally made fools of themselves. The Catholic Sisters, Bridgeman claimed, were the only

Religious nursing

nurses who were dependable. When the secular ladies and hospital nurses finally left the Balaclava General Hospital and Bridgeman and her nuns were the only nurses there, all cross purposes, gossiping, and complaints vanished and things finally ran smoothly. In what was obviously an effort to defend himself against what he thought were Nightingale's slanders, Sir John Hall asked Bridgeman to meet with Andrew Smith when she returned to England, which she was more than happy to do. Smith, who was himself a Roman Catholic, asked her opinion of his plan of appointing a Catholic and a Protestant matron to each of the large military hospitals. Bridgeman thought it inexpedient. She said the only nurses who were fit to work in military hospitals were well-chosen religious Sisters, presumably not Sisters like the Bermondsey Sisters who condoned Nightingale's supposed total lack of system. Well-chosen Sisters would be a great spiritual and temporal blessing, but otherwise Bridgeman thought the soldiers were better off without female nurses.[56]

Bridgeman's assessment of Nightingale's nursing was obviously partly a result of her bitter hatred of the English ascendancy – she described Nightingale as an insidious, dangerous enemy, 'propped [up] as she is by human power and English infatuation and bigotry.'[57] A good deal of what she said about Nightingale was completely untrue. Colonel John Henry LeFroy whom the War Department sent out specifically to investigate the hospitals, many members of the various parliamentary commissions that investigated the hospitals, as well as doctors and sanitary engineers became lifelong friends and supporters of Nightingale. Dr Peter Pincoffs, a civilian doctor who arrived in Scutari at the end of April 1855, found Nightingale's hospital arrangements admirable. The hospital floors were newly paved, there were no patients in the corridors, and wooden partitions prevented cold draughts from blowing through the wards. The wards were scrupulously clean except for vermin in the summer, and the patients had clean linen, books, newspapers, writing materials, and games, while Alexis Soyer was supervising improvements in the kitchen. The female nurses took care of the worst cases and Nightingale herself, together with her 'clever aide-de-camp, skilful Mrs Roberts,' checked every critical case. The hospital was well staffed with doctors, and well equipped with drugs and instruments for scientific examination, air cushions, water beds, hot water bottles,

Mother Francis Bridgeman and her Sisters of Mercy

baths and so on. Pincoffs praised the splendid dissecting room and all the excellent instruments, microscopes, and chemical apparatus which the government so liberally provided for the doctors in Scutari at Nightingale's request. In direct opposition to Bridgeman, Pincoffs commented that Nightingale was impartial where different religious denominations were concerned. Of course, had Pincoffs come in December when Bridgeman arrived, he would not have found such excellent order and facilities, but by April Nightingale had the two Scutari hospitals running smoothly. Pincoffs acknowledged that female nurses in military hospitals were still controversial but those who had seen the Catholic Sisters at work strongly supported them. In addition, he thought the female nurses had a very beneficial effect on both patients and orderlies. There was a better tone in the wards with less swearing, and medical orders were better carried out. He thought there were few medical men who did not prefer female nurses for both their hospital and their private patients. It was a different question with the working-class nurses. Some were less efficient and their behavior toward the orderlies and general conduct unsuitable, but, as he rightly pointed out, this was because they lacked the training the religious Sisters had.[58]

Despite her hostility and gullibility in believing anything that discredited Nightingale, one should not underestimate Bridgeman's competencies as a nursing superintendent. In Balaclava the nuns eventually had three large prefabricated huts to themselves. They partitioned them so that each Sister had a cell, and they made an oratory, a community room, and a little infirmary. After the secular ladies and working-class nurses left, the Sisters were at last living entirely as an independent religious community in what Bridgeman considered more appropriate housing. Then she abandoned her combative approach. 'All went smoothly and graciously. We made it a point,' she wrote:

> never to complain of an orderly or risk getting any one into trouble. We tried to win those who went wrong by patience, remonstrance, etc. etc., and this course seldom failed. We never might try authority, but found our way must be to success by establishing our influence gently and imperceptibly. Thank God in this we have been wonderfully successful. We should certainly have failed by any other route.[59]

Bridgeman's and Nightingale's systems contrasted

There were indeed significant differences between Nightingale's and Bridgeman's systems but there were equally important similarities. Religious commitment drove both women to their nursing work. Nightingale believed she was working for God, while Bridgeman aimed to save souls. Both were trying to follow the instructions they had been given, Bridgeman from her bishop and Nightingale from the War Department. From a nursing point of view Bridgeman's description of what she called the 'temporal care' her Sisters gave could just as well have been written by Nightingale for her nurses. The doctors seemed to feel, Bridgeman said, that the nuns were needed more for care after surgery rather than during it. Apart from Nightingale herself, who did attend operations, this also applied to her nurses: there is no reference anywhere to any of Nightingale's nurses assisting at operations. Bridgeman and her Sisters saw that doctors' orders were carried out punctually; they monitored post-operative patients for hemorrhage; they informed the doctors of any important changes in the patients' status; they received the extra diets and saw that they were properly prepared and given out at the right time and in the right amounts; they took charge of the stimulants; they tried to teach the orderlies to discharge their duty faithfully; and finally they preserved needful tranquility and order in the wards. All of this was precisely what Nightingale expected of her nurses, but if both women agreed on nursing procedures, there were still very important differences in their nursing systems.

Bridgeman believed the most important difference was that she had a well-organized system while complete chaos reigned in Nightingale's hospitals, and reigned with Nightingale's approval. This was simply not true and Bridgeman must have known that, because she visited the Scutari hospitals at least once a month from February through September 1855 when all other observers agreed that Nightingale had succeeded in bringing excellent order out of the general chaos she found on her arrival. A second major difference was that Bridgeman immediately managed to work her way around the system of signed and countersigned requisitions. This was easier for her because by the time she arrived in Koulali supplies were arriving and beginning to be properly distributed. The Sisters, Bridgeman said, distributed the Free Gifts that Nightingale faithfully sent them as they were needed rather than leaving them to spoil or accumulate as she claimed Nightingale did. The Sisters themselves gave out stimulants, bypassing the orderlies, which made the orderlies more sober, and Bridgeman noted, 'not the less devoted to the Sisters.' The Sisters of Mercy gained a great deal of autonomy in hospital administration but they always strictly obeyed doctors' orders. Although they did away with the signed and countersigned requisitions, they never gave out anything without either general or specific permission from the doctors. At first, some of the doctors objected to the bypassing of requisitions, but when they saw how obediently and precisely the Sisters carried out doctors' orders and how well the Sisters' system worked, they soon came to cordially approve of it.[60] The Sisters were indeed very obedient, in fact so much so that they sometimes carried obedience to extremes. For example, a civilian doctor at Koulali decided to experiment with the Turkish treatment of dysentery, which consisted of starving the men. He used the most extreme form of starving, and more men died in his ward than in any other. The lady nurses refused to work for him, but so attuned were the Sisters to literal obedience to medical orders, that they were willing to carry out his orders[61] even though they knew they were harmful.

Actually Nightingale was very unhappy with the requisitioning system, and once she was better established, began sidestepping it. She apparently made good headway in Scutari, for when she was in the Crimea in 1856 she asked Hall if she could continue her standard practice at Scutari of sending in her requisitions for the men without the signatures of the medical officers. Hall replied absolutely not.[62] Bypassing the requisitions was certainly superior to the system that Nightingale so conscientiously enforced when she first arrived in Scutari, which at its worst meant refusing dying men fluids. However, Bridgeman had the advantages of a smaller hospital that was not being used as a depot, as well as a principal medical officer and staff who were friendly and welcoming. Dr Tice, one of the chief doctors, was a Roman Catholic and Lady Superintendent Mary Stanley was in the process of becoming one.[63] Nightingale had blazed the path: female nurses had been performing well for three months when Bridgeman started at Koulali so there was far less suspicion of them. In addition, at Koulali Bridgeman had a team of nine experienced and expert clinical nursing nuns, while Nightingale struggled with many incompetents.

The issue of religion was another area where the two ladies took different approaches. As instructed, Nightingale left religious matters to the chaplains. The physical care of the sick is the duty of nurses, she wrote right after the war. 'The care of their souls is the great province of the clergy.'[64] By contrast, both parties of Sisters of Mercy believed religious instruction the most important part of their work. Bridgeman felt the Protestants, and Nightingale in particular, persecuted the Sisters because of their Roman Catholic faith – there was persecution in all quarters she said.[65] In fact, Nightingale never discriminated against Catholics as such. She had no problem working with a number of Roman Catholics; she maintained cordial and respectful relations with Moore and her nuns throughout the whole campaign and Moore became one of her closest, lifelong friends.[66] However, after her unsuccessful dealings with Bridgeman she did become quite violently anti-Irish. Completely overlooking the fact that Moore was Irish, at the end of 1855 she said she would never have dealings with Irish people again because '*they can lie & I cannot.*' Nevertheless, she claimed, 'I am the best personal friends with the Revd. Brickbat.'[67] Bridgeman would never have endorsed her assessment of mutual friendship but it does show that Nightingale maintained polite relations with her.

Bridgeman and Nightingale also had different ideological approaches to health care. Nightingale was thoroughly dedicated to the most modern scientific care. As a committed sanitarian, she believed dirt was the cause of disease and therefore emphasized the principles of fastidious cleanliness, fresh air, good ventilation, sunlight, and where possible the prevention of disease rather than simply treating it. The Sisters of Mercy took a gentler approach. Within two weeks of the Sisters arriving in Balaclava, Sister Joseph Croke wrote, the orderlies began looking more cheerful and the patients said they were getting comforts they had never had before. In fact, Croke said, at that point they were getting little more than they had previously except kind words, cheerfulness, and conscientious observation. When on night duty the Sisters went up and down the wards with their lamps every half hour. Bridgeman urged her Sisters to make what she called 'pretty speeches' when they could do nothing else,

Mother Francis Bridgeman and her Sisters of Mercy

and kind words proved most soothing to the patients. When a doctor told Croke she should not listen to the patients every time they asked her for something she replied, 'Sisters of Mercy always listen to their patients.'[68]

The Sisters' less scientific and kinder approach came out very clearly at the Balaclava General Hospital when Bridgeman resigned in April 1856 and Nightingale took over the hospital. Although she sometimes spoke disparagingly of Bridgeman to her friends, Nightingale did not attack her nursing, but at this point, as a committed sanitarian, she attacked it vigorously as unsanitary. She claimed Bridgeman left the hospital in the most disgraceful state of dirt and filth, the patients grimed with dirt, infested with vermin, and with bedsores like Lazarus. Nightingale reported 'quantities of extra bedding, clothes, carpenters' tools, boots, shoes and slippers cumbered the wards. A frostbitten patient named McDonald in a state "indescribably horrible."' The orderlies were never sober and it was customary for men from the Irish regiments to talk and drink in the kitchen.[69] Bridgeman later explained that there was no space in the hospital to store the cleaning equipment except under the orderlies' beds and there was nowhere to store clothes because anything put in the stores was likely to be eaten by rats. The orderlies were indeed often intemperate but there were many exceptions; she only remembered one who had ever come into the diet kitchen drunk.[70] It took two days of whitewashing and cleaning and three days of washing and dressing the patients, Nightingale said, before the hospital was in what she considered a satisfactory sanitary condition. Roberts had to spend six hours daily dressing McDonald's five bedsores.[71] These dressings, or debridements, are an excruciatingly painful process but Eliza Roberts thought nothing of taking hours to do them.[72] Her thoroughness in this nursing skill had always impressed Nightingale.

Dressings were a much larger part of nursing care in the mid-nineteenth century than they are in our age of antibiotics and sophisticated diagnostic imagery. As well as cleaning the wound and changing the dressing itself, they usually involved applying poultices. These were most often filled with cooked ingredients such as linseed or bread and then the pots had to be washed afterwards, all of which was time-consuming, but even with the five different dressings McDonald required, six hours was an extraordinary amount of time. Masquelez's

Religious nursing

surgeons spent an hour and a half twice a day trying to remove shell fragments from his wound. Since nearly all wounds became infected in pre-antibiotic days they produced enormous amounts of pus so the dressings had to be changed more often than do those in our time. Gunshot produces a contused wound and at that time it was believed the resulting tract must suppurate before it could heal. Contused wounds heal only by suppuration and granulation George Macleod explained. One sees rare exceptions, when there is a superficial wound of the muscles and the wound will close by first intention, but there were very few records of this kind of healing.[73] 'Freakish' wounds, as Macleod termed them, healed quickly but wounds which we would now call infected took much longer and sometimes never healed. Bedsores are different in that they are not contused wounds, but they also became infected and suppurated and sloughed off dead tissue. In the 1850s the most up-to-date theories of disease proposed that dead tissue exuded a poison that diffused throughout the body – or put in a slightly more modern way, breakdown products of gangrenous tissue spread infection through the body – so it was essential that these materials be removed before they could diffuse further.[74]

Bridgeman had specifically mentioned McDonald to Nightingale as a difficult case when she left the Balaclava General Hospital. He had been bedridden from the time he was admitted several months previously; the slightest move tortured him. At first Dr Murray had dressed his bedsores twice a day but then he decided the benefit of the second dressing was more than counterbalanced by the agony it caused him, so he did the dressing only once a day. Bridgeman pointed out that in any case, except with express permission of the surgeon in charge, the nurses had been forbidden to do dressings ever since the dressers arrived in December 1854. However, she knew that the dressings had been faithfully done because a Sister always assisted the doctor. She cut the linen to the sizes required for each wound and prepared the poultices. The doctor then applied two dressings to his back, two to his feet, and one to his hip, with McDonald moaning piteously the whole time. It was indeed true that McDonald's bed had not been changed for a week, or perhaps even two weeks, but when frequent changes caused great suffering or exhaustion, the Sisters used all the standard nursing methods to avoid changing the bed: a waterproof cover over his mattress, and over this sheets folded and placed so that they could be removed with the least possible amount of suffering, and many soft pillows. When one of the Sisters asked Dr Murray if she might change McDonald's bed he told her to wait until he was more able to bear it. 'I did not know before that any nurse however clever,' Bridgeman commented, 'might put a patient through the ordeal described by Mrs Roberts without the express consent of the surgeon in whose charge he was.' She wondered, and with good reason, how long McDonald survived Mrs Roberts's six-hour ministrations.[75]

By contrast, in a letter to the family of Major Ellis who died in the Balaclava General Hospital, Nightingale described his care under her direction:

> He pressed my hand when he could not speak. The last words he said were "Turn me on my right side" & we turned him. He had milk every hour, arrowroot when he could take it, and port wine put between his lips every quarter of an hour. He required constant changing and I took care that he should have a continual supply of dry sheets, sometimes many times a day.[76]

It would appear that Ellis was given meticulous care and may well have been kept cleaner with all the changes of sheets than was McDonald although undoubtedly, knowing Bridgeman's emphasis on proper feeding, McDonald received as careful feeding. We do not know Ellis's diagnosis or whether he had wounds to dress, but it apparently caused him no pain to be moved or he would not have asked to be turned. For Nightingale cleanliness trumped causing the patient horrible pain. When germ theory was later introduced Nightingale, as did many other well-informed people, at first resisted it. But as she came to accept it she tended to identify germs with the filth and decomposing matter which the sanitarians had believed caused disease. For example, when discussing teaching hygiene in the 1890s she wrote,

> Above all, avoid in a class of the comparatively uneducated, the doctrine of 'germs', 'bacilli', 'bacteria' – all that fashionable farrago & way of explaining disease' but rather describe it as caused by 'dirty air, dirty water, dirt any where.[77]

The Sisters may not have maintained the immaculate cleanliness Nightingale insisted on, but the Balaclava General Hospital could not have been the disaster area she claimed or the doctors and patients would not have been so pleased with the nuns' work.[78] It is noteworthy that Bridgeman complained of the coarse nursing, the deplorable state of the fourteen huts that comprised part of the Balaclava General Hospital, and the filth and disorder in the kitchen when she and her nuns arrived in October 1855.[79] Vermin infestations were omnipresent in Turkey and the Crimea, and Nightingale knew this when she complained about the rats in the Balaclava General Hospital. There was vermin in the Scutari hospitals in the summer. Shortly after arriving in Scutari Nightingale started using bear's grease, shaved her head, and wore a wig to escape the fleas in her hair. She would continue to do so throughout the war.[80] Her description of the condition in which Bridgeman left the hospital was obviously written in a fit of pique and grossly exaggerated.

Perhaps the biggest contrast of all between Nightingale's and Bridgeman's military nursing was the scope of their missions. Nightingale was keenly aware of the political aspects of her assignment, whereas Bridgeman paid no attention to the difficult diplomatic and administrative problems within the military hospitals. As Moore pointed out, Bridgeman wanted to establish her nuns as a regular religious community and carry on exactly as they did at home in Ireland. It speaks to Bridgeman's ability that she partially accomplished this at Koulali and completely achieved it in Balaclava. Nightingale, on the other hand, was dealing with three different organizations – the doctors in the civilian medical department, the War Office, and her very heterogeneous team of nurses – as well as nursing the patients. She was supervising up to seven hospitals, hundreds of miles apart in Russia and Turkey, while Bridgeman was unofficially in charge of two if we count Koulali as two rather than one hospital, and then officially superintended one, the Balaclava General Hospital. The Barrack Hospital alone was larger than either the Koulali or the Balaclava hospitals. Eliza Mackenzie, although brand new to the nursing world, appreciated immediately the enormous scope of Nightingale's challenge. Furthermore, Nightingale, with her holistic approach to health care, understood her mission as having a wider range than simply the hospitals. She considered her mission not simply humanitarian, but as an experiment of the War Department in introducing women into the British army medical department. She understood that better nursing was dependent not only on skilled nurses and the resources the government provided for them but also relied heavily on good medical practice. The splendid arrangements for the medical staff which Pincoffs praised are one example. It would never have occurred to Bridgeman to ask the government for fine surgical instruments, microscopes, or a dissecting room. Nor did Nightingale confine herself solely to the hospital-bound soldiers. She arranged to have any soldier who so wished send his money home to his family. She organized recreational activities, established a coffee house, and helped the senior chaplain set up a library and school rooms, and arrange evening lectures for the men.[81] Nightingale also took upon herself purveying in the first months of the war when so few supplies were getting through to the hospitals.

Bridgeman, on the other hand, started work in Koulali when the armed forces were finally getting the distribution of supplies sorted out. She had a second major advantage that Nightingale never enjoyed: her nurses were all experienced and professionally trained. This is not to say that her Sisters always worked together harmoniously. But, she said, when there was a problem, 'God has enabled me to crush it.' She got rid of one nun and 'waged war against the wrongful spirit of two others.' Some of her Sisters were a comfort, she continued, 'but one *rotten* sheep is sufficient to corrupt a flock.'[82] There can be no question that by the end of her first year in the East, Nightingale's hospitals were just as well run as Bridgeman's and delivering as good, if a somewhat different kind of, nursing care. Bridgeman provides an example of an individual who could not take a transnational view. She never tried to understand what Doyle called Nightingale's difficult position, and she genuinely believed she could not provide a good nursing service until she had replicated the conditions under which she worked in Ireland. Once she had a kind of conventual accommodation – cells for each nun, an oratory, community room and so on, and had no working-class or lady nurses on her team – and the Sisters were living entirely as an independent religious community, she believed the nursing ran smoothly and graciously.

Bridgeman had her limitations but we must not underestimate her accomplishments and those of her nuns. They indiscriminately took care of men of all religious callings, and Mother Mary Clare Moore,

Religious nursing

whom they treated very badly, wrote that they were greatly beloved by the soldiers and had laboured efficiently among them.[83] They gave top flight nursing care that was considerably kinder to the patients than the more up-to-date scientific care Nightingale and Roberts sometimes administered.

Notes

1 A decoration Queen Victoria instituted in 1883 to recognize exceptional work of military nursing Sisters.
2 Luddy, *Crimean Journals*, pp. xxvii–xxviii.
3 Doyle, 'Memories,' p. 28.
4 Chadwick, *Victorian Church*, vol. I, pp. 271–309; Gilley, 'Roman Catholicism,' p. 33.
5 For example see Bridgeman, 'Account,' p. 230; Croke, 'Diary,' p. 107. Croke liked to regale her fellow Sisters with stories of the Crimean campaign. They were the subject of 'evening recreations.' Luddy, *Crimean Journals*, p. xxivfn.
6 Croke, 'Diary,' p. 81.
7 Doyle, 'Memories,' pp. 10, 56.
8 Bridgeman, 'Account,' p. 124.
9 Bolster, *Sisters of Mercy*, pp. 49–51; Bridgeman, 'Account,' pp. 127–9.
10 BL 43393, Nightingale to Herbert, 10 December 1854, fols 22–5; 15 December 1854, fols 36–7.
11 BA 1854, pp. 227, 242–3.
12 BL 43393, FN to Herbert, 10 December 1854, fols 26–7.
13 Cook, *Nightingale*, vol. 1, pp. 155–6.
14 Bridgeman, 'Account,' pp. 130–4.
15 BA 1855, pp. 242–3; Bridgeman, 'Account,' pp. 135–7.
16 Bridgeman, 'Account,' pp. 141–2.
17 Ibid, p. 176.
18 Bostridge, *Florence Nightingale*, pp. 286–7.
19 Croke, 'Diary,' p. 77.
20 Bridgeman, 'Account,' pp. 133, 213–14.
21 Stanmore, *Sidney Herbert*, vol. 1, pp. 371–2.
22 Bridgeman, 'Account,' p. 223.
23 BL 43397, FN [to Col. LeFroy], 16 March 1856, fol. 225.
24 Goldie, '*I Have Done my Duty*,' p. 54; Bostridge, *Florence Nightingale*, p. 242.
25 A novena usually consisted of attending Mass on nine successive days.
26 Neither Nightingale nor Bridgeman were aware that there was a second hospital in Scutari, the Scutari General Hospital, until they were actually in Scutari.

Mother Francis Bridgeman and her Sisters of Mercy

27 Croke, 'Diary,' p. 71. Bridgeman's Sisters often referred to Nightingale as 'the Nightingale' or 'the bird,' and Nightingale would refer to Bridgeman as a 'brickbat.'

28 Goldie, '*I Have Done my Duty*,' p. 157.

29 Bridgeman, 'Account,' pp. 137, 139, 238; Doyle, 'Memories,' p. 19.

30 BA 1854, pp. 242–3.

31 Bolster, *Sisters of Mercy*, pp. 102–3.

32 BL 43393, Nightingale to Herbert, 3 April 1856, fols 229–30.

33 BA 1855, pp. 245–7.

34 Bolster, *Sisters of Mercy*, pp. 49–51; Bridgeman, 'Account,' pp. 122–3.

35 BA 1854, pp. 218–19.

36 Bridgeman, 'Account,' p. 138.

37 Doyle, 'Memories,' pp. 44–5.

38 BA 1855, pp. 245, 250–2.

39 Bridgeman, 'Account,' pp. 146, 154, 156.

40 WI Ms 8895, Nightingale to 'My dearest friends' [Selena and Charles Bracebridge], 7 August 1855, Letter 26, [8–9].

41 Bridgeman, 'Account,' pp. 154, 177–8.

42 Bolster, *Sisters of Mercy*, pp. 97–8.

43 Doyle, 'Memories,' p. 50.

44 Bridgeman, 'Account,' pp. 137–8, 143–4.

45 WI Ms 8995, Nightingale to [Charles Bracebridge], [October–November 1855], Letter 58; Croke, 'Diary,' p. 94.

46 Bridgeman, 'Account,' pp. 219–20.

47 LMA/H01/ST/NC3/SU15, Unsigned letter to Mary Jones, 4 December 1854; BA 1854, pp. 252–3.

48 Bridgeman, 'Account,' p. 219.

49 Ibid, pp. 138, 171, 219–20; Taylor, *Eastern Hospitals*, vol. 1, p. 93.

50 Bridgeman, 'Account,' pp. 141, 144, 219–20.

51 Penney, 'Letters from Therapia,' p. 417.

52 Bolster, *Sisters of Mercy*, p. 198. Catherine McAuley founded the Sisters of Mercy in Dublin in 1831.

53 Doyle, 'Memories,' p. 35.

54 Ibid, p. 24; Bridgeman, 'Account,' p. 141.

55 Bridgeman, 'Account,' pp. 142–5, 153, 169.

56 Ibid, pp. 157, 201, 220, 239.

57 Ibid, p. 145.

58 Pincoffs, *Experiences of a Civilian*, pp. 30–1, 55–6, 80–1, 84, 180–3.

59 Bridgeman, 'Account,' pp. 201–2.

60 Bolster, *Sisters of Mercy*, p. 265.

61 Taylor, *Eastern Hospitals*, vol. 1, pp. 247–51.

62 Nightingale to Sir John Hall, 27 March 1856, BL 39867 fols 101–4; Goldie, '*I Have Done my Duty*,' pp. 277–8.

Religious nursing

63 BL 43393, Nightingale to Herbert, 15 February 1855, fol. 160; Nightingale, *Crimean War*, p. 336fn; Smith, *Reputation and Power*, p. 31.

64 Nightingale, 'Introduction of Female Nursing,' p. 7.

65 Bridgeman, 'Account,' p. 154.

66 Sullivan, *Friendship*, p. 16.

67 WI Ms 8995, Nightingale [to Charles Bracebridge], [October–November 1855], Letter 58.

68 Croke, 'Diary,' pp. 81, 84, 87.

69 BL 45792, Nightingale to Uncle Sam Smith, 17 April 1856, fols 29–30; Nightingale Report to the War Office, cited in Bolster, *Sisters of Mercy*, p. 260.

70 Bolster, *Sisters of Mercy*, pp. 266–7.

71 BL 45792, Nightingale to Uncle Sam Smith, 17 April 1856, fols 29–30.

72 See for example WI Ms 8995, Nightingale to the Bracebridges, 7 August 1855, Letter 26.

73 Macleod, *Surgery in the Crimea*, pp. 107–8; Macleod, 'Surgery of the War,' pp. 989–91.

74 Worboys, *Spreading Germs*, pp. 33–7.

75 Goldie, '*I Have Done my Duty*,' p. 254.

76 Nightingale [to mother of Major Ellis], 25 November 1855, Columbia-Presbyterian School of Nursing, Nightingale Papers, C14.

77 BL 45811, Nightingale Memorandum [1890?], fol. 20.

78 Hall to Bridgeman, 28 March 1856, cited in Bridgeman, 'Account,' p. 225.

79 Bridgeman, 'Account,' pp. 196, 201.

80 WI Ms 8995, Nightingale to her family, 28 July 1855, Letter 25; Nightingale to Charles and Selena Bracebridge, 7 August 1855, Letter 26.

81 Pincoffs, *Experiences of a Civilian*, pp. 30–1, 78; Bostridge, *Florence Nightingale*, pp. 283–5; Cook, *Nightingale*, vol. 1, pp. 276–82.

82 Luddy, *Crimean Journals*, p. xx.

83 Sullivan, *Friendship*, pp. 70–1.

6

The other British religious Sisters

Introduction

The Sisters of Mercy, who made up twenty-three of the Roman Catholic Sisters, produced the largest number of highly efficient nurses in the British army hospitals. There were a number of reasons why the religious nurses were so outstanding. Sisterhoods had a special appeal to ladies who wished to make better use of their talents because they provided a way for competent women to respectably reject the doctrine of female subordination and break out of the domestic sphere. As religious Sisters, ladies could work full time because they were not paid, and at the same time the schools they ran, their social work, and nursing the poor qualified as traditional Christian philanthropy and was appropriately feminine. Married ladies often did part-time volunteer work but there was an enormous difference between this kind of work in philanthropic organizations, where ladies remained subordinate to the men who ran the charities, and the philanthropic work which religious Sisters organized themselves and did independently. And, as well as running their own affairs in their convents, under the protection of the church, Sisters could actually work in slums, prisons, or hospitals.

As a result there was a tremendous surge in the founding of sisterhoods throughout Western Europe during the nineteenth century. In France alone 400 Roman Catholic congregations and convents were established between 1800 and 1880.[1] The possibility of having a real career which the Catholic sisterhoods offered is one reason why Nightingale considered converting to Roman Catholicism.[2] In the Church of England, where convents and monasteries had been dissolved during the Reformation, the first Anglican sisterhood was

131

Religious nursing

established in 1845. Susan Mumm calculated that between that date and 1900 approximately 10,000 women passed through more than ninety religious communities, staying for anywhere between a few months to a lifetime. By 1900 she estimated there were between 3,000 and 4,000 women living in approximately sixty convents.[3] Nearly all of these sisterhoods, both in England and on the continent, were not enclosed but active communities which provided social services and nursing. Most sisterhoods in both the Anglican and Roman churches were self-governing and, like the Daughters of Charity discussed in the next chapter, relatively autonomous. Anglican communities did not report directly to their bishops. Their relationship with the bishops was, as Owen Chadwick wrote, 'delicate and doubtful,'[4] and this was true of most of the new nineteenth-century sisterhoods. Mother Francis Bridgeman complained that her fourteen nuns came from six different convents in Ireland and England. Only two came from her own convent in Kinsale, and the different rules and views of the six Mercy convents made it difficult for her to coordinate her team.[5]

The Bermondsey Sisters of Mercy: a more transnational approach to nursing in the East

With the passage of Catholic Emancipation in 1829 Roman Catholic sisterhoods began establishing convents in England. Founded in Dublin in 1831 by Catherine McAuley, the Sisters of Mercy formed an uncloistered order dedicated to the consolation and service of the sick and the instruction of poor children and ignorant persons.[6] In 1839 the sisterhood sent Moore to Bermondsey, an area of London, to establish the first Convent of Mercy outside of Ireland. Moore was highly talented: she became the Superior of the Mercy Convent in Cork when she was only 23 and was 25 when she arrived in London. She would eventually found eight other autonomous convents in England. She was incredibly able, extremely diplomatic, and a superb administrator – it was said that she could have ruled a kingdom.[7] She was a skilled financial administrator, handling dowries and seeking exemption from the income tax.[8] She used a constructive rather than authoritarian style of management in working with her nuns. She would tell her Sisters, 'Experience is the best teacher – we grow wise

132

The other British religious Sisters

through our blunders,' 'never look back,' and faults and mistakes could be 'remedied by quiet patience and cheerfulness above all.'

Moore and her nuns also took a very different political and social stance from that of the redoubtable Bridgeman.[9] Moore did not try to recreate the same conditions under which she and her Sisters worked in London; she believed the best way to accomplish the mission to help the soldiers was to cooperate with Nightingale. On first meeting Nightingale in Paris in October 1854 Moore wrote that 'her simple demeanour & unaffected kindness was a source of comfort' to the nuns in their new and trying position of being associated with both Protestants and working-class nurses. And, she said, Nightingale was most grateful for our readiness to take any job she assigned us.[10] Nightingale later wrote that 'It was impossible to estimate too highly the unwearied devotion, patience, & cheerfulness, the judgement and activity, & the single-heartedness with which these "Sisters" … have labored in the Service of the Sick.'[11] Moore remained loyal to Nightingale throughout her stay in Scutari. 'The resolution which Mother M. F. Bridgeman had taken to return to Ireland, rather than remain in the Military Hospitals subject to Miss Nightingale's super-intendence, was regretted by all parties,' she wrote in 1856.[12] Despite contending feelings all around them, she and her Sisters tried to press on with the work humbly and simply. Our chief grievances arose, she wrote, 'from the angry way in which both Priests and Religious looked on Miss Nightingale's superintendence and their submission to her in the hospital work.' She thought the only place where there was peace and joy was in her nuns' one room, and reported that the other nurses admired her nuns' conduct.[13]

In the East Moore had three significant advantages which Bridgeman did not enjoy. One reason for Bridgeman's successful nursing was that twelve of her fourteen nuns were ladies, educated women who could understand the principles underlying nursing care and medical orders. Moore's party was smaller and her Sisters were all ladies,[14] and she was able to choose four Sisters 'of whose ready com-pliance with her wishes she felt assured.' They all came from her own convent and had worked together over a period of years. Sister Mary de Chantal was professed in 1853 and was the only one with less than five years' experience.[15] Moore never had the problem of the 'spirit of dictation and faultfinding' that Bridgeman experienced. Second,

Moore's Sisters had been living and working in England and did not have the same hostile feelings toward the English. Furthermore, their bishop, Thomas Grant, was himself English and at least two of the five original Bermondsey nuns had originally been Anglicans.[16] Both Moore and Grant understood the complex political position of Roman Catholics in the United Kingdom and were prepared to work with or around it. Grant had a political as well as humanitarian goal in sending nuns to Scutari. He thought the expedition would give Roman Catholic nuns a chance to demonstrate publicly 'how earnest and charitable nuns are and how much they excel all other nurses.'[17] Moore and Grant would never have thought it possible to place a team of Roman Catholic Sisters in charge of a military hospital as Bridgeman hoped to do when she first arrived in the East. A third important advantage which Bridgeman did not share was that Grant was very supportive of Moore. It was Grant who originally proposed sending Roman Catholic nuns to the military hospitals and it was he who carefully worked out the agreement with the War Office. Bridgeman thought the most difficult part of her expedition to the East was that she never had an assigned ecclesiastical superior.[18]

At home in London the Bermondsey Sisters did many different kinds of work as well as nursing: visiting the sick poor in their homes and in St. Thomas's and Guy's hospitals, instructing and converting Protestants, teaching, and running an infant school.[19] They were highly skilled nurses who, unlike the Daughters of Charity of St. Vincent de Paul, did provide hands-on care to men as well as women. For example, Moore took care of Bishop Griffiths, Grant's predecessor, when he was dying; she dressed the blisters on his abdomen twice a day.[20] Sister Mary Aloysius Doyle applied all the standard remedies for cholera patients while the orderlies rubbed their viciously cramping muscles. When the orderlies were too tired to go on she herself took over and kept on massaging until the soldiers died. 'While there is life, there is hope,' she said, and she kept up the warm applications to the abdomen and massaging until the last moment. Bridgeman, who was so shocked by Nightingale attending operations on naked men, also gave physical care to the soldiers. She was especially noted for the skillful way she applied chloroform poultices to the abdomen. Moore and her nuns were equally as professional as Bridgeman's nuns. They arrived in Paris ahead of

The other British religious Sisters

Nightingale, where they bought aprons and sleeves and shortened the trains of their habits to make them more suitable for hospital work.[21] They went to hospitals and other institutions in Paris seeking information about military nursing. The Daughters of Charity were especially helpful, urging them to buy cases of surgical instruments, which they did and which later proved invaluable.[22] On first meeting the Bermondsey Sisters in Paris, Anglican Sister Sarah Anne Terrot was impressed by their pleasing manners, cheerfulness and simple, affectionate ways. After working with them for some weeks she was even more impressed. 'However these nuns may have erred in faith and practice,' she wrote:

> the deepest impression their conduct left was one of affectionate admiration; their invariably patient, cheerful, gentle manners, their constant considerate kindness, left a very pleasing remembrance, a beautiful picture of true and practical Christianity which those who boast a purer faith would do well to emulate.[23]

When the Bermondsey Sisters first started work Nightingale showed considerable bias against them, but very quickly revised her opinion.[24] She came to rely heavily on them and almost immediately requested more because they were such efficient and helpful nurses. 'Miss N. is very kind to us and prefers us to all the rest,' Sister Mary Gonzaga Barrie told the nuns at home in Bermondsey a few weeks after arriving in Scutari. 'Revd Mother [Moore] is a favorite with all parties & is invaluable for keeping peace, rather a difficult thing in these parts. The Nurses are always wrangling with each other ...' The Bermondsey Sisters were so able that Nightingale eventually made four of them superintendents although she had to do so unofficially because they were Catholic: Barrie at the Scutari General Hospital until Tebbutt came, Moore in charge of the Barrack Hospital when Nightingale was in the Crimea and her Aunt Mai was officially in charge, Sister Mary Stanislas at the Balaclava General Hospital after Bridgeman left, and Sister Mary Helen in charge of one of the Land Transport hospitals. Despite Moore's strict enjoinder not to discuss religious matters with anyone except Catholics, Barrie told the Sisters at home she hoped to convert a few people. 'I am not without hope,' she wrote, 'we may convert some, about five seem inclined, thanks to the misrepresentations that have been made, and which seeing us has

Religious nursing

opened their eyes to.'[25] Whether these five soldiers followed through is not recorded.

The first nurses Nightingale sent into the wards were three Devonport Sisters (Sarah Anne Terrot, Bertha Turnbull, and Margaret Goodman), two Bermondsey Sisters, and eight or ten hospital nurses. One day Sister Jean de Chantal, the second Bermondsey nun, told Terrot that Barrie was in charge of the Scutari General Hospital. Although Terrot realized that Barrie was in fact directing the nursing service, she was not certain Nightingale had actually placed her in charge. Thinking it wrong to have a Catholic superintendent, she told Nightingale that while she admired and respected the Catholic nuns, she did not wish to be under their direction. Nightingale replied that Barrie's direction only concerned the outward conduct of the working-class nurses and did not apply to the Anglican Sisters. Barrie was 'inclined to take rather more authority than this,' Terrot wrote, 'though on the whole she exercised it with gentleness and wisdom, and was very considerate and yielding.' She noted that the Catholic Sisters did not differentiate with regard to faith although some soldiers, especially the Scots, felt antipathetic to their traditional black habits while some of the Irish preferred them. Nevertheless, in general, Terrot said, 'the gentle, cheerful manner of the nuns overcame all such dislike.'[26]

In her first months in Scutari, Moore's quiet patience and cheerfulness were severely tried. When Nightingale sent the Norwood Sisters home two of the Catholic chaplains, Father Cuffe and Mr Maloney, accused Nightingale of treating them unfairly. When the Bermondsey nuns tried to justify Nightingale's decision the two chaplains became very angry. Chaplain Maloney, 'with enthusiastic zeal for the dignity of the Religious State' as Moore put it, wrote to influential persons in Rome complaining about her. When Father Ronan pressed Nightingale for better domestic arrangements for the nuns in Mary Stanley's party, Moore thought he produced a complete misunderstanding between Nightingale and Stanley. Cuffe called Moore a plotting woman who had misled him. He thought she also misled Nightingale in a way so harmful to the Catholics that he asked Bishop Grant to recall her. Moore did not entangle herself in these disputes. We did not take part in the disagreements with the priests, she said, but she refused to accept Ronan as chaplain for her team.[27]

The other British religious Sisters

It speaks well of Moore and her nuns, and later of Bridgeman and her team, that they never let these unpleasant quarrels interfere with their nursing practice. Everyone reported that they treated Protestants and Catholics with the same kind care. Later, in 1856, the Jesuit chaplains in the Crimea made life even more difficult for the Bermondsey Sisters. A number of lay individuals also treated the Sisters very badly. When Mrs Clarke was sent home, Miss Inglis succeeded her as matron for a short time before being invalided home. Miss Polidori, who was very anti-Catholic, replaced Inglis. Her conduct was less repulsive than that of Clarke but far more trying and difficult. When Nightingale fell ill in May, Mr Bracebridge, who was also very anti-Catholic, took charge for many weeks and lost no opportunity of annoying the Sisters and preventing them from working in the hospitals. This changed in August 1855, after the Bracebridges had gone home and the new matron, Miss Clarke, arrived. She was very kind to the Bermondsey nuns and gave them the largest and best room in the whole building for their chapel. The majority of the Protestant chaplains were always friendly but there were some who interfered in the most tiresome way. Still, the nuns were cheered in their everyday work, Moore said, by the Catholic soldiers' response to Christian instruction.[28]

When Moore was invalided home in April 1856, Nightingale acknowledged her immeasurable support in a much quoted letter:

> Your going home is the greatest blow I have had yet. But God's blessing and my love and gratitude go with you … You were far above me in fitness for the general superintendency, both in worldly talent of administration, and far more in the spiritual qualifications which God values in a superior … Dearest Rev Mother, what you have done for the work no one can ever say.[29]

And indeed, Nightingale, who was prone to hyperbole, was not exaggerating in this instance. Moore had been her mentor and greatest support during her time in the East.

The Anglican Sisters

Of the ten Anglican Sisters who went to the East four did not work out and were sent home, but the remaining six built quickly on their lesser experience and made enormous contributions to Crimean War nursing. They were less experienced nurses than the Sisters of Mercy and fewer in number because they were such new communities, the first founded only nine years before the war started. The Anglican bishops were suspicious of the sisterhoods and did not offer them any real support. They tried to make sharp distinctions between them and the Catholic sisterhoods by insisting they be called Sisters, not nuns, and forbidding them to take lifelong vows or bring dowries. They were nevertheless real religious communities. They took annual or biennial vows, had set religious offices or devotions, and almost all wore nuns' habits which were indistinguishable from those of Catholic Sisters. St. John's House was unique in that its Sisters did not wear traditional nuns' habits, and in that it was completely devoted to nursing and was actually a nurse training school. St. John's House Sisters were all trained nurses themselves, and unlike the Catholic sisterhoods who trained only their own nuns as nurses, St. John's House trained lay women, both working- and upper-class.[30] All but one of their nurses who went to the East were working-class. The one lady was Miss Bartlett,[31] who went to the naval hospital in Therapia. St. John's House also differed from other sisterhoods in that it was Broad Church when nearly all the others were High Church, which attracted hostility from large segments of the anti-Catholic public which identified them with the Roman Church.

The interest in finding an area where ladies could develop their own abilities and escape subordination to men is especially clear in the case of the Anglican Sisters. Most came primarily for the opportunity to do meaningful work, not for the religious life, and while most of the new Sisters were conventionally religious, most were not interested in developing spirituality. When the chaplain enquired after the spiritual life of one of these Sisters she thought to herself, 'I really don't know. I am interested in my work; I am always at office; I have my time of devotion. What more does he want me to do?' Mother Harriet Brownlow Byron, the founder of the All Saints Sisters of the Poor, one of the largest, most successful, and also most fashionable of the sisterhoods, exemplified the Anglican Sisters' standard belief that work must come first. As one of her Sisters explained, Byron repeatedly said, '*Work* and Pray – or that work must come first, and Meditations, Devotions, etc., must make way if the work

The other British religious Sisters

came.' Sister Sarah Anne Terrot, one of the three original members of the Park Village sisterhood, joined because she was seeking what she called 'greater usefulness.' After helping the Devonport Sisters in the cholera epidemic in 1849 she transferred to their sisterhood because they were less austere than Park Village and she liked their greater emphasis on work. She enjoyed the nursing but disliked the religious aspects of the community; in fact she often ignored the conventual rules.

As would nearly all the new sisterhoods, the oldest sisterhood, the Park Village Sisters, did social work and some domiciliary nursing. They visited the poor in their own homes, ran a ragged school, and rescued 'distressed women.'[32] The sisterhood had been designed with an emphasis on asceticism which would not combine well with the hard physical work of military nursing. Nearly all of the Anglican sisterhoods began as little groups of ladies who had been helping their vicar with parochial duties and then decided to expand their sphere of action into a sisterhood.[33] By contrast, the Park Village sisterhood was primarily the inspiration of Edward Bouverie Pusey, who atypically placed more emphasis on the spiritual life. This famous Anglican cleric became essentially its superior as well as its spiritual advisor. He developed its rules himself, using those of Catholic sisterhoods on the continent as his model. The original 1845 rule had the Sisters observing the Benedictine canonical hours – Matins, Lauds, Terce, etc. – although Pusey abridged the eight offices into seven by merging the midnight Matins and 3 a.m. Lauds into one office which the Sisters observed at 5:20 in the morning. Pusey later became the leader of the High Church party, most famously reviving auricular confession. He was a real ascetic, fasting rigorously and wearing a hair shirt. Mother Lydia Sellon visited the Park Village sisterhood in 1848 and was appalled by the strictness of Pusey's rules. Some of the Park Village Sisters tried to emulate Pusey's ascetic lifestyle, and in 1854 one Sister died, according to the death certificate from tuberculosis. Her sister, however, thought she did not die of disease but from being 'worn out by the bodily austerities of nine years.' In 1850 another Sister died from starvation trying to follow Pusey's rule for Lenten fasting. Sister Etheldreda Pillans was a bright, gay lady who helped Pusey with his translations but she became very ill with smallpox in 1848 and never really recovered her health, which may have been partly a result of

Religious nursing

the asceticisms the sisterhood practiced. She had no clinical experience and was acting as Mistress of Orphans in 1854 when she left for Scutari. Already in frail health, she became so ill from seasickness on the voyage to Turkey that she never recovered and had to be sent home, having done no nursing.[34]

Mother Emma Langston had some clinical experience helping the Devonport Sisters during the cholera epidemic but she was a failure as a manager. She was close to 50 years old and working as a governess in Dublin when Pusey appointed her Mother Superior. He was impressed by her 'fervid desire to engage in more devoted service to God ... and still more by her anxious self-trust,' which he mistakenly interpreted as humility. In her ten years as Mother Superior, although pious and hard-working, she was always indecisive. Pusey soon realized his error and thought he should have waited to establish the sisterhood until a better candidate for Superior had appeared.[35] Nightingale placed Langston in charge of the seven nurses who went to Balaclava in January 1855 because she assumed that as a Mother Superior she would know how to manage. Nightingale soon found she showed 'a lack of brains'[36] and feared she was becoming senile.[37] When she was invalided home in April 1855, Nightingale said Langston had lost 'her money, her head & her health.' The money consisted of the funds Nightingale gave her for hospital expenses, all of which disappeared except for £1. Langston thought it possible that Martha Clough had stolen it.[38] Sister Harriet Erskine accompanied Langston and a hospital nurse home. Erskine, who was really not a Park Village Sister but only visiting when she volunteered, was a 'certificated nurse.'[39] Later in the century this term meant a nurse who had completed a certain amount of time working in a hospital, but what it meant in 1854 is hard to determine. It could have meant only two or three weeks observing in a hospital. Nightingale considered Erskine invaluable. After delivering her patients to England Erskine returned to the East but went to the naval hospital at Therapia, not to the army hospitals.[40]

Pusey was also the spiritual director of the Devonport Sisters and a close friend and spiritual director of Sellon. At the request of the Bishop of Exeter Sellon went to Devonport in 1848, starting work there with only one helper. Within two years she had established in Devonport and Plymouth an orphanage, a home for delinquent

The other British religious Sisters

boys, two refuges for training girls for domestic service, an industrial school, six model lodging houses for poor families, five ragged schools, a soup kitchen, a home for old sailors, and a naval training school. She later set up a printing press which was run by young women.[41]

During the 1849 cholera epidemic the Devonport Sisters and their medical officer set up a hospital of sixty beds in a temporary wooden building with a shed for the medical officer, a marquee for the Sisters, and another marquee for children orphaned by the disease. There the Sisters worked in shifts around the clock. Sellon benefitted from the fact that she founded her sisterhood in 1848, three years after Park Village, and Pusey had learned a great deal from his experience there.[42] In any case, Sellon was too practical and also too experienced from nursing in the cholera epidemics of 1849 and 1853 to expect her Sisters to endure severe austerities when they were doing such hard physical work as nursing. Like Bridgeman she appreciated that nurses had to maintain their own health if they were to be able to help the patients. She specifically told her five Sisters when they left for the Crimea that they were not to fast. 'Do not fast, and take all the care you can of your health,' she instructed them. She ordered them to take an hour off every day for exercise in the fresh air. Sisters Bertha Turnbull and Margaret Goodman always did, and they attributed their being two of the few women who were never sick once during the entire campaign to this practice.[43] Successful Mother foundresses like Sellon were usually well-educated women with strong character and the ability to command. Like Nightingale's father, many of their fathers had given them boys' educations.[44] Sellon tended to be more authoritarian than most foundresses but she is an excellent example of this type of very competent woman. After seeing the temporary hospital she organized in an unused factory in Spitalfields during the 1866 cholera epidemic, Charles Wood, later Viscount Halifax, became one of her ardent supporters. He had always had a prejudice against her, he said, and she may have had her faults, but he thought her energy and power of organization were marvellous and the work she and her Sisters did impressive.[45]

Of the five Sisters Sellon sent to the East two, Sisters Bertha Turnbull and Margaret Goodman, were highly successful. Both had clinical experience and their stamina and commitment to the nursing, as well as their religious discipline, made them first class nurses. When Shaw Stewart left the Castle Hospital to take over as superintendent of one of the Land Transport hospitals, Turnbull took her place as superintendent. Nightingale had complete faith in her judgment – she knew she would always make the right decision. She considered her the most valuable superintendent after Jane Shaw Stewart and Mother Mary Clare Moore.[46] Sister Mary Gonzaga Barrie, who became a close friend of Nightingale, felt rather superior to the three Anglican Sisters, Turnbull, Goodman, and Terrot, who worked under her at the Scutari General Hospital; she of course, as a Roman Catholic, did not consider them real Sisters. She thought the working-class nurses, who she said were always fighting with each other, only made common cause to abuse the Anglican Sisters and resist their authority. She characterized the Sisters as 'thoroughly self-relying sufficient Protestants' who were very proud of themselves. At first, she said, they talked of '"us Nuns," but I suppose, finding they could not establish their character as such, they always now speak of us as "the Nuns."' One of the three Anglican Sisters working under her paid her the compliment of saying how well they had all gotten on together. In less than a month Barrie felt she had her team working reasonably well together, although, she said, 'nothing here is *very settled*.'[47] The Bermondsey and Anglican Sisters did work well together despite some reservations on both sides.

It is interesting that Bridgeman, who spent more than half her time in the East in Koulali, never mentioned an Anglican Sister, Sister Anne Thom, an outstanding nurse and a major force in the Koulali hospitals. She came from a professional family and was 39 years old when she arrived in the spring of 1855 but we have no information about what she had done beforehand. She always wore her Sister's habit, which suggests that she came from a High Church sisterhood. She had worked as a surgical nurse at the Middlesex Hospital where the matron pronounced her a skilled, sensible, and very useful nurse. She had a good deal of experience in nursing, was very devoted to the work, and was much and deservedly loved by her patients. She also helped organize clothing and other necessary items for the soldiers' wives, who were often desperate for clothes for themselves and their children, when they went home to England. Thom was just as kind to the orderlies as to the soldiers, training them and teaching them not

The other British religious Sisters

to swear or drink excessively. The most malignant cases of cholera were put in her wards and yet she always had them in perfect order. It was Thom who organized the night nursing which was to save so many lives at Koulali. Some of the dehydrated and feverish patients required a spoonful of wine or beef tea, or if an ice ship had come in, a bit of ice, every five minutes through the night, another indication of how labor-intensive rehydration was in the days before intravenous therapy and why nursing became such an important part of medical care. Thom was briefly superintendent when Miss Hutton left in early November 1855. She apparently was willing to transfer to Scutari and work under Nightingale, but Nightingale did not have a suitable opening for her so in December 1855 she went home.[48]

In summary, of the nine Anglican Sisters who worked in the British army hospitals, one, Langston, was incompetent, one, Pillans, was too ill to ever do any work, Sharpe was sent home as unsuitable, and Wheeler, whose colleagues considered her an excellent nurse, was dismissed for political reasons. Terrot's colleagues considered her an excellent nurse but Nightingale claimed that, although she was a good and conscientious nurse, she was not skillful.[49] Four, Sisters Bertha Turnbull, Ann Thom, Harriet Erskine, and Margaret Goodman, were first class nurses. The tenth Sister, Miss Bartlett, worked in the naval hospital in Therapia, where Harriet Erskine joined her after taking Langston home. So of the ten Anglican Sisters, five were outstanding nurses.

Notes

1 O'Brien, 'French Nuns in Nineteenth-Century England,' p. 143.
2 Bostridge, *Florence Nightingale*, pp. 173–4.
3 Mumm, *Stolen Daughters*, p. 3.
4 Helmstadter, 'Robert Bentley Todd,' pp. 306–8; Chadwick, *Victorian Church*, vol. 1, pp. 509–10.
5 Bridgeman, 'Account,' p. 246.
6 BA 1839, p. 1.
7 Sullivan, *Friendship*, pp. 5–11.
8 Bermondsey Archives, Moore to Bishop Grant, 1 July 1850, 400/2/221; Moore to Grant, 9 May 1854, 400/2/183.
9 Sullivan, *Friendship*, pp. 9–10.
10 BA 1854, p. 219.

Religious nursing

11 BL 43402, Nightingale Report No. II, 16 June 1856, fol. 10.

12 BA 1856, p. 293.

13 BA 1855, pp. 247–8.

14 Bridgeman, 'Account,' p. 185.

15 BA 1854, p. 210.

16 Terrot, *Reminiscences*, pp. 7–8.

17 BA 1854, pp. 218–19.

18 Bridgeman, 'Account,' pp. 245–6; Sullivan, *Friendship*, pp. 6–8, 51–2.

19 Sullivan, *Friendship*, p. 5.

20 Bermondsey Archives, Letter of Moore to Sister M. Aloysius, August 1846, 27/400/2, 1–2.

21 Lady nurses generally had trains on their dresses so that when they bent over their patients their ankles would still be covered.

22 BA 1854, p. 222.

23 Terrot, *Reminiscences*, pp. 7–8, 44.

24 BL 43404, Nightingale Note, [October] 1854, fol. 1.

25 BA 1854, pp. 229–30.

26 Terrot, *Reminiscences*, pp. 46, 70–1.

27 BA 1855, pp. 231–2, 242–4; Luddy, *Crimean Journals*, p. xix; Bolster, *Sisters of Mercy*, pp. 102–3.

28 BA 1855, pp. 247–8, 252–5.

29 Bermondsey Archives, Nightingale Collection, Nightingale to Moore, 29 April 1856.

30 Helmstadter, 'Robert Bentley Todd,' pp. 299–300.

31 Because St. John's House was a Broad Church community and the bishops were so worried that they would be identified with the Anglican High Church or the Roman Church, originally the St. John's House Sisters were not given names in religion or the title of 'Sister,' hence 'Miss Bartlett.'

32 Mumm, *Stolen Daughters*, pp. 14–15; Williams and Campbell, *Park Village*, pp. 22, 36, 56, 108.

33 Chadwick, *Victorian Church*, vol. 1, p. 506–7.

34 Williams and Campbell, *Park Village*, pp. 15–16, 27, 67–9, 96, 100–2; Cobb, 'Pusey.'

35 Williams, *Sellon*, pp. 22–3.

36 BL 43393, Nightingale to Herbert, 15 February 1855, fol. 155.

37 Pusey House, Nightingale to Sellon, 5 December 1854 and 5 March 1855.

38 WI Ms 8995, Nightingale to her family, 22 April 1855, Letter 12.

39 Williams and Campbell, *Park Village*, p. 91.

40 WI Ms 8895 Nightingale Report, 30 November 1855, Letter 78.

41 Cobb, 'Sellon.'

42 Williams, *Sellon*, pp. 37, 51, 69–75, 93.

43 Williams and Campbell, *Park Village*, p. 94; Goodman, *English Sister of Mercy*, p. 187.

144

The other British religious Sisters

44 Mumm, *Stolen Daughters*, p. 57.
45 Williams, *Sellon*, pp. 229–30.
46 BL 43402, Nightingale Report No. IV, 26 June 1856, fols 19–20.
47 BA 1854, Barrie to Sister Mary Ignatius, Advent Sunday 1854, pp. 229–30.
48 Taylor, *Eastern Hospitals*, vol. 1, pp. 226–7, 256, 276–8, 281–90; vol. 2, pp. 59, 173; ibid (3rd edn, 1857), pp. 136–7; LMA/H01/ST/NC8/4, Register of Nurses, p. 20; Columbia University School of Nursing, Nightingale to Sister Anne, 8 December 1855, C-15.
49 Pusey House, Nightingale to Sellon, 5 December 1854; WI Ms 8895, Nightingale Report, 30 November 1855, Letter 78.

7

The Daughters of Charity of St. Vincent de Paul

Introduction

Florence Nightingale received an enormous amount of press for her work in the Crimean War, at first often critical but later highly laudatory. In an age when class was so rigidly delineated and social status meant so much, the lady of high estate who nursed working-class soldiers and who organized the first official British army female nursing service became a national heroine. By contrast, despite the high profile the Daughters of Charity of St. Vincent de Paul enjoyed in the British press at the beginning of the war, French military nursing has received little attention in the English-speaking world. Yet the achievements of these Sisters were a major reason why the British government sent female nurses to the East and the Daughters were also one of the models on which the Grand Duchess Elena Pavlovna based her highly successful Russian nursing sisterhood. The Daughters, or Sisters of Charity as they were also called, had a long tradition of trained nursing. Founded by St. Vincent de Paul in 1633, they were one expression of the Catholic Counter-Reformation, forming the first unenclosed order of women in the church. Although they wore traditional nuns' habits and were called Sisters, the Daughters were not strictly speaking nuns for they did not take lifelong vows – they took only private annual vows – and they did not have to bring dowries. Their rule eschewed the ascetic life, placing work ahead of prayer and daily offices. 'Prefer the service of the sick poor to all other corporeal or spiritual exercises,' St. Vincent instructed the Sisters in 1659. Their work, he explained, extended principally to the soul but they should never let spiritual care compromise physical care.[1] Already by 1700, Colin Jones stated,

146

the Sisters had become 'an archetype – patient, saintly, laborious, discreet, committed – and tough.'[2] By the end of the *ancien régime* the Daughters, or nursing sisterhoods like them, had taken over the nursing in nearly all the hospitals in France. They signed contracts with the hospitals which, in return for a fixed sum of money, gave them complete control of the pharmacy, housekeeping, and kitchens as well as the nursing. They themselves, not the doctors, prescribed the diets for the patients, a key part of medical treatment at that time.

The Daughters formed a highly centralized order which was not accountable to the bishops of the various dioceses within which their convents were located. Rather they reported to the mother house in Paris and to the Vincentian Order (also called the Lazarists), an order of secular clergy which St. Vincent established a few years prior to founding the Daughters. The Sisters were first tested for their vocation for nursing over a period of months in a provincial house. If successful they were then sent to the mother house in Paris for more advanced training, which included elementary surgical work. When they went out to new hospitals they always took lancets and other surgical instruments with them. In the women's wards they did the bleeding and minor surgical procedures, dressed wounds, and applied poultices. They considered their skills superior to those of apprentice surgeons. Although the Daughters' rule forbade them to do corporeal work in the men's wards,[3] they had been nursing in the French army almost since their founding in the seventeenth century when they were sent out in groups of two and four to take charge of military hospitals.[4] Their long tradition of military nursing meant that they were not only widely accepted in the army hospitals but widely welcomed. They never met the antagonism and resistance which Nightingale and the other lady superintendents encountered in the British military hospitals.

The Daughters of Charity in the Crimean War: professionally trained nurses

In 1854 the sisterhood had a network of 12,000 Sisters throughout Europe. The Daughters who held the original contracts with the French army came from local convents in Constantinople, Smyrna, and Pera. The eleven French military hospitals in and around

Constantinople over which they presided were, in Helen Rappaport's words, 'havens of calm, order, neatness, cleanliness and harmony among the nurses,' while the Sisters themselves were always cheerful and gay.[5] Gaiety was a fundamental part of the Sisters' approach to nursing from the very beginning of their order. When training the early Sisters in 1642 St. Vincent urged them to greet the sick with a 'modest gaiety.'[6] Herbé paid tribute to their cheerful approach. After being severely wounded at the Battle of the Tchernaya he spent two months in a divisional hospital in Kamiesch. In October 1855 he was transferred to Constantinople to the Sisters' hospital for officers, which was housed in the beautiful Russian embassy overlooking the Golden Horn. Herbé was thrilled with his new accommodation. He had a beautiful view of the Bosphorus, an excellent large bed with two mattresses, and most wonderful of all, a pillow, something he had not had for eighteen months. He found the hospital and its regimen perfect: chocolate in the morning, lunch at 10 a.m. and dinner at 5 p.m.; the doctors made their rounds at 10 a.m. and 4 p.m. He enjoyed the wonderful food, which the Sisters cooked themselves and served on the embassy's fine china. They were first class cooks and their cuisine was very varied. For example, one day for lunch there was first a very good soup with tapioca, then lamb chop jardinière, roast chicken, fried potatoes, and for dessert, fresh grapes and soft biscuits, all served with a carafe of excellent Bordeaux which Herbé drank from the embassy's crystal glasses. 'This menu,' he declared, 'seasoned by the sea breeze which comes through our large windows is, as you can see, most reviving, and should promptly restore the strength which we lack.'[7] It was a very different meal from the crushed hard tack and raw bacon[8] (because there was no firewood) which he had had to eat at times during the preceding harsh winter. In addition to all these luxuries Herbé said the Sisters of Charity encouraged the men to have patience and charity.[9]

Nightingale considered the Daughters' rule forbidding physical care of men prudish and incompatible with efficient nursing.[10] Herbé felt differently. He considered the Sisters well-educated women who nursed the men with a delicacy of feeling which fortified the body, restored courage, and softened the sadness of being so far from home when ill. 'It is above all when one is suffering, when one is sick or wounded,' he wrote, 'that one appreciates the true worth and courage

The Daughters of Charity of St. Vincent de Paul

of these brave Sisters.' 'Every officer waits impatiently for their arrival,' he said,

> and uses every ruse to keep them at his bedside as long as possible. They do not do the dressings; this service is for convenience and respect assigned to the male nurses; but they provide all the little cares so necessary for the wounded, with a grace and good humor which almost heals their wounds! Also they are very much obeyed, very much cherished, loved and blessed!

One of the Sisters assigned to Herbé's room was a close friend of the sister of a comrade who had been killed at Herbé's side during an attack on a Russian redoubt. Despite being very wealthy this Sister, inspired by patriotic devotion to the army in which her brother was a captain, took a vow of five years with the Daughters of Charity. She came almost every afternoon to sit with Herbé and talk about mutual friends and his family.[11]

Other patients were equally complimentary. Captain Montaudon, who arrived in the hospital with severe bowel disease, spoke of the Sisters' great kindness, their wise and intelligent care, and their anticipation of every detail.[12] Lt. Masquelez, who was wounded on the escarpment above the Alma, would never forget the emotion he felt on seeing a Sister of Charity with a smile on her lips coming towards him when he first arrived in the hospital. She brought to mind our consoling religion, he wrote, our beautiful country which he had not seen for such a long time, his family, and the care they gave him. In the days before diagnostic imagery Masquelez had to undergo probings and dressings of the enormous wound in his foot twice a day. Each procedure took an hour and a half and was excruciatingly painful. The surgeon would seize the shell fragment with forceps and then, using scissors, cut it away from the muscle or tendon to which it adhered. They often had to twist the muscle as when pulling a tooth, which was even more agonizing. It took eight days to get one fragment out, and then, even worse, the wound closed over some of the splinters and the doctors had to cut it open and dig about again to find them. They urged Masquelez to cry out because it would relieve the pain a bit, thus making their job a little easier. Sometimes one of the Sisters would hold Masquelez's hand while they probed and say 'Courage, courage,' which he said he certainly needed. Since almost every wound became infected, Masquelez suffered from fever. At the end of September his fever became violent and his sufferings redoubled. He did not sleep for the next three months despite all the opium they gave him but sometimes, he said, the door to his room would open and a saintly Sister would come in to console him. Sister Josephine, the Sister Superior, was empathetic and had an exquisite tact. She knew how to make religion amiable without being too evangelical and gave the men medals of the Virgin which they wore around their necks. We were all so grateful to her, Masquelez wrote. Later he often thought of her and thanked her for helping him overcome the despair that prolonged suffering engenders. Her sweet sympathetic voice awakened memories of childhood, religious sentiment, and mothers, families and friends in France.[13] One must keep in mind that Herbé was a St. Cyr trained veteran soldier and Montaudon and Masquelez were Zouaves, the toughest soldiers in the French army.

All their patients admired the Sisters but not all welcomed their religious instruction. Henry Clifford met a French cavalry officer who had been wounded and nursed by what he described as 'a pretty little Sister of Charity.' He told Clifford, 'I believe her looking at the wound did it more good than anything else. I'm not a good man, but I always thought of the Blessed Virgin when I saw that pretty face, and what my mother used to tell me.' Like the Sisters of Mercy, the Daughters did not give religious instruction when the men were acutely ill, but when the fever finally left him and he was feeling better this Sister asked him, 'How is your poor soul?' and urged him to see a priest, which he refused to do. From that moment until he was discharged from the hospital she never gave him a moment's peace, and when he left she told him 'You will be sorry for this someday.'[14] Nevertheless, even if some men did not appreciate religious counsel, the Sisters clearly offered a great deal of moral support and consolation as well as a professionally run nursing administration. Admiral Slade agreed with the patients' evaluation of the Daughters. He thought the soldiers derived inappreciable solace from the Sisters, who cared for the critical cases themselves, fed those unable to feed themselves, and cheered the desponding with their gaiety. In addition, he said, the Sisters treated Russian soldiers, who were in the same wards as the French, with the same care and kindness.[15]

The cantinières: entrepreneurs and sutlers

Another group of women who helped the French soldiers was the *cantinières*, literally canteen ladies. These women were descendants of the camp followers and female sutlers who followed the old royal armies. In 1794 the Republic gave them the official title of cantinière. They wore colorful uniforms consisting of a loose red petticoat over red Turkish trousers and they carried attached to their belt a flask of wine or brandy with the number of their regiment on it. They travelled with the army selling food, drink, and various other small items from their mobile canteens. The army rated cantinières who married soldiers as corporals and assigned eight to each regiment. When the French troops came up to support the British at the Battle of Inkerman, one British officer said, the cantinières were riding with them as if at a review. On the battlefield they provided drinks and first aid for the wounded gratis but they were basically entrepreneurs who sold alcohol and other provisions from their canteens or on horseback. The British soldiers found their tents a great attraction because they could get 'most gloriously drunk' there, as one British officer put it.[16]

The cantinières were highly respected by the troops and very much a part of each regiment. For example, when the officers in Algeria were selecting soldiers for the Crimean campaign a venerable cantinière named Marie desperately wanted to go. She had been very beautiful in her youth and was a legend in the regiment. For twenty years she had accompanied it on all its African campaigns but she was not chosen for the Crimea because of her age and infirmities. Disguised as a soldier she tried to embark but was caught and turned back. Following the Battle of the Alma, the Colonel of the 2nd Zouaves sent one of his cantinières, Dumont, back to Varna to buy extra food. She paid for it partly out of her own money and partly with money the officers advanced to her. Worn out by three successive such voyages, she died from incipient cholera soon after her husband was wounded at the Alma.[17] The cantinières were in much the same position as Mary Seacole although the British army gave Seacole no official recognition or rating. But, like the cantinières, she was essentially an entrepreneur and sutler who helped injured soldiers on the battlefield cost-free. She gave some nursing care to officers who paid to stay on the second floor of her 'British Hotel' in

Kadikoi, a town a few miles from Balaclava, but her primary activity was running the store on the ground floor which supplied every kind of article, both edible and otherwise.[18] Seacole is sometimes called 'the black Florence Nightingale' but that is really a misnomer. She called herself a 'doctoress', never ran a nursing service, and had no impact on the development of the new nursing as Nightingale did.

The French army medical department: professional soldier nurses and outdated administrative arrangements

Totleben considered the French army the most professional of the five Crimean War armies,[19] and indeed the 30,000-man Army of the East which landed in the Crimea in 1854 had many advantages over those of its allies, the British and Turks, as well as over the Russians. It incorporated veteran soldiers, battle-hardened in the Algerian campaigns, and included four regiments of the famous Zouaves. Originally native tribesmen commanded by French officers, by 1854 these elite troops were almost all Frenchmen although they kept the colorful Zouave uniform of baggy red trousers and blue jackets. They were all armed with the new Minié rifle before leaving for the Crimea, and although there was little in common between warfare in Africa and that in the Crimea, they quickly adapted to European-style combat. In Algeria we fought fanatics who were audacious and brave, one of the Zouaves' most experienced officers, Colonel Montaudon, wrote later, but they had no military organization or esprit de corps. They were incoherent masses who did not understand the art of war or the science necessary when fighting well-disciplined, well-organized soldiers. Nevertheless, he said it was a good preparation for the Crimea because our generals learned what was necessary for the well-being of our soldiers – the importance of provisions, means of transport, how not to use excessive force when dealing with subordinates, how to build camps, and how to guard against surprises. Above all, battle-hardened by incessant fighting, accustomed to hunger, thirst, privations, and marches in all kinds of temperatures, our officers and men developed an uncomplaining spirit and esprit de corps. They understood, Montaudon proclaimed, that 'the difficulty in war is not to know how to die with honor: it was to know how to stay alive for the greatest good of the fatherland.'[20]

The medical department illustrated the professional nature of the army. It was extremely well organized and well supplied with bread and biscuit bakeries, appropriate transport, and hospitals for the sick.[21] British officers were impressed by its efficiency. 'The French are far superior to us in everything but fighting,' Clifford wrote in late December 1854. 'They have learned much by the long war in Africa and are quite at home in the field.' He thought the French medical, engineering, and commissary departments perfect but deemed the Zouaves and the Chasseurs de Vincennes, an elite cavalry unit, the only good French fighting men.[22] (British officers would often make derogatory comments about the French army's fighting abilities and vice-versa.) Admiral Slade supported Clifford's view of the French medical department. He thought the French hospitals had all the improvements modern science could offer.[23] By modern science he meant the dramatic change in therapeutics as depleting practices gradually went out of use with the advent of the new scientific doctors. 'The first and most essential remedy in the treatment of pleuritis and pneumonia from [gunshot] injury is bleeding,' Napoleonic War surgeon G. J. Guthrie wrote. Bleeding should be done 'in every case, whenever the febrile excitement is really inflammatory.' Guthrie's preferred practice was to bleed the man until he fainted. The bleeding should be repeated every four hours or more often – as long as pain or difficulty in breathing remained, and 'under this improved practice,' Guthrie declared, all his patients recovered. He also recommended two internal heroic remedies, tartar emetic and calomel, a powerful purgative, for chest infections. Guthrie was too old to take part in the Crimean War himself but he corresponded with younger surgeons in the East and included a good deal of the information they sent him in his sixth edition of *Surgery of the War*. He thought bloodletting less serviceable in the Crimea because of the climate and the impaired vigor of the soldiers.[24] Although bleeding and drugs with violent effects were going out of use at mid-century George Macleod, who finished medical school in 1853, thought bleeding still efficacious. 'It is well known,' he wrote,

> that in sieges generally, soldiers do not show their usual tolerance of bleeding, and when their health is so much undermined as it was at Sebastopol, the surgeon is often placed in a most unpleasant dilemma. That many most excellent recoveries [from wounds of face and chest] were made without

having recourse to the lancet is undoubtedly true; but not a few, I fear, died from want of it.[25]

The new scientific medicine encouraged the use of painkillers, more cleanliness, and liberal diet and stimulants. As a result it had to rely heavily on nurses who would faithfully administer these measures.[26] From the surgeon's point of view, the most wonderful new modern scientific treatment was chloroform, and anesthetized patients required close post-operative monitoring. We used chloroform constantly, Dr Gaspard-Léonard Scrive, chief medical officer in the French Crimean army, stated. He soon found his fears that it would depress the nervous system or weaken the vitality of the wounded were groundless; in fact, it did just the opposite, he said, and although we used it thousands of times, there was not a single accident.[27]

The French soldier nurses particularly impressed Slade. They had, he said,

> high professional knowledge joined with extensive practice. The familiarity of everybody with his duties rendered their performance easy. The intelligence of the attendants, a trained body, saved the surgeons much time and trouble: they made the preliminary arrangements for operations, and were adept in the art of assuaging pain with pad and pillow.[28]

In former times, hospital nurses had largely only cleaned up after all the bleeding, purging, and vomiting which Guthrie's generation ordered, but the new supportive therapeutics made trustworthy, competent trained nurses a major component of successful medical treatment.[29] The intelligent trained attendants who so impressed Slade were what the French called *infirmiers militaires* or *soldats infirmiers*, military or soldier nurses. Baron Pierre-François Percy was the surgeon in charge of the regimental hospitals when the Revolutionary Wars started in 1792. Appalled by the barbarous way in which the sick and wounded soldiers were abandoned on the field, he developed a special field corps of stretcher-bearers who, as soon as the battle began and soldiers were wounded, went onto the field, administered first aid, and then brought the men back to a field hospital. For this special corps he chose several hundred of the bravest, most adroit, and strongest soldiers, just the opposite of Col. Sterling's suggestions for these men. They saved many lives and, equally important, when the men knew they would not be abandoned if wounded, the new system was excellent for morale.

At the same time Baron Dominique Jean Larrey developed what he called 'flying ambulances.' Inspired by the horse artillery which moved the field artillery around the battlefield so efficiently, these were light carriages on springs which carried soldiers off the field. In 1797 Bonaparte asked Larrey to organize flying ambulances for the Army of Italy. In 1824 a royal decree also formally established a standing corps of soldier nurses who worked in hospitals. The system was perfected in the ensuing years and the results were outstanding.[30] The army gave these nurses higher status, additional pay, and opportunities for promotion, although promotion only extended through non-commissioned ranks. All had to know how to read and write and they were what one English doctor called 'perfect nurses.'[31] The doctors were highly dependent on the trained nurses but complained bitterly that there were always too few. In the Crimean War, men commandeered from the troops and from convalescents outnumbered the specially trained nurses: the French used 2,000 commandeered soldiers to make up for their lack of soldier nurses.[32] Sir James McGrigor, Director of the British Army Medical Department through 1855, observed these men at work in the Peninsular War and made repeated efforts to introduce a similar ambulance corps in the British army but without success.[33]

At the end of the war Scrive recommended expanding the number of soldier nurses to 800 in peacetime and 1,200 in wartime[34] but, even if the government had agreed to these numbers, it was unlikely the army could have recruited so many. Nurses volunteered, were assigned to the nursing corps by the recruiting officer, or were commandeered from other army units. The French also considered nursing a feminine pursuit: few volunteered, because most young men wanted to be fighting men, not nurses, and the same was true of the young drafted soldiers. Assigning draftees to the nursing corps was a poor method of staffing, declared Dr Jean-Charles Chenu, chief doctor of the army medical corps in 1865. 'Is it right to have the recruiting officer make the decision as to whether a man is to be a soldier or a nurse?' he asked in his 727-page statistical study of the army's medical service in the Crimean War. He included a whole chapter demonstrating that understaffing among both doctors and nurses was largely responsible for the dreadful mortality in the hospitals in the second winter of the war. It was also difficult to recruit nurses because, Chenu said, their prospects were so inferior to those of other soldiers. The recruiting officer has two zealous young men, he hypothesized, from the same town with the same intelligence, equal aptitudes, and equally irreproachable conduct. He sends one to the cavalry or infantry, and the other to the nursing corps. The nurse could only become a sergeant while the other man could become a commissioned officer and had many other opportunities as well. (Promotion from the ranks to officer level was infrequent in the British army but common in the French.) Commandeering men was the worst system of all. As in the British army, the regiments sent very bad soldiers and these men made equally bad nurses. They had as little vocation for nursing as for soldiering. Drafting a man from another army corps only worked when the colonel of his unit appreciated the value of nursing and sent competent men. The work of the private military nurses was not generally appreciated or respected, not even by the sergeants or the doctors who were so dependent on them. We must give more recognition to the soldier nurses, Chenu advised.

In wartime doctors improvised many things but they could not improvise a nurse because nurses had to know their métier and the apprenticeship was long. Also a nurse had to inspire confidence in his patients and the patients must be able to trust him to help them, especially during the night. 'Ten auxiliary nurses do not replace one nurse who knows his job,' Chenu declared. He went on to make suggestions for improving the recruitment system. There should be more incentive for drafted men to choose nursing for their military career. Military nurses should have the same rights and opportunities as regular soldiers; they must be able to advance from private to corporal to sergeant to officer. Whether a volunteer draftee or a man officially assigned to nursing, the military nurse's service was no less honorable than that of the highly respected volunteer ladies whom Nightingale directed. There should be more sergeant nurses (*infirmiers-major*) and they should be better recompensed. In fact Chenu thought there should be Guards in the nursing service just as there were Guards in the artillery and engineer corps.[35]

The French medical department suffered as much from the chain of command as it did from its shortage of doctors and nurses. In

1794 the Revolutionary government created a Council of Health for the Armies (*Conseil de Santé des Armées*) and placed it within the commissariat. The Council directed and superintended everything which had to do with the health of the army. French military doctors had held officers' commissions since 1834 and in 1852 were made into a medical corps [*corps de santé*] which was fully integrated into the army, but like the British doctors they could only advise their superiors in the commissariat and had no military authority. In 1854 the Council of Health consisted of three doctors who were called *intendants* or inspectors, or sometimes referred to collectively as the *intendancy*.[36] The Council of Health's superiors in the commissariat paid little attention to its requests.

Scrive strongly believed his superiors were incompetent to direct the army's health care, and this was equally obvious to outsiders. Nightingale identified this problem after being in the East only three months. The French give too much power to their commissariat, she told Sidney Herbert, with the result that the medical men are its slaves.[37] Longmore, like Chenu and Scrive, believed the subordination of the medical department to the commissariat was responsible for the horrendous death rate from disease in the second year of the war.[38] Macleod, who had worked in the French hospitals, thought the French made a terrible error giving those in the commissariat higher rank and hence control of the surgeons; their very promotion depended on the intendants, he said. He liked the idea of the purveyors doing hospital administration so the doctors could concentrate entirely on medical matters, but thought the people who were responsible for food and equipment should be subordinate, not superior, to the doctors.[39] From the point of view of the medical corps and its patients, this arrangement had never worked. Percy was constantly fighting with the Council of Health, which turned down almost every improvement he suggested. Ideally Percy thought the medical department needed to be more heavily staffed and should be a completely independent unit like the engineers or artillery. The generals and the soldiers strongly supported Percy but he and the commissariat soon became enemies. By contrast, as a professional soldier Napoleon I saw at once the great benefits to the army which Percy's suggestions made and later, when he came to power, encouraged his work and showered him with honors.[40]

When the Geneva Convention was being worked out in 1864, the financially appealing system of volunteer female nurses was suggested. The military doctors of all nationalities were adamant that they had to have trained nurses. The French doctors pointed out that volunteer nurses were simply not practical. The British nurses and the French Sisters of Charity did excellent work but could not work on the battlefield, the very place where nurses were most needed. There were other things female nurses could not do. The Sisters of Charity were not allowed to undress a sick or wounded man. Women did not have the muscular strength to turn and position a soldier, lift him into bed, or sometimes even carry him a significant distance.[41] In the harsh mountainous terrain of Algeria where the French army had been operating since the 1830s, Larrey's flying ambulances were impractical. The medical corps therefore devised wicker litters and chairs which were called *cacolets*, carried by mules and led by a specially trained group of muleteers.[42] On the battlefield, Chenu pointed out, nurses had to have the strength to carry a wounded soldier and know how to place him on a stretcher and put him in a *cacolet*, things which were not easy to do and required a great deal of practice. Nurses had to be familiar with pain and the sight of blood. Equally important, Chenu continued, they must have devotion, discipline, obedience to orders, and know how to work in a team, something which all soldiers were trained to do. Volunteer men would not do either. They might have the strength required, but only soldiers who were used to the dangers of the battlefield – the gunfire, chaos, and smoke – could be expected to retrieve the wounded from the field under fire.[43]

The French encountered severe medical problems almost from the start of the campaign when cholera struck in Bulgaria. Scrive tended to take bowel disease in the East for granted and reported that, although there were quite a few sick, the health of the army and its morale were reasonably good in September and October 1854. The weather was mild and favored surgical practice: wounds healed quickly.[44] Scrive had to send reports to his superiors in the commissariat every ten days, and beginning in October, he was able to include good statistics. When reading his figures one must keep in mind that the 452 men who died from enemy fire did not include the men who died on the battlefield. The 452 deaths include only those who made it into the hospital and died there. In November the situation became

The Daughters of Charity of St. Vincent de Paul

Table 7.1 Outcomes for patients admitted to French medical department hospitals, October 1854 (46,000 effectives)

	Admitted to hospital	Died in hospital
Wounded by [enemy] fire	370	45
Cholera	820	289
Wounded by accident,[a] itch, venereal disease, fevers	2,618	118
Total	**3,808**	**452**
625 cured		
1,934 evacuated to Constantinople		
787 remaining in hospital[b]		

Source: Scrive, *Relation*, p. 127.

[a] 'Wounded by accident' referred to the many accidents which occurred in handling munitions, digging trenches, etc. as opposed to those struck by enemy fire.

[b] I have added this line, 'remaining in hospital,' to Scrive's tables. It consists of the total admitted to hospital minus those who died, were evacuated to Constantinople, or were discharged as cured.

less favorable as harsh weather set in and became much worse as the winter progressed. The commissariat was not providing enough vegetables, and in January frostbite became a major problem. There were not enough ships to transfer the men to Constantinople expeditiously so the hospitals quickly became overcrowded and typhus appeared, which was attributed to the resulting foul air.[45]

The war was going badly for the allies in January. The British were making no headway against the Malakhov on the allies' eastern flank and the Russian defenses at the Flag Staff and Central Bastions were successfully repulsing every French attack on the western flank. Bitterly disappointed by the costly fighting and the inability of the allied commanders to agree with each other, Napoleon III sent his chief engineer, General Adolphe Niel, to the Crimea to develop a new strategy. Niel concluded that it was impossible to break the defenses at the Central and Flagstaff batteries and ordered the army to make the Malakhov, which he identified as the key to Sevastopol, their primary focus.[46] The French therefore took over the eastern flank and British troops were moved to the central part of the line. When the Russians saw the change in the allies' strategy they responded vigorously. Totleben began extending the Malakhov's defenses. In early March

Religious nursing

he built two redoubts armed with cannon on the eastern flank close to the Tchernaya River. Because the soil there was whitish the allies called them the 'White Works.' Later in March he designed a lunette which the French called the *Mamelon Vert*. These fortifications enfiladed the French trenches and batteries and halted their advance to the Malakhov.[47] The Russians also mounted more fierce and successful sorties, causing many more French deaths and wounded and a great deal more work for the French doctors and nurses. On the night of 23 February there was a tremendous fight in the trenches, with terrible losses. Ninety-four Zouaves were killed, and 200 officers and soldiers wounded, many very seriously. The soldiers were now so weakened and pale from living on campaign rations that Scrive feared hospital gangrene might set in. The Russians suffered major losses on the nights of March 14, 15, and 17 when they launched ferocious attacks on the French trenches. Then on the night of 22 March they launched their largest and most effective sortie ever.[48] It was a terrible and bloody fight forcing the Russians, who always carried all their wounded and dead back into the city, to leave many behind.

March briefly brought better weather and Scrive thought the sanitary situation more satisfactory because he was able to see that the camp was cleaned up. The earth on which the tents were pitched was believed to have become infected so every tent was moved to new ground, all filth and garbage was brought to one place, distant from the camp, and burnt, the latrines were renewed frequently, and dead animals were buried as deeply as possible. If the ground was too rocky to bury the horses, they covered them with lime. Scrive ordered fresh meat and conserved vegetables and instructed every soldier to pick dandelions to put in his salad. During the brief stretch of warmer weather in March he moved many of the sick into tents to get them out of the poisoned air of the barrack hospitals, but the cold and snow soon returned and he had to bring them back into the barracks.[49] Out of 96,258 effectives, in March 1,484 died in hospital from enemy fire and 5,243 suffered from accidents and disease as compared to 370 and 2,618 in October.[50]

Throughout the spring the French continued very actively pushing their siege works forward but they had to capture the White Works and the Mamelon before they could launch an assault on their ultimate goal, the Malakhov. The capture of these three fortifications was

The Daughters of Charity of St. Vincent de Paul

a horrific battle with a tremendous number of losses but Scrive had prepared carefully for the fight. He expanded the nursing service with non-combatant soldiers and musicians, allocating eight to twelve of these basically untrained men to collect the wounded and transport them to the field hospitals. There one of the doctors inspected the wounds and decided whether they needed immediate attention or could be sent on to the divisional hospital. He assigned two nurses to each doctor to do dressings, and four, preferably the trained and experienced nurses, to each operating table. He was very proud of the performance of his doctors and nurses who worked under fire and some of whom were wounded. The signal for the attack was given at 6 a.m. on 7 June and by 2 p.m. the trench hospitals had cared for over 2,000 wounded and sent them on to the divisional hospitals.[51]

In May, with the arrival of the Sardinians to support the British, and the White Works and Mamelon in French hands, the allies were ready to launch what they hoped would be the final assault on Sevastopol. Raglan chose 18 June as the date because it was on that day that Waterloo was fought. The Russians put up a fierce resistance and repulsed the attack successfully, inflicting hideous wounds on the French. In the middle of these terrible events, as well as dysentery, intermittent and remittent fevers, cholera struck again. A total of 21,449 men were admitted to hospital during the month of June.

Table 7.2 Outcomes for patients admitted to French medical department hospitals, June 1855 (121,887 effectives)

	Admitted to hospital	Died in hospital
Wounded by [enemy] fire	6,062	433
Cholera	4,756	777
Scurvy	630	4
Typhus	0	4
Wounded by accident, itch, venereal disease, fevers	10,001	2,588
Total	**21,449**	**3,806**
2,929 cured		
10,453 evacuated to Constantinople		
4,261 remaining in hospital in Crimea		

Source: Scrive, *Relation*, p. 211

Religious nursing

Although there were more wounded in the final assault on Sevastopol in September – 8,665 wounded as opposed to 6,062 in June – only a total of 14,548 men were admitted to hospital in September as compared to the 21,449 in June. The hospitals were jam packed, with 4,261 remaining in hospital at the end of the month as compared to 787 in October. One can see why there was simply not enough suitable accommodation or doctors and nurses to deal with this huge influx.

The Piedmont-Sardinian Daughters of Charity

The arrival of the first of the Piedmont-Sardinian contingent of 18,000 men[52] under the command of General Alfonso de la Marmora[53] on 5 May 1855 gave the British army a major boost. Piedmont-Sardinia was a small country which no longer exists. It consisted of Nice and Savoy in southeastern France, which it would cede to the French a few years later, northwestern Italy, and the island of Sardinia. Contemporaries referred to it as Piedmont-Savoy as well as Piedmont-Sardinia and often called it simply Piedmont or the Savoy or Sardinia for short. Although Italy did not yet exist as a nation, contemporaries also referred to its citizens as Italians because those living on the Italian peninsula all spoke Italian of one kind or another. When the Aberdeen government began searching for mercenaries Lord Palmerston, then Home Secretary, asked Lord John Russell, the Foreign Secretary and later Minister without Portfolio, 'Might we not get six thousand men from Portugal, ten thousand from Spain, and ten thousand from Piedmont?' Enquiries were made and the Piedmontese government responded positively, promising as many as 15,000 men but with strings attached. It is a tribute to the skillful realpolitik of Count Camillo Cavour, the Piedmontese Prime Minister, that rather than providing mercenaries, in January 1855 he managed to negotiate a treaty to enter the war against Russia as an ally of Britain and France. Cavour's aim in making this arrangement was to bring the question of Italian unification into mainstream European diplomacy.[54] Within the next fifteen years Piedmont-Sardinia would lead the unification of Italy. Napoleon III wanted to use the Sardinian troops as a part of his army, but Lord Panmure insisted that because the British had raised the soldiers and were paying them, the British would command them. The Emperor is very anxious to direct the

Sardinian army, Panmure wrote to Raglan, and we must be very firm that we alone are to direct them. At the end of April the *Croesus*, the ship bringing stores for the Sardinians, sank. 'I hope you will send stringent instructions to Raglan and Filder [the chief purveyor], that they must feed the Sardinians,' Lord Clarendon, the Foreign Secretary, wrote to Panmure. 'Otherwise we will have to give them ships for fetching their provisions. Indian corn, beans and vegetables will probably be required. They have a horror of our salt provisions.'[55]

The Daughters of Charity had been working in Piedmont-Sardinia since 1833 when, at the suggestion of the Minister of War, Giacomo Durando, and his brother, Marcantonio Durando, the local Superior of the Vincentians, King Carlo Alberto invited the Sisters to take over the monastery of St. Salvario in Turin. The Piedmontese army was closely modeled on the French and adopted nearly all the French regulations for its medical service, including contracts with the Daughters of Charity to direct their military nursing, a good example of the transnationalism of both the Piedmontese army and the Sisters of Charity. The Sisters immediately took over the military hospitals in Genoa and Turin as well as a number of civilian hospitals.[56] In 1855 they established two base hospitals in Turkey and seven hospitals, including a base hospital of 400 beds and a field hospital of forty, in Balaclava. The French Daughters did have a hospital in Bulgaria which they called a field hospital, probably because it was under canvas, but it was fifty or sixty miles from the Danube front. Otherwise the French Daughters and the British nurses worked only in base hospitals, but the Piedmontese Daughters were more daring and had a real field hospital. Like the French medical department, the doctors reported to their commissariat but, unlike the French, some of their soldier nurses were officers. The nursing corps originally consisted of 451 male soldier nurses of whom nineteen were officers, with twenty-eight Sisters of Charity to supervise and coordinate them.[57]

The campaign got off to a bad start when cholera struck the army a few days after it landed in Balaclava. 'Cholera is making sad havoc in the Sardinian camp,' Raglan wrote to Panmure in June.[58] On the three-week voyage on British ships from Genoa to the Crimea the soldiers were fed the standard British rations of salt meat, hard biscuit, dried peas, and rum. When they reached Balaclava the British had made no preparations for them so they had to spend almost another

Religious nursing

three weeks on the same rations before their own supplies arrived. British rations were a major change from the normal Sardinian army diet with its freshly baked bread, daily doses of lemon juice, and meat twice a week. The first Sardinian camp was overcrowded, housed in inadequate tents, and constructed on the cemetery where British and French soldiers were buried so the ground was believed to be infected. Chief Dr Antonio Commissetti did indeed have a horror of the British salt rations: he attributed the high mortality and morbidity rates in his army to scurvy resulting from the British salt provisions as well as the poor location of the camp. In addition to all the illness, there were problems in the nursing department with the distribution of food and with theft. In the first month in Balaclava seventy-four nurses were sent home to Piedmont sick, while fifty-five more died later, and two officers and two soldiers were removed after being court-martialed. As a result there were not enough soldier nurses so, like the French, the Sardinians were forced to use soldiers who were unfit for combat and convalescents.

The Minister of War kept requesting more Sisters, so four more parties of Sisters went to the East, making a total of sixty-four Piedmont-Sardinian Daughters who served in the war. Twenty of the Sisters died, fifteen in the Crimea and five on board ship. The Sisters ranged in age from 23 to 46 and were carefully selected for their physical fitness, dedication, obedience, courage, and discretion. All had to have had training in military hospitals, and all had to be able to read and write in both Italian and French.[59] They were well trained. As novices, training lasted from seven to twelve months and included learning the catechism, the rules of the sisterhood, and handicrafts such as shoemaking and needlework as well as nursing, which was taught entirely on the wards. St. Vincent had opened the sisterhood to all social classes, and an hour of reading and writing classes each day was needed for some of the Sisters. The Sisters were not allowed to speak their native Italian dialects because they differed so radically that a southern Italian dialect could be incomprehensible to a northern Italian. 'We have to speak French because we have to make everyone understand each other,' the Sisters explained. As with most Catholic sisterhoods, etiquette was strongly emphasized. Treating the other Sisters politely and good table manners were seen as ways of expressing 'exquisite charity.' Finally, the Daughters were always

The Daughters of Charity of St. Vincent de Paul

sent to Paris at the end of their novitiate for further training and also to give them a wider awareness of the mission of their worldwide community.[60]

The Piedmontese Daughters were directed by an outstanding and gifted superintendent, the Countess Cordero de Vonzo Éléonora Maria Giulia. Noted for her spirituality and warm and generous nature, she spent two years, from 1847 to 1849, in the Daughters' convent in Constantinople so she was somewhat familiar with the East. Aged 39 when she volunteered to go to the Crimea in 1855, she was then Bursar for the whole province.[61] In Balaclava she became a close friend of Florence Nightingale, who considered her 'one of the most remarkable women it has ever been my good fortune to know.' She spoke of her 'with the warmest affection and respect … a woman of high rank, of the most captivating manners, but of the utmost simplicity of character, and of unfailing devotion to right and to God.'[62] Nightingale was very impressed by the Piedmontese hospitals when she visited them and it was probably she who recommended to Queen Victoria giving medals to the Sisters. In June 1856 the Queen awarded medals to eight Sardinian Daughters.[63] Like Nightingale, the Italian Sisters were strictly ordered never to become involved in anything political. As in France the war was not popular; Cavour had had a difficult time convincing his government and the public to take part in a war which offered no immediate reward. The terrible sufferings of the British and French soldiers and the inadequacies of their medical departments had been well publicized in Piedmont and Father Étienne, the General Superior of the Confraternity,[64] was very worried that the Sisters might write home about the difficult conditions or the political situation in the Crimea, making the war even more unpopular at home as well as being helpful to Cavour's opponents in the government. He therefore ordered the Sisters never to talk, even to each other, about politics, and they were never to write home about them. So concerned was he about this that he arranged to have their letters censored at the central house before being sent on to the addressee.[65]

After working with French, Italian, and English Sisters of Mercy, Dr Pincoffs rated them nurses *par excellence*. It would appear he conflated the Daughters of Charity with the Sisters of Mercy for there were no French or Italian Sisters of Mercy and there were no English

165

Daughters of Charity. In Scutari Pincoffs worked with Moore and Gonzaga, and he worked with Daughters in the French hospitals, so more accurately, he rated Roman Catholic Sisters as top-notch nurses. He considered them 'thoroughly conversant with the practical part of their business,' and characterized by their cheerfulness and strict obedience to doctors' orders. Pincoffs himself had not worked with Protestant Sisters but he heard that they were less enthusiastic and obedient than Catholic Sisters.[66] One must keep in mind that at this time one of the greatest problems with secular hospital nurses was their failure to implement doctors' orders, so it is understandable that Pincoffs was pleased to find nurses who cooperated with the medical men and implemented rather than ignored their orders for the patients.

Nightingale is the only contemporary who made adverse comments about the Daughters of Charity. As a thoroughly committed sanitarian she was dedicated to preventing disease and was disappointed in what she considered the Daughters' lack of interest in preventative health care. In all the camps there were canteens where liquor was freely available and where the men often got very drunk. Every night both Nightingale and Cordero saw patients in their hospital gowns and slippers sneaking out of the hospital huts, slipping past the conniving sentries, and making their way to the canteen to buy liquor. Nightingale tried to convince the countess to join her in complaining about the canteen to their respective chiefs of staff. She thought they would readily support them in stopping this source of drunkenness in the hospitals, but Cordero refused to join Nightingale in the complaint. Nightingale was frustrated because she was completely unable to convince her to take any proactive measure against drunkenness or, for that matter, against any other problem. The Sisters, Nightingale said, not completely fairly, believed they should 'console the suffering which evils produced – They are not to remove the causes of those evils.'[67] It is more likely that the Sardinian Sisters were trying to obey their enjoinder to be strictly obedient and not to stir up trouble.

Nightingale identified another weakness in the Daughters' system: she thought it was unclear whether the Sisters or the chief nurses (non-commissioned officers) were ultimately responsible for the nursing care, although she thought the Sardinian Sisters had more control of their military nurses than did the French. While she considered their housekeeping and cooking superb, she believed that the rule forbidding physical care of men meant the Sisters gave only 'the finishing touch' to the nursing and made them largely consolers as opposed to real nurses. The Daughters' failure to give corporeal care, Nightingale said, also caused an epidemic of 'bed-sores and such like.' French officers and men complained to her about bedsores while both French and Sardinian Sisters came to her to learn how to treat them as well as to borrow air pillows and water beds.[68] On the other hand, Slade commented on the French soldier nurses' skill with pad and pillow, which suggests that they were careful to reposition their patients. However, by the end of June 1855 there were not very many trained soldier nurses left in the hospitals and it may be that the untrained men paid little attention to preventing bedsores, or with the understaffing, they simply did not have the time to reposition the patients.

Notes

1 St. Vincent de Paul, *Conferences*, vol. 4, pp. 274, 287.

2 Jones, *Charitable Imperative*, pp. 15, 89.

3 Hickey, *Local Hospitals*, pp. 140–1; Jones, *Charitable Imperative*, p. 15; Nelson, *Say Little*, pp. 17–23.

4 St. Vincent de Paul, *Conferences*, vol. 3, p. 173, vol. 4, p. 165; Jameson, *Sisters of Charity*, pp. 59–60.

5 Rappaport, *No Place for Ladies*, pp. 94–6, 172–3.

6 St. Vincent de Paul, *Conferences*, vol. 1, p. 58.

7 Herbé, *Français & Russes*, pp. 341–3.

8 The word *lard* in French means bacon, fat, or lard. It may have been lard that the men were eating raw.

9 Herbé, *Français & Russes*, p. 342.

10 Nightingale, 'Introduction of Female Nursing,' p. 7.

11 Herbé, *Français & Russes*, pp. 342–3.

12 Montaudon, *Souvenirs*, pp. 361–2.

13 Masquelez, *Journal*, pp. 129, 135–7, 140–3.

14 Clifford, *Letters*, p. 168–9.

15 Slade, *Turkey*, pp. 371–3.

16 Taylor, *Journal*, vol. 1, pp. 77, 301.

17 Cler, *Reminiscences*, pp. 112–13.

18 Rappaport, *No Place for Ladies*, pp. 14, 56–8; Cler, *Reminiscences*, pp. 112–13, 197–8; Blackwood, *Residence on the Bosphorus*, pp. 262–3.

Religious nursing

19 Totleben, *Défense*, vol. 1, Part I, pp. 39–40.
20 Cler, *Reminiscences*, pp. 199–201; Montaudon, *Souvenirs*, pp. 216–17.
21 Figes, *Crimean War*, p. 179.
22 Clifford, *Letters*, pp. 132, 185.
23 Slade, *Turkey*, pp. 369–71.
24 Guthrie, *Surgery of the War*, pp. 411, 413–18.
25 Macleod, *Surgery in the Crimea*, p. 237.
26 Helmstadter and Godden, *Before Nightingale*, pp. 6–8.
27 Scrive, *Relation*, pp. 120–1, 123.
28 Slade, *Turkey*, pp. 369–71.
29 Helmstadter and Godden, *Before Nightingale*, pp. 6–8.
30 Longmore, *Ambulance Transport*, pp. 20–8; Rochard, *Chirugerie Française*, pp. 81–3, 870.
31 Pincoffs, *Experiences of a Civilian*, pp. 178–9.
32 Chenu, *Rapport*, pp. 707, 710–11.
33 Dodd, *Pictorial History*, pp. 295–6.
34 Scrive, *Relation*, p. 479.
35 Chenu, *Rapport*, pp. 709–11, 713–15.
36 Meynen, 'Hôpitaux militaires,' pp. 92–109; Scrive, *Relation*, p. 312.
37 BL 43393, Nightingale to Herbert, 28 January 1855, fols 117–18.
38 Longmore, *Sanitary Contrasts*, p. 27.
39 Macleod, *Surgery in the Crimea*, fn, pp. 48–9.
40 Rochard, *Chirugerie Française*, pp. 28–32, 81–2; Chenu, *Rapport*, pp. 696–7.
41 Chenu, *Rapport*, pp. 688–9, 692, 715–16.
42 Rochard, *Chirugerie Française*, p. 871.
43 Chenu, *Rapport*, pp. 688–9, 692.
44 Scrive, *Relation*, p. 126.
45 Ibid, pp. 136–7.
46 Curtiss, *Crimean War*, pp. 372–3.
47 Curtiss, *Russian Army*, pp. 344–5.
48 Pirogov, 'Historical Survey,' p. 34.
49 Scrive, *Relation*, pp. 144–8, 183–5.
50 Ibid, p. 148.
51 Ibid, pp. 204, 205–7, 241–3.
52 The first contingent of Piedmontese is usually reported as 15,000 men, but in fact it was 18,000. See LaTorre and Lusignani, 'Sardinian-Piedmontese Army,' p. 239.
53 The general's name was actually della Marmora but the British always referred to him as de la or de le Marmora.
54 Baumgart, *Crimean War*, vol. 1, pp. 32, 88–90.
55 Panmure, *Panmure Papers*, vol. 1, pp. 105, 142–3, 173.
56 Baudens, *Guerre de Crimée*, pp. 106–7; LaTorre and Lusignani, 'Sardinian-Piedmontese Army,' pp. 237–42.

The Daughters of Charity of St. Vincent de Paul

57 LaTorre and Lusignani, 'Sardinian-Piedmontese Army,' pp. 239–41.
58 Panmure, *Panmure Papers*, vol. 1, p. 234.
59 LaTorre and Lusignani, 'Sardinian-Piedmontese Army,' pp. 239–41; Colli, 'L'Organisation Sanitaire,' pp. 624–5, 627–8.
60 San Salvario Convent, Rules of the Sisters of Charity, 1842.
61 Ibid, 'Ma Soeur Éléonore Cordero,' pp. 165–6; Minutes of Council, 22 February 1855.
62 WI Ms 8997, Nightingale to Lady Canning, 23 November 1856, Letter 11; Nightingale, 'Introduction of Female Nursing,' p. 21.
63 Ministry of War, Turin, Hospitals Section, 17 December 1855 and 16 June 1856, Nos. 9628 and 3295.
64 Because the Daughters reported ultimately to the Vincentian Fathers, the two orders together were called a confraternity.
65 San Salvario Convent; Colli, 'L'Organisation Sanitaire,' pp. 621–2; Minutes of Council, 22 February 1855.
66 Pincoffs, *Experiences of a Civilian*, pp. 80–1.
67 WI Ms 8997, Nightingale to Lady Canning, 23 November 1856, Letter 11.
68 Nightingale, 'Introduction of Female Nursing,' p. 21.

8

The financial costs of war

The summer campaign and sickness among the doctors

Following the unsuccessful assault on 18 June, sickness wreaked havoc among the doctors. One to three doctors was sick in each field hospital and the medical department deteriorated rapidly. Scrive asked the Intendant-General to send doctors from the Constantinople hospitals and he did send a few, but because they had to work in burning heat and often under fire, Scrive feared that soon half would be ill and he would no longer be able to provide an acceptable medical service. The army had been on field rations for such a long time, and there was so much scurvy, that the soldiers were very susceptible to disease. In the spring they had dandelions, but even dandelions could not grow in the hot, dry Crimean summer. Scrive asked incessantly for preserved vegetables but got none.[1] Scurvy was especially disastrous because it chiefly attacked the valuable veteran soldiers since they had been on field rations the lengthiest time.

Despite the severe setback, on 18 June the French pressed on, moving the trenches forward toward the walls of Sevastopol. It was slow and back-breaking work: they had to burrow foot by foot in stony or rocky ground, which often required mining; they used their pickaxes more than their muskets and rifles. In the daytime an unseen enemy kept them under constant fire, and at night there were sudden, unexpected, vicious Russian sorties.[2] At the end of July the French trenches were 80 meters away from the Malakhov so that the Russian musket fire became far more effective. We have as many guns in action now as the Russians, staff officer Captain Henri Loizillon reported, but their fire gets sharper and sharper as we draw closer to their walls – bombs, shells, grenades, grapeshot – and we

170

The financial costs of war

are now close enough so that their muskets have enough force to kill a man. Seventy to a hundred men were wounded every day and the doctors were doing five to six urgent amputations daily in the field hospitals. In the daytime about one in seven men was killed and two seriously and four lightly wounded. About half the fever patients had scurvy and Scrive kept begging the commissariat in vain for preserved vegetables. The sanitary state of all the army camps was unsatisfactory and the doctors continued to suffer from overwork and the terrible heat as well as from disease. Scrive had to evacuate sixteen surgeons to Constantinople.[3]

In August came the Battle of the Tchernaya in which Herbé was wounded. His experiences in the field and divisional hospitals provide a good illustration of the deterioration in medical care. Herbé had visited several of his men in the field hospital the previous fall and noted that they were being very reasonably cared for. The hospital consisted of well-pitched large tents and the patients lay on straw mattresses which kept them completely off the ground. The wounded were separated from the sick and there was no cholera or typhus fever and very few bronchial conditions. When the bad weather set in in November and it became difficult to bring provisions up to the camp from the harbor the army often had to make do with biscuit and lard, but the medical department managed to feed their patients somewhat better. By contrast, when Herbé visited the field hospitals the day before the Waterloo Day attack he found the hospitals inadequate for ordinary siege times and definitely insufficient for the press which the upcoming battle would cause. There were only three doctors to look after 300 wounded and as many sick – in other words, one doctor for 200 men. The doctors were utterly exhausted and were using their nurses for both dressings and surgical operations. They could only look after those wounded who seemed to have some chance of getting better. Certainly, Herbé thought, many were dying who would have lived if the staff could have been tripled.[4]

At the Tchernaya Herbé was first hit in the calf by shrapnel. His leg felt numb but he was able to carry on. However a few minutes later, just as his colonel was coming to give him the order to retreat because the Russians had broken the French line, a ball struck him in the hip, knocking him off his horse. Four of his men were carrying him back to the dressing station, using two rifles under his arms and two under

Religious nursing

his hips as a stretcher, when he was struck by another ball. He thought he was dying so he told the men to put him down and go back to the front to fight. However a little later, as the Russians made further inroads into the French lines, one of his men came back, threw him over his shoulder and carried him off the field. The chief doctor of his regiment staunched his wounds in the trench hospital and after leaving him lying for several hours under a very hot sun, sent him on to the field hospital. There the doctors were horribly overworked – three doctors for 500 wounded patients – and Herbé had to wait nine hours before they could find him a place – and 'What a place!' he exclaimed. The very narrow bed in which he was put already held another officer who was delirious, and thinking Herbé the enemy, punched and kicked him in an effort to kill him. The nurse rescued Herbé by knocking the man to the floor and the poor man died a few minutes later.

Several hours after he arrived at the field hospital, the French muleteers transferred about 200 wounded men including Herbé into cacolets and took them to the divisional hospital. But in the divisional hospital there were so few doctors with so many patients that they also had to ignore those they considered hopeless cases. Assuming Herbé could not survive, they passed his bed without stopping every morning. Herbé, as an officer, did much better of course than the private soldiers because he had his batman who could bring him food and water, help him turn and so on. After five days, when the doctor came in Herbé attracted his attention by making some jokes which made the doctor smile so he went over to his bed and examined his wounds. They badly needed cleansing so the doctor, whose name was Félix, asked the nurse to wash and dress them. Herbé considered Dr Félix an admirable doctor. With only two other surgeons to look after more than 500 wounded, he was sleeping only four hours out of the twenty-four, eating while he was dressing wounds, and, in order not to lose any time, put his bread and piece of meat down on the bed of the man he was dressing. A large number of men had just been evacuated to Constantinople and the doctors were planning to send more, after which Herbé hoped Félix would have more time to give to the remaining patients.

Herbé's wounds healed quickly, in fact Dr Félix said too quickly, for there was one small area which was still suppurating and refusing

The financial costs of war

to close. Félix opened the wound and found a piece of Herbé's little leather purse. As soon as it was removed the wound healed properly. A few days later, when Félix was away, one of his junior doctors came to dress Herbé's wounds. Feverish and in a very bad mood, Herbé took an instant dislike to this doctor with his great blood-stained apron and quite rudely refused to let him do the dressing. The doctor was kind enough to ask a nurse to dress the wound. The next day Dr Félix returned and told Herbé he should not regret having been rude to that doctor; gangrene had developed in every wound he had dressed, and for Herbé's safety Félix was going to move him into a tent by himself, and would send him to Constantinople as soon as possible. When Herbé left the Crimea on 13 October he had spent almost two months in the divisional hospital, which he considered a short time for such a serious wound to heal.[5]

As with the British, one of the biggest problems the French doctors faced was an inadequate number of hospital ships. The navy therefore hired commercial ships, which were obviously not designed to handle sick and wounded men. John Codman, the captain of an American steamer that the French had chartered, took horses and cattle up to the Crimea and on the return voyage brought wounded and sick men back to the base hospitals. They bedded the men with straw, just as they did the animals. There were no nurses on board and if there was a doctor, he had absolutely no linen or dressing supplies. If there was a doctor's assistant he was often helpless due to sea-sickness. The patients were turned out from the camp hospitals and brought down to the beach by 8 or 9 a.m.; hundreds of patients lay in the hot sun for hours while the tenders were got ready to take them out to the ships. Some were in the critical stages of fever or cholera and many died on the beach, or on the tenders, as they were being carried up the ladders on the ship's side, or on the voyage to Constantinople. Codman thought many might have survived if they had remained in the camp hospitals, but the camp hospitals were so overcrowded that in order to make room for new admissions Scrive had no choice but to ship men out who were not ready to be moved.[6] Herbé's sea voyage lasted only a day and a half but he left the hospital on 13 October, the ship did not sail till the next day, and the men remained on board overnight after arrival in Constantinople, so he was on shipboard for four days. There were two or three nurses, one administrative sergeant,

173

and no doctor for 133 sick or wounded men and officers, so the men's wounds were not washed or dressed for those four days.[7] As did the British soldiers, the men arrived in a pitiable state, terribly weakened and covered with vermin, their clothes containing evacuations from the beginning of their voyage. Combined with the smell of gangrene, it was so horrible that the patients had to be washed and provisional dressings done before they were allowed inside the hospital.[8]

The Russian assault on the French and Sardinians at the Tchernaya was a surprise attack so Scrive had little time to prepare his teams. Yet despite their understaffing and Russian projectiles falling amidst them, the doctors and nurses worked cool-headedly throughout the battle. Eight hundred French wounded, as well as 1,750 Russian prisoners of war, were rapidly given first aid or an urgent operation and transported to the divisional hospitals. In less than three hours the doctors and nurses had emptied the trench hospitals of the wounded and were ready to receive new casualties if the Russians launched a new attack. The medical service, however, would not have been able to continue if the admiralty had not sent twelve doctors who stayed for two weeks, working day and night caring for the Russian soldiers. The field hospitals were so short-staffed that Scrive had to send divisional hospital doctors to work in them in the morning. Then when they returned to their own hospitals, they had to perform their own urgent operations, which they often could not finish until the middle of the night. When the naval doctors left, Scrive desperately pleaded with the intendancy for forty more doctors. He had only eighty, which was simply not sufficient for sixteen hospitals when the army was fighting. He was especially short of senior doctors because the replacements he received were junior men. He also complained that the surgical instruments the government supplied were of mediocre quality. At the same time disease soared in August.[9]

The fall of Sevastopol and the typhus epidemic

In the midst of all these demanding activities Scrive had to prepare for what was to be the final and successful attack on 8 September. He provisioned the three field hospitals, and assigned a flying ambulance and a senior doctor who, aided by two junior doctors and three nurses, was to dress the wounded. The first nurse was responsible for the dressings and surgical equipment, the second helped the doctor, and the third wrote down the necessary information about the patient – his name, regiment, nature of his wounds etc. The soldiers were then transported immediately to the divisional hospital on litters or in cacolets. Soldiers who needed immediate surgery were taken to a barrack where Scrive had another team of doctors at work. The final assault resulted in colossal casualties, which the medical teams treated efficiently with generous help from the Sardinian doctors.[10] On visiting the French hospitals in 1856, Nightingale was impressed by the accuracy and completeness of their medical statistics. How, she wondered, with so few doctors could they find the time to keep notebooks recording the complete history of each case, the diet, medical treatment, and daily medical observations of every patient?[11] The duties of the third nurse explain how: there was one nurse who did nothing but keep records.

The medical department performed well on 8 September, but Scrive's fears that he would soon be unable to provide an acceptable medical service were realized the following winter. In his view the French soldiers had suffered no more than the ordinary amount of disease for an army on campaign in the first winter, but their incredible rates of sickness and mortality in the winter and spring of 1855–56 were worse than those of the British in the preceding winter. The department had been on a downhill path since the disastrous assault on 18 June when Scrive reported that one out of every three of his doctors was ill and the soldiers were suffering dreadfully from untreated scurvy.[12] In November 1855 Nightingale and a number of British doctors visited the French headquarters and their chief divisional hospital. Nightingale was shocked by the state of the hospital. The French openly admitted that they had lost proportionately more men from dysentery than the British, and said they had not saved even one sixth of their amputations, while Nightingale believed a quarter of the British amputations had survived.

Among the French doctors with whom Nightingale spoke was Baudens, one of the intendants in Paris. He made two trips to the East, one in October and November 1855, and again in March 1856. He strongly supported Scrive's requests for more hospital beds and other resources, and he impressed Nightingale immensely. 'His behaviour to & moral influence over his Patients was not to be

Religious nursing

Table 8.1 Outcomes for patients admitted to French medical department hospitals, November 1855 (143,250 effectives)

	Admitted to hospital	Died in hospital
Wounded by [enemy] fire	287	53
Cholera	177	126
Scurvy	717	25
Typhus	10	6
Wounded by accident, itch, venereal disease, fevers	7,417	544
Total	**8,608**	**754**
4,033 cured		
3,250 evacuated to Constantinople		
4,816 remaining in hospital in Crimea		

Source: Scrive, *Relation*, p. 240

mentioned in the same day with anything we are able to exercise,' she wrote.[13] Today, 'moral' is almost always used to mean having to do with ethics or right and wrong, but it also means pertaining to character or conduct, as distinguished from a person's intellectual or physical nature. We still speak of 'moral support' as opposed to physical or material support. In nineteenth-century medical parlance 'moral' was frequently used in this sense to distinguish physical treatments such as medication, diet, or surgery, from a general approach to the patient. Hence Samuel Tuke's famous 'moral treatment' at the York Retreat consisted of a humane and affectionate concern with individual patients' needs, not the kind of character raising which Nightingale and Morton attempted.[14] The French soldiers shared Nightingale's view of their doctors. Despite the excruciating pain they inflicted, Masquelez admired the devotion and skill of his surgeons,[15] while Herbé considered Félix an admirable doctor. Non-patients also noted the kind and cheerful way the French doctors treated their patients. For example, an English visitor to a French hospital in 1854 was impressed by the compassionate, pleasant way the doctors approached their patients; the patients' faces lit up when they spoke to them, addressing them as 'mon garçon' or 'mon brave.'[16] Fanny Taylor visited the French hospital in Pera on her way home from Koulali in November 1855. She thought the hospital was less clean

176

and had fewer comforts than those at Koulali, but found the medical officers 'a very superior class of men.' She was surprised when one of the doctors spoke very courteously to a Sister who was not a lady either by birth or education, which would never have happened in a British hospital. She concluded that the French system worked better than the British.[17]

Scrive described what Nightingale called moral influence as the excellent relationship between the doctors and their patients. All our doctors agreed, he wrote, that in the overall treatment of our patients the most important factors were rest for the body and the spirit, pure air, suitable drinks, and diet. Our soldiers' morale was never in jeopardy: we addressed them with kind, consoling words, and the men, Scrive wrote, 'trusted and loved their doctors who gave them affectionate and devoted care.' But by November 1855 the other conditions Scrive listed – rest for body and spirit, pure air, suitable drinks and diet – were no longer available. The men's bedding consisted of straw mats or only blankets, and men were put on shipboard with open wounds. The problem, Scrive thought, was that a few of the medical department's chiefs did not accept the recommendations of the doctors in the field; he thought they were more interested in habits of command than in the successful treatment of severe wounds.[18] This was a structural problem, not simply one which arose when supplies were so severely limited.

The French public had never been enthusiastic about the war, tending to think they had been dragged into a conflict which did not serve French interests but rather supported the imperial ambitions of their traditional enemy. Furthermore, by November 1855 the political position of Napoleon III was shaky.[19] As more and more men were killed, the war became increasingly unpopular in France. The soldiers were so demoralized by the lack of supplies that by January 1856 there were rumors of possible uprisings in the field army as well as at home. The government could afford to generously supply and equip its original army of 30,000 who landed in the Crimea in September 1854, but as the Russians put up such tough and skillful resistance Napoleon had to keep sending more soldiers. In October 1854 there were 46,000 effectives, in March 1855 96,258, and in June 121,887, four times the size of the original army. The number of soldiers peaked in November 1855, after the fall of Sevastopol, when there were 145,120 men.[20] The

French economy, which had seemed to be booming in 1854, was suffering badly from the war effort. Trade diminished and, with 310,000 men drafted into the army, the agrarian workforce was hard hit, resulting in food shortages in the cities. By contrast, the flourishing British economy was able and prepared to pay for expensive sanitary and medical improvements as well as all the other costs of the war. In 1853 the British government spent £15.3 million on its army and navy, or 27.7 percent of the central government's budget including debt interest. In 1856 the cost of the armed forces was 50.2 percent of the budget or £46.7 million. The French Treasury did not have such resources, and as it cut back on army funding the situation of a horrifically under-supplied British army and a well-supplied French army in the fall of 1854 was reversed. Furthermore, the French were running out of experienced veterans. As in the British army, a large proportion of replacements now were young recruits who had no idea of life in the field; they were all very green, some undisciplined, and some very homesick. The Emperor, who had come to power by less than legitimate methods, was very sensitive to public opinion and began to fear his position could become untenable. At the beginning of November he brought some of his best troops, the Imperial Guard, back to France. A little later, he ordered more regiments home and sent some back to Algeria. The Emperor has recalled 20,000 of his best soldiers, Goodlake noted on 10 January 1856.[21] Napoleon III became thoroughly committed to ending the war.[22]

The number of sick increased prodigiously in December 1855. In addition to all the hardships of the soldier's life, the second winter was exceptionally bitter, with temperatures from 7° to 24° Celsius below zero. Then typhus appeared. In the Crimea seventy-five doctors, of whom thirty-nine died, contracted the disease. It was almost impossible to evacuate men to Constantinople because the bitter weather prevented the men being left lying on the beaches for several hours while boarding the ships, and storms on the Black Sea prevented ships from sailing.[23] The sanitary state of our camp is poor and the medical staff are dying off at a frightening rate, Loizillon reported in February 1856. Indeed, in each of his ten-day reports at this point Scrive was reporting three to seven doctors dead of typhus. The soldiers were eating all kinds of unconventional food. Loizillon had a little Russian cat who disappeared. Then a very beautiful Russian dog adopted him

The financial costs of war

and he got a second very intelligent and pretty cat, but despite all the precautions he took, they also vanished. He was certain that soldiers had seized and eaten them. We continue to destroy Sevastopol, he wrote, but watching his brave common soldiers build the siege works with their incredible gaiety and insouciance as enemy fire picked them off made him absolutely desperate. The doctors were more and more tried but he thought the field officers in good health. They had neither scurvy nor typhus simply because they were not subjected to the dreadful conditions under which the soldiers and doctors had to live and work.[24]

In the four months from December 1855 through March 1856 the French hospitals were in a horrifying state. As Scrive put it, despite the superhuman efforts of the doctors typhus reigned, transforming every illness, even a minor one, into a typhoid form.[25] That diseases could transform from one to another was a principle of medicine in the days before bacteriology. In 1855 typhus had a very different meaning from that of today. Now it means a louse-borne rickettsial disease which we distinguish from typhoid fever, a completely different illness caused by salmonella. But in 1855, before the advent of laboratory medicine, fevers were a disease not a symptom, and had to be defined by their symptoms rather than their causes. Typhoid fever then meant any fever which caused stupor and debility, confusion, and frequently hallucinations. There were basically two kinds of fever: intermittent and continued. Intermittent or remittent fevers were usually what we now identify as clinical malaria. Most other fevers fell into the category of continued fever. Continued fever was subdivided into inflammatory and nervous or low fever. Inflammatory fever was characterized by a strong pulse, high temperature, and vigorous body reaction; because it was believed it was caused by too much blood, the proper treatment was bleeding. Patients with low or nervous fever had a weak pulse, were prostrated, and had a severely disturbed intellect. Typhus was originally a Greek word meaning smoke or vapor; in medical terminology it came to mean confusion and stupor and was applied to any disease, including apoplexy, which produced these symptoms. Nineteenth-century doctors often used the adjectival form 'typhoid' as well as typhus to describe this condition. Therefore, when earlier nineteenth-century doctors spoke of typhoid fever they could have meant either what we now call typhoid fever or typhus. From the late 1830s on, leading doctors began discriminating between the two diseases, but it would be many years before the specificity of the two was widely accepted.[26] Nightingale demonstrated the belief that even minor illnesses could be transformed into typhus when she stated in 1859 that 'Diseases are not individuals arranged in classes, like cats and dogs, but conditions growing out of one another.' Overcrowding was also believed to be a major cause of disease because it depleted the supply of pure, uncontaminated air. A healthy person exhales about three pints of moisture a day, which nineteenth-century people believed was loaded with organic material ready to putrefy; a sick, feverish person exuded even more lethal material in perspiration, and their hot, humid, heavily infected breath spread disease through the air to the other patients.[27] Hence Scrive's orders to air the tents and bedding and take the patients outside into the fresh air.

'The sufferings of the French are so frightful,' Nightingale wrote in March 1856 after visiting their hospitals,

> They are suffering more than we were last year. They have now 16,000 sick, one in eight, 10,000 down here [in Constantinople]. Typhus alone kills 50–60 per diem in these hospitals alone [*sic*]. The medical men are dying, three in one day. So are the sisters. They themselves tell the same story that we did last year, that want of food and clothing sends down the patients in a typhoid state, which is propagated by the overcrowded state of the hospitals.[28]

So many soldiers were suffering with typhus that the French had to establish three new hospitals in Constantinople – an additional 5,460 beds – making a total of fourteen French hospitals on the Bosphorus.[29] Pincoffs was helping in a French hospital at this time. He thought scurvy was the main cause of the typhus epidemic, and certainly the cause of its enormous mortality. Nine out of ten patients were scorbutic and four out of nine deeply affected with sloughing ulcers, gangrene of the mouth, dropsy, and chronic diarrhoea – all of which, without the proper diet, would ultimately kill them.[30] We were completely overwhelmed by typhus, Scrive reported: despite our incessant efforts to fight it, medical treatment was totally ineffective. He summarized the incessant efforts as airing the barracks three times a day, when possible taking the bedding out into the fresh air where the nurses shook and beat it, sprinkling the infected soil with iron sulfate solution, fumigating and whitewashing, constantly disinfecting the latrines, taking better care of the nurses, and when weather permitted taking the patients out into the fresh air.[31]

Baudens, who was then in Balaclava, approved of Scrive's work and tried to convince his superior, Marshall Vaillant, the Minister of War, that the medical department must have 2,500–3,500 more beds, more medical personnel, and better supplies. He was allowed only 1,000 more beds, and as a result Scrive had to continue evacuating diseased men to France. Many sailors and officers on the ships caught typhus from them and died. Vaillant replied to Baudens that he was sending several Daughters of Charity, 200 nurses, and twenty doctors.[32] Whether they arrived is not recorded. Scrive was most concerned about the humid, muddy earth on which the hospital tents were pitched, but he could not get permission from his superiors to change the location of the tents so as to give the men better air, nor was he able to get more tents so that he could isolate the typhus patients. All he could do was put down lime to absorb the humidity. In April typhus finally began to slowly disappear but Scrive was still unable to convince the authorities to let him change the site of the camp. He commented sadly that doctors could only advise; they could not act on their own authority. However, as the soldiers were sent home and various hospitals were closed, the medical staff recovered and there were enough men to look after the few patients who remained. In May Scrive finally succeeded in getting the hospital tents moved and believed it made a great improvement in the health of the men.[33]

Throughout these terrible four months the medical staff continued to make superhuman efforts, but at great cost to themselves. We always had enough medicines and medical supplies, Scrive wrote, and, given the circumstances, did well by the patients. Medicines and dressing materials probably were the two most important medical supplies during the Napoleonic Wars and commissariats seemed to think this was still the case, when the new supportive therapies required much more expensive proper accommodation, clothing, and better diet. Even so, Scrive still considered his biggest problem in these harrowing times the lack of zeal and aptitude of the nurses who were commandeered from the troops, and who made up the majority of his nurses. The commandeered men more often fell sick, and were the cause of the most complaints. By contrast, the small number

Table 8.2 Outcomes for typhus patients admitted to French medical department and regimental hospitals,[a] December 1855 through March 1856

Month	Effectives	Admitted with typhus	Cured	Evacuated to Constantinople	Died in hospital
December	145,120	12,953	4,844	4,461	1,336
January	144,512	13,418	4,044	6,258	1,763
February	132,793	13,454	1,358	9,781	2,846
March	120,000	8,028	1,883	7,281	2,841
Totals		**47,853**	**12,129**	**27,781**	**8,786**
Remaining in hospital					
1 December 1855 4,695					
1 April 1856 3,964[b]					

Source: Scrive, *Relation*, p. 278

[a] Scrive's preceding tables did not include regimental hospitals and were only for the medical department's hospitals. They also covered all patients, not just typhus patients.

[b] For the numbers remaining in hospital I get 1 January: 7,007, 1 February: 8,360, 1 March: 7,829, and 1 April: 3,852, not 3,964. I cannot explain the discrepancy, but given the conditions he was working under it would not be surprising if Scrive had made a mistake.

of trained soldier nurses were full of energy and devotion to their patients. Scrive was very concerned about their health. He changed their tents and moved them further away from the hospital, increased their wine ration, gave them alcoholized tea or coffee every morning, shortened their night duty hours, and finally took them out of the hospitals when they exhibited the slightest sign of typhus.[34]

There are never enough doctors when a battle is raging or when an epidemic strikes, Baudens explained, and this was also true of the trained soldier nurses. To compensate for this lack in both Constantinople and the Crimea, the medical corps experimented with a new category of nurse that they called *soldats panseurs*, or dressing soldiers. They took non-commissioned officers and also well-educated young convalescents – men with baccalaureates, or some were even lawyers – and private soldier nurses who were intelligent and experienced in minor surgery, and trained them to prepare fracture materials, dress wounds, feed the soldiers, and give out medicines. This is what the Russians do, Scrive explained, and they have been very successful. The dressing soldiers proved crucial in saving the medical service because the department was then able to let go those commandeered soldiers and convalescents who were not reliable. Furthermore, the new duties actually sped up the recovery of the convalescents who acted as dressing soldiers.[35]

During this second winter Scrive visited the British hospitals many times. He agreed that the French hospitals were notoriously inferior but, he said, their inferiority was easily explained by the completely different situation of the two armies. Unlike the British army, the French did not originally have regimental hospitals, but to take the pressure off the field and divisional hospitals, following the fall of Sevastopol Scrive introduced this third kind of hospital. He replaced the tent hospitals with prefabricated huts as quickly as he could, but the French huts were not designed to be hospitals, or intended for the harsh Crimean climate. They were unheated, inadequately ventilated, and none had floors, so the earth on which they were built quickly became muddy and the soil infected. The patients' cots were also badly maintained. As a result, the hospitals became seedbeds of infection and the infection spread to the hospitals in Constantinople. By contrast, the English had huts and tents with wooden floors, heated barracks, real beds with sheets, lots of hot water, excellent latrines, and agreeable distractions such as reading and writing rooms. Furthermore, British surgical instruments were far superior to those the French commissariat supplied.[36] In addition, until the peace was signed at the end of March 1856, the French army was differently deployed. In order to pin down the Russians on the north side of the city and prevent them from rejoining their forces on the Belbek River, the French army was defending a 21-league[37] area from Sevastopol to the Belbek. While the French troops marched and counter-marched, in Scrive's view, the British put war service completely aside. They remained in their old camp, preparing for the winter: maintaining roads, improving their railway, and building barracks. Furthermore, they used Turkish and Greek laborers and also imported civilian workers to do the manual work, so Scrive believed they practically had a second army, almost half as big as the real army.[38] Loizillon thought the English did nothing but take their ease: they built nice barracks, made music, and took exercise all day long.[39]

In March 1856 Nightingale reported that the French were actually starving.[40] The doctors told her that many doctors and Sisters had died and each doctor was now responsible for 200 patients. They needed port wine, arrowroot, beds and blankets, preserved meats, and sugar. Nightingale officially offered to give them some of these supplies, either as a gift or, if they preferred, they could pay for them. The French army had generously given the British a great deal of help in the first winter – a little food, men to work on the roads and carry ammunition up to the camp, and especially the use of their muleteers to convey the wounded down to the port in Balaclava[41] so it seemed appropriate that Nightingale should reciprocate. The medical staff, including Baudens, accepted the offer but their superiors declined because they were afraid the gift might get into the newspapers. The French press was strictly censored and the Ministry of War had recently reminded the doctors that they could not publish any medical details without prior approval. However, the doctors were willing to accept all these items privately so Nightingale borrowed government steamers and sent them as much as she could spare.[42]

At the end of the war Scrive summarized the service of the medical department. The hospital service, he said, was put to severe and painful tests due to lack of resources and overwork. The regimental doctors lived and worked with the regular army officers, who knew

The financial costs of war

and supported them. By contrast, the medical department's field and divisional hospital doctors were isolated and could only make requests to their administrative chief in Paris, who was a stranger and often did not have time to bother with them. The lack of support from our chiefs has had a terrible impact, Scrive declared. Deprived of the most important resources despite urgent requests for them, doctors and patients in the field hospitals lived miserably in leaky tents pitched on a sea of mud. A doctor usually had to oversee at least 100 sick or wounded men each day with no one to help him. He had to write prescriptions himself and often had to stay up late into the night working. He also had to toil in the trenches every third day and work on the beaches when the men were being put on board ship. Nevertheless, the doctors kept working, giving the same generous and efficacious help to the Russian prisoners as to their own soldiers. Eighty-three doctors, including Dr Félix, paid for this service with their lives. The doctors in the base hospitals in Turkey had fewer privations but they treated 116,000 patients and suffered as badly from disease and death as did those in the Crimea; 422 soldier nurses contracted typhus, of whom forty-two died, as did thirty-one Daughters of Charity. Finally, Scrive concluded, the whole medical corps deserved more respect and recognition. It suffered all the same privations, miseries, pains, and dangers as the army officers. Some were killed by gunfire but most died of disease, which they suffered at a much higher rate than the regular soldiers.[43] Scrive, like Percy before him, believed the medical department should have the same status as the other scientific corps of the army, the engineers and the artillery.[44] Scrive and Baudens both survived the war but Baudens died in 1857 and Scrive in 1861, both from diseases contracted in the Crimea.[45]

Ideological vs practical considerations

At the beginning of the war the French medical department appeared to be in a much better position than that of the British. The British department was a civilian department, as was the commissariat on which it depended for its supplies. The commissariat did not control the medical department as the French commissariat did, but it was so inefficient and bound by bureaucratic red tape that in the earlier months of the siege it was incapable of distributing the ample supplies which it actually had in Balaclava. As civilians, British doctors had no military authority and had to do as the army officers ordered, and they had to rely on untrained orderlies for nurses. By contrast, both the French commissariat and medical department were integrated into the regular army, doctors were officers, and they enjoyed the services of trained soldier nurses and the Daughters of Charity. However, by the end of the war the position of the two medical departments had reversed. The British learned from their mistakes, and before the fall of Sevastopol the army's administrative arrangements had undergone significant reform and were more coordinated. The commissariat became a military department and Panmure consolidated the army command. In the French army the eighteenth-century arrangement of placing the medical department under the direction of the commissariat persisted. The French doctors had no more military authority than the British, and their situation was made much worse as the war progressed because the French Treasury could not support the constantly enlarging army with the necessary resources on which medical and nursing care are so dependent. The Minister of War did send a member of the intendancy, Baudens, to the Crimea for two visits but he was unable to convince the minister to send adequate supplies. The new war correspondents were partly responsible for pushing the British government into its military reforms, but the French press was censored and could not run the kind of sensational news which so stirred public outrage in Britain. Furthermore, even if the press had been able to sway the government, there was not enough money in its coffers to pay for the needed resources.

However, even when the French sick and wounded were starving in the second winter, there can be no question that their nursing service was superior to that of the British, much improved as the British department was by the end of the war. The British did have some excellent clinically experienced religious nursing Sisters, but they had many secular ladies and hospital nurses who were incompetent, while the French soldier nurses and Daughters of Charity were all trained nurses. Using the Russian idea of dealing with the shortage of nurses, the French doctors developed the highly successful dressing soldiers. The doctors showed extraordinary devotion to their patients, who trusted them implicitly. Although the British soldiers and officers spoke of how hard their doctors worked, they did not seem to have the trusting – or affectionate, as Scrive described it – relationship with them. In their field and base hospitals in Balaclava and Constantinople, the Piedmontese Daughters of Charity offered first class nursing services, and the French Daughters did the same in Constantinople. However, the Daughters could never have accomplished this without the soldier nurses who gave much of the basic nursing care. Nightingale criticized the Sisters for not being proactive enough in preventing poor health practices but their patients and the doctors thought the Daughters superb nurses.

The French doctors spoke as highly of their trained soldier nurses as they did of the Daughters of Charity. Yet one does not find patients talking about these accomplished male nurses in the same way as they did of the doctors and Sisters. Why was this? Perhaps the soldiers took them for granted while the Daughters of Charity were a novel experience for them. Or was it because the soldier nurses were less caring and tender-hearted than the women, as the doctrine of woman's mission claimed? Although there were many complaints about the commandeered nurses there do not appear to have been any about the trained soldier nurses, nor did anyone report them as rough and unfeeling. Was it the theorized inherently feminine qualities of tender-heartedness which made the Daughters of Charity such outstanding and well-loved nurses? Neither the doctors who worked with the soldier nurses nor the Sisters' patients ever mentioned tender-heartedness. Masquelez was heartened by the sight of the Sisters and by their tactful religious care. Montaudon spoke of the Sisters' kindness, their wise intelligence, and their command of detail. Herbé was heartened by their professionalism and also appreciated the way the Sisters taught patience and charity. Rather than tender-heartedness, the doctors and patients spoke of the Sisters' courage, bravery, grace, good humor, their attention to detail, and their ability to inspire obedience, love, and blessing.

Gender does not determine any of the above-mentioned qualities, but gender was involved in that the Sisters reminded the officers of their mothers and families at home and of the solace of religion. Everyone enjoyed the Sisters' feminine company after living in an all-male society for long months of campaigning in mud, tents, and trenches under constant fire. Russian civilians treated British

Religious nursing

prisoners of war very kindly as they marched across Southern Russia, usually to Odessa, to be exchanged. One such prisoner, Colonel Atwell Lake, was entertained at dinner by Princess Dondukoff whose husband commanded a regiment of dragoons. 'There was something strangely pleasant, after the horrors of war, and our long banishment from female society,' Lake wrote, 'to be in the company of a clever and kind-hearted woman.'[46] Class may also have played a role in what appears to be a lack of appreciation for the male nurses. Herbé was impressed by the wealthy young Daughter of Charity who came from the same society as he did, while the soldier nurses were separated from the officers both by rank and social class. Herbé could not have had conversations about his family and mutual acquaintances with the soldier nurses. The Sisters' education, intelligence, and competence, which impressed the officers, are all characteristics which the advantages of belonging to the upper class can develop more highly. It is noteworthy that the officers also made no mention of the working-class cantinières who rode out to the Inkerman battlefield to help the wounded as if on parade. Religion also played a central role in producing excellent nurses. Their long tradition and experience in military nursing were key factors in producing the accomplished French and Sardinian nursing Sisters. Sisterhoods, as we saw in the case of the British Sisters, tended to attract enterprising women and gave them discipline, training in nursing, and experience in independent living. Religion could have a divisive effect as it did in Britain with its religious pluralism and its intense dislike and suspicion of Roman Catholics, but in France and Piedmont-Sardinia where there was not the multiplicity of denominations this did not obtain.

Finally, the French and Sardinian doctors approached military nursing from a practical rather than ideological viewpoint. They needed trained nurses and they wanted men for the battlefield and the Daughters of Charity for their professional hospital administration. The British were more hamstrung by the separate spheres ideology. Macleod, for example, had worked in French hospitals, and commented on how excellent the trained soldier nurses were. They were, he said, steady soldiers of character, specially recruited, forming a distinct corps with promotion granted for merit. He thought they were well paid and well fed and had a military spirit and the military idea. Yet, writing two years after the war, he did not mention them as a possibility for the British medical department. In his view women were naturally endowed with more patience and it was their mission in life to attend to trivial details. 'To the surgeon a good nurse is of incalculable service,' he wrote:

> His medicines and splints cannot cure unless those many trivial and insignificant points connected with the management of the sick bed, which are more than half the cure, are attended to. The surgeon has enough to occupy all his scant time in the greater and more serious duties of his service; while those nameless constantly-recurring necessities of a sick room, none can minister to like a woman. To perform such duties aright seems part of a woman's mission on earth.

One could not expect, Macleod thought, a strong, vigorous man to have the same patience, gentleness, and sensitive recognition of a sick man's wants.[47] He seems to have dismissed the excellent soldier nurses with their military spirit in favor of what he was accustomed to. In general the British seemed less open to transnational ideas. Bridgeman provides an extreme example. She ran an excellent nursing service but was not prepared to incorporate any new ideas.

Notes

1 Scrive, *Relation*, pp. 207–14.
2 Cler, *Reminiscences*, pp. 199–201.
3 Scrive, *Relation*, pp. 211–16; Loizillon, *Campagne*, p. 142–4.
4 Herbé, *Français & Russes*, pp. 152–3, 274–5.
5 Ibid, pp. 307–10, 313, 323–4, 339–40.
6 Codman, *American Transport*, pp. 85–7, 96–8; Chenu, *Rapport*, pp. 709–10.
7 Herbé, *Français & Russes*, p. 341, 343–4.
8 Chenu, *Rapport*, pp. 709–10.
9 Scrive, *Relation*, pp. 218–22, 225.
10 Ibid, pp. 223–4, 227–30.
11 BL 43397, Nightingale to Col. LeFroy, 9 June 1856, fol. 236.
12 Scrive, *Relation*, pp. 234–7, 273–4, 305–6.
13 BL 43397, Nightingale to Charles Bracebridge, 4 November 1855, fol. 171; Scrive, *Relation*, pp. 273–4, 305–6.
14 Digby, 'Tuke.'
15 Masquelez, *Journal*, pp. 140–3.
16 Figes, *Crimean War*, p. 293.
17 Taylor, *Eastern Hospitals* (3rd edn), pp. 280–2.
18 Scrive, *Relation*, pp. 453–6.

19 Figes, *Crimean War*, pp. 153–5; see, for example, Montaudon, *Souvenirs*, p. 374.

20 Scrive, *Relation*, pp. 127, 148, 240.

21 Goodlake, *Sharpshooter*, p. 166.

22 Hoppen, *Mid-Victorian Generation*, pp. 179–80; Simpson, *Louis Napoleon*, pp. 334–5; Figes, *Crimean War*, pp. 311–13, 402–3; Scrive, *Relation*, p. 238.

23 Scrive, *Relation*, pp. 274–8.

24 Loizillon, *Campagne*, pp. 207, 261–3, 269, 270–1; Scrive, *Relation*, passim.

25 Scrive, *Relation*, pp. 275–8.

26 King, *Transformations*, p. 47, 93–116.

27 Nightingale, *Notes on Nursing*, pp. 6–9, 23, 65.

28 BL 43397, Nightingale to Lady Cranworth, 5 March 1856, fols 97–9.

29 Niel, *Siège de Sévastopol*, pp. 329–30.

30 Pincoffs, *Experiences of a Civilian*, p. 25.

31 Scrive, *Relation*, pp. 274–7, 321–3.

32 Baudens, *Souvenirs*, pp. 98–102.

33 Scrive, *Relation*, pp. 311–12, 315–17, 329–30; Loizillon, *Campagne*, pp. 275–6, 290.

34 Scrive, *Relation*, pp. 331–2, 363–5.

35 Baudens, *Guerre de Crimée*, pp. 101–3; Baudens, *Souvenirs*, pp. 39–40; Scrive, *Relation*, pp. 478–80.

36 Scrive, *Relation*, pp. 361–3, 366–9, 373–8.

37 A league was approximately three miles.

38 Scrive, *Relation*, pp. 300–1.

39 Loizillon, *Campagne*, pp. 125–6.

40 BL 43397, Nightingale to Lady Cranworth, 5 March 1856, fols 98–9.

41 Baumgart, *Crimean War*, p. 142.

42 Scrive, *Relation*, pp. 315–17; Figes, *Crimean War*, p. 311; BL 43397, Nightingale to Lady Cranworth, 5 March 1856, fols 96, 98–9.

43 Baudens, *Souvenirs*, pp. 37, 100, 102; Scrive, *Relation*, pp. 472–8.

44 Scrive, *Relation*, pp. 477–8.

45 Baudens, *Guerre de Crimée*, Note des Éditeurs, no pagination.

46 Lake, *Captivity in Russia*, p. 250.

47 Macleod, *Surgery in the Crimea*, pp. 48fn, 50–1.

Part III
Doctor-directed nursing

9

Turkish military hospitals: An absence of trained nurses and basic resources

Part III looks at nursing services which doctors directed successfully in two British civilian hospitals, one British naval hospital, and the Russian army. In the Ottoman army there appears to have been no effort to organize a nursing service. What little nursing was done was carried out by doctors and untrained orderlies. A recent book in both Turkish and English, *Sağlik Ordusu/The Medical Forces*, indicates that modern trained nursing in Turkey did not begin until the twentieth century.[1] Interestingly, the book begins with a brief survey of military nursing from the time of Suleiman the Magnificent but makes no mention of the eighteenth- and nineteenth-century Russo-Turk Wars until the war of 1877–78. The section for the Ottoman Empire in the Turkish government archives lists no entries for the Crimean War. Most of what we know about the Turkish medical department comes from the writings of two British observers, Rear Admiral Adolphus Slade and Dr Humphry Sandwith. Slade spent many years in Turkey: in 1849, retaining his rank in the Royal Navy, he entered the Ottoman service as administrative head of the navy. Known to the Turks as Mushaver Pasha, he served for seventeen years – until 1866 – introducing many improvements.[2] Sandwith qualified as a doctor at University College Hospital in 1846. He first visited the East in 1847 and two years later moved to Constantinople and set up practice there. In 1853 he volunteered to help the Turkish army in Bulgaria, and in July 1854 the Ottoman government officially made him an army staff surgeon. The following year he became chief medical officer for the Turkish forces in the Transcaucasus.[3] Slade and Sandwith both spoke fluent Turkish and both admired the Turkish private soldiers. 'Ill- treated and abandoned by their officers,

193

Doctor-directed nursing

plundered of their dues, wretchedly clothed and armed,' Sandwith wrote, 'many were twenty-four months in arrears of pay.' He found their patience and long-suffering under these dreadful conditions incredible and beyond all praise.[4]

The Ottoman army as a whole reflected the pre-industrial and backward nature of the empire. The sultan's government had been making efforts to introduce European military techniques since the abolition of the Janissaries in 1826, but his reforms met with strong resistance and were only very partially successful. He did establish a military medical school and a military academy in the early 1830s, and in the late 1830s he brought a small team of Prussian officers, including a young lieutenant named Helmuth von Moltke, to train his troops. However, the army could not be basically reformed without a complete restructuring of its funding system as well as a radical change in its method of drafting the men, and this massive undertaking did not take place.[5] The Ottoman system of drafting soldiers often consisted of simply arresting them. They were then assigned to either the army or the navy, where they served for life. For example, in August 1853, 14,000 Egyptian soldiers were brought in chains to Alexandria and shipped off to Constantinople to be sent to the Caucasian and Danubian fronts.[6] As a result of this less than ideal system of recruitment, soldiers deserted by the hundreds and thousands, especially when they had not been paid or fed and were starving to death.[7] The problems with the Ottoman Treasury stemmed in large part from not being run in a businesslike way. Ottoman bureaucrats had no concept of government finance in the Western sense; rather they concerned themselves primarily with collecting taxes and seeing that their own salaries were paid. European observers believed embezzlement and corruption was the rule; it was very difficult for an honest man to rise to high rank and keep his position without resorting to bribery. Budget deficits were chronic in the 1840s, and in 1851 the Treasury went bankrupt, making the government dependent on foreign loans.[8]

When the Crimean War began there were a few very effective army units which had the most modern European weapons, but as a whole the army was poorly trained, had archaic tactics, and ignorant and often illiterate commanders. For example, the commander-in-chief on the Caucasian front had been educated in Vienna but his chief of staff was illiterate. Exacerbating this problem was the fact that there was always jealousy and antagonism between the educated and the uneducated officers. The army also incorporated irregular troops such as the Bashi-Bazouks, the infamous Cossack cavalry. The government supplied these men with ammunition but nothing else; it did not pay them a salary. The Bashi-Bazouks fought independently and were primarily interested in looting and killing or mutilating enemy soldiers. In the regular army corruption and graft, as in the government, were rampant.[9] Shortly before the Battle of the Alma Lt. Masquelez visited the Turkish camp. There he saw officers brutally mistreating their men and observed that the army was utterly unable to supply its medical corps. He spoke with the medical officer, whom he characterized as 'a kind of renegade.' This doctor told him that no one knew exactly how many soldiers were in the camp and that he did not have any of the necessary medicines. When a sick man consulted him all he could offer was to tell him to go and lie down.[10]

In addition to all these structural problems, the allies treated the Turks disgracefully. Both the British and French High Commands assumed that they were not adequately disciplined or brave enough to fight alongside European troops. However, those who knew the Ottoman soldiers appreciated their fighting abilities. Slade pointed out that the Ottoman army had a great deal of potential but did not have disciplined officers, a regular commissariat, or organized hospitals.[11] Still, the Turks had more than held their own against the Russians in Bulgaria. Baudens wrote that 18,000 Turks had defended Silistria heroically against 100,000 Russians. The British, however, attributed the Turkish success to a few British officers who were with the Turkish troops. The allies lowered their valuation of the Ottoman troops even more after the Battle of Balaclava when 1,400 Ottoman soldiers manned the four redoubts north of Sevastopol. The 500 men in the first redoubt, who had never been in action before, put up a valiant resistance for about an hour during which more than a third of them were killed. When they ran out of ammunition, realized that no support was coming from their allies, and saw 1,200 Russian soldiers preparing for a bayonet charge, they fled. The men in the other three redoubts then followed them. Most of the British and French officers interpreted their flight as cowardice. In fact, John Blunt, Lord Lucan's Turkish interpreter[12] who spoke with them, said that most of the men were not Turkish but Tunisians who had just arrived and were inadequately trained. They were starving because as Muslims they could not eat the standard British campaign rations of salt pork and rum and the British gave them only an extra half pound of biscuit as a replacement. They had been in the redoubts for two or three days with very little water and only biscuit to eat, and were parched with thirst and completely exhausted. They also told Blunt that some of the ammunition they were given did not fit their guns and asked him why no British troops had come to their support.[13]

After the Battle of Balaclava the British and French not only looked down on the Ottoman soldiers but treated them cruelly. They used them largely for night working parties digging trenches, carrying supplies, and maintaining roads. They subjected them to all kinds of humiliation. When they started stealing food because they were starving, the British had them flogged, and flogged well beyond the prescribed number of lashes. Soldiers kicked, slapped, and spat on them and allied officers would not sit at the same table with their Ottoman peers. Of the 4,000 Ottoman soldiers who fought at Balaclava, half died of malnutrition within the next two months and many of the others became too weak for active service. Throughout the winter of 1854–55 the Turkish death rate soared as a result of overwork. Slade could not understand why the allies were so indifferent to their sufferings unless, he wrote, 'one might trace it to the habitual bearing of Anglo-Saxons towards an "inferior race."'[14] The French, however, who were not Anglo-Saxons, treated them just as badly.

Slade described the Turkish hospital in Balaclava as a deplorable hovel. It had originally been a holding place for Russian prisoners and when they all died of cholera it was made into a hospital. There were up to 400 men strewn across damp mud floors with one Armenian doctor struggling to help them. The doors and windows were all closed to keep out the cold, so the atmosphere was awful. The doctor told Slade he had plenty of medicines but they were no help because he had no food to give the men; he had not been able to save a single life. He did not even have utensils to make hot drinks, much less for purifying water. Many died every day and were buried in shallow graves; dogs dug up the corpses and ate them.[15]

In December 1854, following a defeat by the Russian army in the Transcaucasus, the Turkish Anatolian army withdrew into Kars, the most important Ottoman fortress in Eastern Anatolia. The Russians were besieging the town when Sandwith arrived as chief medical officer in February 1855. The Ottoman Anatolian army was then under the command of British General William Williams who had, not entirely legitimately, taken it under his control. The soldiers were suffering terribly because their Turkish commander and his senior officers were fleecing and plundering them. (Sandwith considered peculation and plunder the only things in the Turkish army that were well organized.) The Turkish commanders were using the standard Ottoman practice of muster-roll fraud. They reported the army in Kars as 40,000 men when in fact Williams found only 18,340. The commanders pocketed the money for the pay and rations of the fictional 21,660. The army accepted these practices: Williams reported three commanders who were arrested and tried but, despite the hard evidence he provided, two of the three were acquitted and reinstated. There was an Ottoman saying that an embezzler 'describes his peculation as if it was an accomplishment or an act of bravery.' The majority of the private soldiers in Kars were men who had been arrested and torn from their families in the villages. During the winter 20,000 of these men died of disease and hunger. When Kars was reinforced in the spring it was with similar men, who sought every opportunity to desert.

On arrival, Sandwith found the hospitals in a terrible state with insufficient bedding, few or no medicines, and men suffering from fever and scurvy. Conditions, he said, were too disgusting to publish. The medical staff was feeble and incompetent, but nevertheless tried to do their best for their patients.[16] The purveyor was completely dishonest. Many of the doctors and apothecaries had gained their positions by bribing him. He supplied the hospital in a very capricious way: there were huge amounts of purgatives and enough chloroform for 100,000 operations, all kinds of dainties, cosmetics, and gynecological instruments, but few of the necessary medicines and those which were there were of poor quality.[17] This method of supplying was not atypical: on the Danubian front in the spring of 1854 the surgeons in one Turkish camp of 7,000 men had no instruments for extracting musket balls.[18] Sandwith had a staff of about fifty physicians, surgeons, and apothecaries. When he took over, the medical department was functioning at a very low level because of his

Doctor-directed nursing

predecessor's shortcomings. He had indulged in all the standard graft and peculation typical of army officers and the department was split into factions which intrigued against each other. Most of the doctors were Turkish but there were some from France, Poland, and Italy. The foreigners were mostly what Sandwith called 'ignorant pretenders,' men who had no diplomas or very doubtful ones. Sandwith considered the Turkish medical doctors the only educated men in Anatolia. The surgeons knew only how to bleed, pull teeth, and dress wounds, but some of the physicians had studied in Paris, spoke French, and knew something about the world outside Turkey. What made them the best of Sandwith's doctors was their eagerness to learn more about their profession. While supplies were still getting through, Sandwith organized an ambulance corps for the field and introduced modern standards of cleanliness and water dressings for the wounded. He was pleased that he never had a case of typhus or gangrene.[19]

Sandwith gradually came to admire the Turkish surgeons, who were just as eager to learn as the physicians. He attributed much of his success to 'the noble little band of ill-paid and ill-treated Turkish surgeons. Though less well educated than their colleagues in the West, their love of their profession, and their industrious attention to the wounded soldiers, both Turkish and Russian, in the midst of our crowded hospitals, and in the face of frightful difficulties' were admirable. They adopted any improved method of treatment Sandwith suggested. He esteemed their devotion to their patients and their enlightened views. Yet, he said, their government never rewarded them with promotion or decorations: theirs was a 'despised and unappreciated calling.' The Turks put up a valiant defense over the summer and fall of 1855, but by October the troops had been living on bread and water for months and were no longer what Sandwith described as 'the stout and hardy men who fought for seven hours against overwhelming odds, and drove back a magnificent Russian army.' Sandwith's hospitals began filling daily with men whose only disease was exhaustion from the deficient diet. By November there were about 2,000 men in the hospitals and about 100 died every day. Many soldiers were so enfeebled they could not even make their way to the hospitals, and as heavy snow fell they lay dying and dead in every part of the camp. On 21 November 1855 Williams surrendered to the Russians.[20]

Turkish military hospitals

In April 1855 a large number of Ottoman soldiers landed in Balaclava, causing a great stir. Everyone seems pleased with the Turkish infantry who have just arrived, Assistant Surgeon Frederick Robinson declared enthusiastically. Well supplied and officered by the British, the men were strong, well clad, and well drilled. A few days later Turkish artillery, cavalry, and even men armed with the new Minié rifle landed and were dispersed throughout the allied position.[21] These soldiers were temporarily no longer in the Ottoman army but rather constituted what was called the Turkish Contingent. This unit consisted of what would eventually be 20,000 Ottoman soldiers who were paid by the British government and trained by British officers. At the end of the war they were to be returned to the Ottoman army. The Ottoman government was not happy about renting out some of its troops but, unable to feed and pay their soldiers properly themselves, in February 1855 they grudgingly agreed to lease them to the British.[22] Robinson thought the Contingent's medical department equally satisfactory. The majority of the doctors were Turkish but there were some Western surgeons and dressers. The British provided good food and the hospital buildings consisted of twenty-four British prefabricated huts which were remarkably clean and well supplied, the *Lancet* reported. The Turkish hospitals allotted two orderlies to the fourteen patients in each hut, a generous ratio.[23] The orderlies were quickly becoming good nurses because the surgeons were spending a great deal of time supervising and teaching them. The orderlies could not, the *Lancet* reported,

> (*as yet*) [February 1856] tell one medicine from another, or read a label as English hospital corporals and serjeants do, and yet by the unremitting personal industry of surgeons, assistant-surgeons and acting-assistant surgeons, hundreds of patients are daily supplied with medicines, and this with regularity and precision, the doses being explained and the administration superintended.

The British doctors believed that the Contingent's hospitals were 'superior in neatness, warmth, and comfort, to any in the Crimea.'[24]

However, the Contingent's hospitals were actually a part of the British army. The hovel that the Ottoman government supplied for the hospital in Balaclava, and the Kars hospitals when Sandwith first arrived were more characteristic of Ottoman military hospitals and

Doctor-directed nursing

their level of medical and nursing care. Lack of resources placed the Turkish doctors in the position of the regimental surgeon who, with no equipment except his amputating kit, purgatives, and a kind word, came every day to see Bell when he lay ill in the kindly peasants' kitchen. In Balaclava the Armenian doctor could not even make his patients warm drinks, much less feed them. It was a deplorable situation but the Turkish doctors were devoted and very kind to both their Russian and Turkish patients. One should never underestimate the importance of kind and encouraging words as a powerful constituent of nursing care, a component which the Sisters of Mercy and the Daughters of Charity understood and exemplified so well. Russian surgeon Nikolai Pirogov (see chapter 12), who directed the Russian nursing, deemed warm drinks and 'propping up the spirits' of the wounded more important than changing their bloody, infected, oozing dressings.

Notes

1 Beyhan, *Medical Forces*, p. 12.
2 Slade, *Turkey*, pp. 192–4; Laughton, 'Slade, Sir Adolphus.'
3 Sandwith, *Siege of Kars*, pp. iii, 118–19; Kennedy, 'Sandwith, Humphry.'
4 Sandwith, *Siege of Kars*, pp. 164–5, p. 78.
5 Ralston, *Importing the European Army*, pp. 52–8, 63.
6 Baumgart, *Crimean War*, p. 86.
7 Ibid, p. 86; Slade, *Turkey*, p. 27.
8 Badem, *Ottoman Crimean War*, pp. 289–94.
9 Ibid, pp. 143–8, 377–8, 408–10; Sandwith, *Siege of Kars*, p. 47.
10 Masquelez, *Journal*, pp. 99–101.
11 Slade, *Turkey*, pp. 192–4.
12 Lt. General George Bingham Lucan, 3rd earl, was commander of the cavalry division in the Crimea.
13 Baudens, *Souvenirs*, p. 61; Figes, *Crimean* War, pp. 183, 242; Badem, *Ottoman Crimean War*, pp. 270–3.
14 Slade, *Turkey*, pp. 331, 335; Badem, *Ottoman Crimean War*, pp. 275–6.
15 Slade, *Turkey*, pp. 192–4, 331; Badem, *Ottoman Crimean War*, p. 276.
16 Sandwith, *Siege of Kars*, pp. 46–8, 49, 71; Badem, *Ottoman Crimean War*, pp. 193, 230–351.
17 Sandwith, *Siege of Kars*, pp. 119–20.
18 Slade, *Turkey*, 198–200.
19 Sandwith, *Siege of Kars*, pp. 118–19, 121–2.
20 Ibid, pp. 164–5, 173–5.

Turkish military hospitals

21 Robinson, *Diary*, pp. 302–5.
22 Shepherd, *Crimean Doctors*, vol. 2, pp. 563–4; Sandwith, *Siege of Kars*, pp. iii, 118–19; Baumgart, *Crimean War*, p. 81; Badem, *Ottoman Crimean War*, pp. 257–60, 263.
23 Radcliffe, 'Turkish Hospital,' pp. 8–9.
24 Robinson, *Diary*, pp. 302–5; Lancet, 'Turkish Contingent,' p. 136.

10

The naval hospital at Therapia

Introduction: health care in the Royal Navy

Nursing in the Royal Navy and the Ottoman army present opposite poles in terms of nursing, systematic and well-resourced medical care, and above all, in the patients themselves. This chapter demonstrates how important all these factors were to good nursing care and the immense difference the treatment the sailors received from their military superiors made in their health care outcomes. Dr John Davidson, who directed the naval hospital in Therapia, worked in a completely different world from that of the Turkish doctors. Davidson and his medical staff were both better educated and better supplied than the Ottoman doctors, but the biggest difference between the Turkish hospitals and the naval hospital was the health status of the patients. The Royal Navy had a long tradition of providing good health care, and although Davidson would have to struggle with many other issues, the better health of his patients gave them a much greater chance of making a good recovery.

Modern medical and nursing care depended heavily on proper supplies and a properly functioning commissariat. The British army suffered grievously in the autumn of 1854 when nearly all the necessary materials were in Balaclava but an incompetent commissariat did not have the administrative structure to transport them to the soldiers in the camp. In the second winter of the war the French commissariat did not have the money to buy supplies, and although the Russian commissariat often had the necessary supplies on site, graft, laziness, and incompetency prevented it from delivering them to the patients. When the Ottoman army purveyors did have money they often bought items such as gynecological instruments and cosmetics,

The naval hospital at Therapia

which presumably their friends wanted to sell and which were totally useless in an army hospital. Material supplies were essential for good nursing care, but equally important was the respect and the spirit with which naval officers treated their men.

We tend to forget the important role the navy played in the Crimean War, partly because the press made so much of Nightingale's heroic efforts in the army hospitals, and partly due to historians of nursing focusing on army nursing. However, as discussed earlier, modern historians have indicated that from the point of view of the British government the Crimean War was essentially a naval war,[1] and the navy entered it far better equipped to deal with health problems than did the army. The navy had a Sick and Hurt Board in the seventeenth century, and in the mid-eighteenth century the Victualling Board started providing fresh meat, vegetables, and fruit. In the 1790s, victualing at sea was first introduced and issuing lemon juice on long voyages became standard. Unlike many British army officers, experienced seamen appreciated the importance of a healthy crew and understood the relationship of diet to physical condition and the impact of overwork on physical fitness. 'The great thing in all military service is health, and you will agree with me,' Lord Nelson wrote, 'that it is easier to keep men healthy, than for a physician to cure them.'[2] During the Napoleonic Wars the navy required better qualifications for its surgeons and gave full surgeons an official uniform and better pay. Unlike the army, by 1815 the navy had a real medical administration, and unlike army surgeons, naval surgeons were officers, an integrated part of the navy. Mortality in the navy fell from 1:8 in 1780 to 1:30 in 1812.[3] In 1833 naval regulations established a sick bay staff for each ship and gave its attendants a distinct rating as Able Seamen, with loblolley boys to assist them. However, as with army orderlies, there was a tendency for the captain to send men who were less good sailors to work in the sick bay.[4] By 1841 naval surgeons had to have a 'certificate of fitness' from one of the London, Edinburgh, or Dublin Colleges of Surgeons, and assistant surgeons could not be promoted to full surgeon unless they had served three years and had medical qualifications.[5]

The navy played a major part in the Crimean War from the very beginning of the campaign. After the Alma, naval surgeons worked with the army while 1,000 sailors carried the wounded and sick to the ships to be evacuated to Scutari.[6] During the first months of the siege the ships in the Balaclava harbor were the most comfortable place to live. A young officer invited on board the *Agamemnon* for a few days luxuriated in the comfort of having a cot and being able to undress at night. He pronounced the ship 'quite a floating hotel, and an asylum for sick officers, amateurs and others.'[7] Frederic Robinson was one such officer. He had suffered from severe dysentery and fever from the time he arrived in Bulgaria. At first he was able to keep the dysentery somewhat in check with large doses of opium, but in October he became so dangerously ill that he had to be moved to a ship. There he recovered and was able to return to work but in November he began suffering from what he diagnosed as a disordered liver resulting from all the opiates he was taking. In mid-December he contracted bronchitis on top of his other problems and general debility forced him to apply for a medical board. The board assigned him to a ship to recover once more. He had no idea how emaciated he had become until he saw his face in a mirror on the ship, but within a month on shipboard he made a solid recovery.[8]

It was standard practice for the navy to provide manpower for the army at landing sites. A detachment of marines protected the army while it was landing at Eupatoria and remained there afterwards to secure the port. In early October 1854, at Raglan's request, 1,200 sailors and a large number of marines landed at Balaclava; by the end of the month there were 4,000 sailors and marines on shore. The marines fought and suffered with the army but, in a unit called the Naval Brigade, the sailors also assisted the Royal Artillery. They would participate in every assault on Sevastopol as well as in the Battle of Inkerman. In the first few months of the siege the Naval Brigade manned 40 percent of the British guns.[9] 'They are a magnificent body of men,' Somerset Calthorpe, one of Raglan's staff, exclaimed as he watched them pulling the ship-guns from Balaclava up to the camp. He was impressed by the way they tossed about the heaviest guns. They also dragged many of the artillery's guns up to the heights.[10] The tars are such jovial fellows and are superior to the soldiers, Henry Bushby, a war correspondent, observed. They did everything to music. 'In camp, where no fiddle was to be had,' Bushby wrote, 'they used to time their steps in hauling up the guns, by making one of their number sing.'[11] Midshipman Evelyn Wood

The naval hospital at Therapia

described getting the guns up to the camp somewhat differently. For six days we did the work of horses, he wrote, dragging the guns a distance of eight miles up to the camp on ship trucks. Wood, who enlisted in the navy in 1852 at the age of 14, has given us one of the best accounts of the brigade. He described how they put fifty sailors on three drag ropes, placed a fiddler or fifer on the gun to keep them in rhythm, and when neither was available, as Bushby indicated, used a singer. The sailors had breakfast at 5 a.m., started work at 5:30, had an hour off for lunch at midday, and then worked through till 6 p.m. Wood thought that no 1,200 men had ever worked harder.[12] The naval officers and their men also exhibited extraordinary courage. Henry Clifford, who spent a good deal of his time in the trenches and batteries with the soldiers, was astounded by the sailors' coolness and bravery. During the Second Bombardment in April 1855[13] he saw eleven sailors in Gordon's Battery killed or wounded by the explosion of one shell about fifteen yards from where he was standing. 'And the men behaved so coolly,' he exclaimed. 'The men who are not killed or wounded at a gun when a shell or round shot comes, go on working just as if nothing had taken place.'[14]

The brigade's officers believed their gunners were more accurate than the soldiers. The Royal Artillery apparently thought the same because they manned their new, long-range Lancaster guns entirely with sailors. Throughout the siege naval losses were disproportionately heavier than those of the Royal Artillery because the Russians also considered the sailors better gunners. For example, during the Second Bombardment the Russian sharpshooters specifically targeted, and with lethal effect, those guns manned by sailors. The navy lost 200 men. Over the course of the war the brigade served forty-nine guns, a little over a third of the total number, but lost 89 men compared to the Royal Artillery's 104, almost three times as many men per gun. Kinglake attributed the heavier naval losses to the reckless bravery of the sailors who, he claimed, skylarked under fire. Wood denied this assertion. He never saw any sailor skylarking; rather, he attributed the brigade's severe losses to the navy's small diameter truck wheels on which they had to haul their guns back into firing position after the recoil. The army's field carriages had large wheels which rolled more easily and quickly so the soldiers were exposed to the Russian sharpshooters for a shorter period of time.[15] Except in the

Doctor-directed nursing

sea bastions and batteries, all the Russian guns were taken from their ships and all their gun-carriages were naval trucks.[16]

In the army on the battlefield, lack of transport to first aid stations or hospitals was the biggest cause of mortality. This problem did not exist on shipboard: the sailors could carry the wounded the few steps down to the surgeon in the cockpit. This did not obtain in the Naval Brigade, which fought on land, but it did mean the doctors appreciated the efficacy of prompt medical aid. The navy had another key advantage over the army: its ships sailed all over the world and its officers and men knew how to deal with harsh sub-arctic and equatorial conditions. Wood pointed out that few British army officers understood that their men had to be appropriately clothed and well fed. Army officers fared much better than the enlisted men because when the commissariat became unable to transport clothes and food from the harbor up to the camp, officers could usually afford the extortionate prices of the shops in Balaclava and had the means of getting from the camp to the port while the private soldiers did not.

'Throughout the long ensuing siege the working parties in the trenches did well or badly in proportion to the efficiency of the officers,' Wood contended.[17] And indeed it would seem that many British officers felt little commitment either to the army or to their men. 'A very great number of Officers have left,' Henry Clifford wrote in July 1855, 'some from ill health, *many from pretended ill health* who are as well as I am, and others from disgust and tired of the long dreary siege.' He predicted that many more would leave before the second winter set in. One of his best friends did exactly this in August 1855. 'Young Clifton,' Clifford wrote to his family, 'has sent in his papers, he is tired of the service and is going home and leaves the Army.'[18] French officers made similar remarks about the British officers' lack of concern for their men. If you asked a British officer how he was going to feed his men, Montaudon later wrote, he would reply, 'Oh that is not my affair, it is up to the commissariat.' In Second Empire France the gulf between the social classes was less rigid and it was considered quite suitable for officers to mix with their men. Montaudon considered it essential because it enabled them to exercise a moral influence and build *esprit de corps*.[19] Clifford agreed that the French looked after their men better than the British. He was one of the few staff officers who visited his men when they were in

206

The naval hospital at Therapia

hospital and the only one on General Codington's six-man staff who visited the trenches regularly. As a result, he often had to do the work of the other five aides.[20]

By contrast, the naval officers fought together with their men and looked after them sympathetically. Captain Stephen Lushington and Captain William Peel, his second-in-command, took assiduous care of us, Wood explained; we seldom lacked for supplies. The officers saw that the men had warm clothes and good food, and when for two days the sailors were on half rations with no biscuit in November and one day during a heavy snowstorm in December did not receive any rations at all, the officers shared their private stores.[21] The sailors had good cooking arrangements, better clothes, and less work than the soldiers. They lived in a sheltered valley in well-drained tents and had a good water supply because they sank their own well. The naval officers made every man returning from the trenches remove his wet clothes before he was allowed to lie down. There were drying sheds for the wet clothes, an advantage that the army officers did not have; they sometimes had to wear wet clothes for several days. The navy did not have store ships so all of its supplies came from Balaclava. A naval officer, who always carried his own load, took a party into Balaclava every day to buy coal and charcoal. The cooks did not work in the trenches but spent their whole time preparing the food and drink for the men when they went on and came off duty. The sailors had coffee, cocoa, quinine, lime juice, and fresh oranges before they set off for the batteries in the morning. In the evening they had hot soup made from salt meat from which the salt had been extracted. And in December, when the soldiers were living on half and quarter rations of hard tack and salt meat with no means of cooking it or water to soak it in to remove the salt, the sailors had fresh meat ten times. The army of course was starving, not because food was unavailable but because they had no way to transport it from Balaclava up to the camp. Sailors were also used to working shifts, which they called watches, around the clock so shift work in the trenches was not new to them. Still another important advantage the sailors enjoyed was that nearly all of them spent only three to four months on shore; then their ships returned home and they were replaced.

In addition, the sailors' isolated wooden world when at sea taught them to be more resourceful and enterprising than army life made the soldiers, and many sailors put their talents to profitable use. As soon as they came off duty many sailors went directly to the army camp where they did odd jobs such as repairing tents for the officers, who unfortunately usually paid them with grog.[22] This is not to say that the sailors had an easy time during the siege – quite the contrary – but their officers and comrades supported them when they faced danger and all the other problems of life in the field. For example, one night when Wood was on duty and it was his turn to sleep he chose a spot which was sheltered from the wind rather than a dry place. When it began to rain he was too tired to get up and move. During the night the temperature fell precipitously and the water froze around him so that when he tried to get up in the morning he could not move. His comrades freed him, carried him back to the camp and placed hot water bottles around him so he would not get frostbite. The naval officers even looked after some of the soldiers: every morning they went out and brought in soldiers who were frozen in place.[23]

The Naval Brigade reached its peak strength in the ill-fated assault on 18 June. The sailors manned fifty-six guns and so many were wounded or killed that the navy was unable to replace its ratings. Peel and Wood, who was his aide-de-camp, were both severely wounded leading a ladder party of sixty sailors. When the brigade was broken up in September 1855, of the 4,469 sailors and marines who served, 100 were dead, 475 wounded, and thirteen sailors had won Victoria Crosses.[24] The mortality rate for the Naval Brigade was 10.5 percent, of which 7 percent were fatal wound cases and only 3.5 percent resulted from disease. The cavalry lost 15 percent, and the infantry 39 percent from sickness alone. In the eight front-line battalions the mortality was 73 percent.[25] By contrast, in terms of British mortality for the whole war, in May 1856 Lord Panmure gave the total British losses as 20,000, with men killed in action at 4,000 and the remaining 16,000 dying of wounds and/or disease.[26] Clearly, the navy's know-how and its superior care of the sailors were the principal causes of its better medical record.

As soon as his crew was landed at Balaclava, Captain Peel's ship, the *Diamond*, was made into a hospital ship.[27] It was rather a makeshift hospital – it was not well equipped, and it had to continue its work as a picket ship, moored so that her remaining guns swept a valley to prevent a Russian assault on the British lines. But her surgeon,

William Smart, was an extremely competent doctor and an excellent organizer.[28] The navy subsequently fitted out three more hospital ships, and by the end of the war the brigade had a hutted hospital near its camp and a larger purpose-built hospital at Eupatoria. However, the female nurses the government sent did not work in any of these hospitals; they were sent only to the base hospital at Therapia. Here the navy had a head start on the army. There had been an Anglo-French fleet in the Black Sea since January 1854 and in February, before war was declared, the navy began making arrangements for a base hospital. The Ottoman government gave them a very dilapidated three-story wooden building in Therapia, a small, pleasant town on the Bosphorus now a part of Istanbul, where a number of diplomats had summer homes. Davidson undertook refitting the building, which was a challenge. He used rags to stop up the cracks through which icy winds blew in the winter. The floors were so rickety that he did not use the top floor for fear it would collapse under the additional weight of patients. The drains were open creeks, constantly blocked and filthy. However, there was a nice garden and a good water supply. Originally there were only forty beds but Davidson planned to expand it to 100, and at one point it consisted of 159 beds.[29]

The Therapia building was not an ideal hospital but Davidson was a very competent person. He would face many of the same problems with accommodation, understaffing, and red tape as did the army doctors. When war was declared at the end of March 1854 he already had forty-five patients, mostly fever cases, and only one marine corporal, three privates as guards, and five male nurses (or orderlies to use army terminology). He had no dispenser, cook, or laundry man and only one assistant surgeon for the projected 100 patients. The navy's medical department was so short of surgical staff that it hired medical students aged 18 to 22 at six shillings a day to serve in the Baltic for six or seven months, thereby releasing more experienced assistant surgeons to go to the Black Sea. There was not enough space in the Therapia building for storing supplies and there were major problems with the victualing system because, apart from medicines and other medical supplies, it was not clear who was responsible for the hospital's stores. A ship's paymaster was the only officer who could issue food and the hospital obviously was not a ship, so it had to buy its own meat, bread, and vegetables locally – a considerable

Doctor-directed nursing

expense but it was probably better food. Davidson's superior, Admiral Edward Boxer, considered his numerous requests a major nuisance and thought they showed he lacked system. Boxer reprimanded him for lack of discipline and reported him to the Admiralty as unfit to be in charge of the hospital.[30] Fortunately the Admiralty thought otherwise. Boxer was born in 1784 and started his career fighting in the 1790s,[31] which probably explains why he was so unsympathetic with Davidson's more modern approach to proper medical care. In any case, Boxer was not a popular figure with the younger generation. Fanny Duberly, the wife of one of the army officers, called him a 'noisy, vulgar, swearing old ruffian' and a bully, but she recognized that he did do good work in cleaning up and organizing the chaotic Balaclava harbor.[32]

The new female nurses in Therapia

Among all of Davidson's problems none was more pressing than the lack of skilled nurses. The five original orderlies were volunteers from the fleet and were utterly incompetent and unhelpful. If Davidson tried to correct them they immediately asked to be sent back to their ships. Malta, the chief supply base for the Mediterranean fleet, had a well-supplied 200-bed base hospital but it also had dreadful problems finding efficient nurses.[33] However, when Davidson decided to give up on the volunteer sailor nurses, it was the only place he could tap for replacements. The six Maltese nurses[34] who arrived were completely illiterate and proved, if anything, worse than the sailors. They neglected their patients and stole hospital stores and rations. Davidson dismissed all of them and began once again drawing men from the fleet. As with the army doctors, he had no authority over the seamen assigned to him; only their ship's captain could discipline them for the standard infractions of drunkenness, insubordination, and patient neglect. Also like the army doctors, Davidson wanted to keep the few men who were competent but was rarely able to do so. In December 1854 his clerical staff consisted of only one marine sergeant, which meant that he had to spend a great deal of his time on clerical matters rather than medical care. Making matters worse, the building work was behind schedule and the patients were suffering from the cold and damp.[35]

The naval hospital at Therapia

Nursing help, however, was soon to come. Davidson and his immediate superior, Dr David Deas, Inspector of Medical Services to the Black Sea Fleet, had been emphasizing the importance of better nursing for some time, and on 27 November 1854 the Board of Admiralty began looking for suitable female nurses for its hospitals. On 10 January Rev. John Mackenzie, a retired Presbyterian minister, his wife Eliza, and a small party of nurses arrived.[36] Eliza was a daughter of Thomas Chalmers, the founder of the Scottish Free Church. The Mackenzies had offered their services to the army in the fall of 1854 when Nightingale was no longer accepting nurses, and were sent to the Admiralty which assigned them to Therapia. There is not a great deal of information about the nursing in Therapia but we are fortunate in having some of the letters Eliza Mackenzie wrote home to her family. 'I shall not need to learn nursing,' she wrote to her sister before leaving for the East, but rather she was to study hospital management. After the first group of nurses left with Nightingale the ladies in London who selected the nurses made it a rule that lady applicants spend at least two or three days to several weeks working in a London hospital as a test of their ability to function in a clinical setting. The Park Village sisterhood and St. John's House agreed to board these ladies and treat them as short-term probationers. Later Lord Shaftesbury set up a third establishment in Upper Charlotte Street for this purpose. Eliza had spent some time at the Middlesex Hospital, for she told her sister that the surgeons at the Middlesex considered her qualified to be 'a kind of Miss Nightingale' in the naval hospital. John was to accompany her as an unpaid chaplain since the hospital already had a chaplain. In fact, the Anglican chaplain fell ill and Mackenzie became a kind of unofficial chaplain for the Anglicans, conducting services in their rite (which would cause some problems). Eliza felt it was a very difficult undertaking for her, 'with such responsibility to the Admiralty, and John as my appendage with no position at all.' If she and her nurses were successful the Admiralty hoped to introduce similar female nursing throughout their hospitals. She continued:

> This responsibility is truly awful, but I have been inclined to undertake it as it appears to be most difficult to get anyone who will go out without settling so much beforehand about creeds and confessions ... even about gowns and bonnets, that time is passing, and wounded sailors and marines

Doctor-directed nursing

are lying in a deplorable state, and the medical men are anxious for female aid.[37]

There had already been significant improvements in Therapia when Mackenzie and her nurses arrived; the Anglican chaplain was there and the medical staff had doubled.[38] The nurses did not experience the initial resistance Nightingale met. On their arrival Davidson welcomed them and immediately distributed them as day and night nurses to each floor. He gave them full hospital rations and made Mrs Mackenzie an honorary member of the Officers' Mess, something Nightingale never was given. Like Nightingale, Davidson did not see the role of the female nurses as replacing the male orderlies, but rather as supervising them. Three months' worth of washing awaited the women when they landed, and only a few days after their arrival ninety men in terrible condition, unfed for four days, disembarked. The nurses fed the men arrowroot and brandy but did not have enough sheets for the beds. They aired the sheets, pillowcases, shirts, and nightcaps they did have, which were still damp from the laundry, before putting the men to bed.

Soon after arriving, Mackenzie visited the Barrack Hospital in Scutari, where she found everything in a state of chaos and could not see how any one person could manage two such huge hospitals. She thought she would be able to manage the much smaller Therapia Hospital, and indeed she did manage it well. Like Nightingale she had full responsibility for the discipline and conduct of the nurses, but unlike Nightingale, she seemed to have more confidence in her nurses, accepting their failings and considering them basically respectable. 'Keeping such a set of good, respectable women [but] with unrestrained tempers and foolish ideas in order, and concealing their most violent rows and absurdities from Dr Davidson' was not easy, she wrote. In the early days she was not certain that she had his full support. She thought that if he became aware of the nurses' sometimes discreditable behavior, he would think nothing 'of blowing the whole thing sky-high and saying it was a failure!' She felt she had to treat Davidson with the utmost tact: she humored him constantly but believed it worth the effort because he did his job so well. She thought his hospital 'the *only* one where there is any comfort at all.' As in Nightingale's case, the military red tape was one of Mackenzie's biggest hindrances. It was so difficult to get anything done, she said, because of the Rules of Service. She often had to go to the storeroom herself to get what she needed. When the *Witness* published a letter asking people to send warm clothes to the sailors, Mackenzie had a reaction similar to Nightingale's when Sister Elizabeth Wheeler's letter was published. Mackenzie was horrified because it reflected badly on the hospital and its doctor; she appreciated that Davidson could not admit publicly that his hospital lacked anything.[39] Fortunately, the naval doctors were not under the gun of the newspapers and did not become distraught as did the army doctors.

At the beginning of February 1855 the hospital was running at full capacity with 159 patients, but by the end of the month there were only eighty.[40] The patients recovered quickly, partly because their underlying health was good and partly because conditions in the Crimea had improved, but Mackenzie's nursing team also made a major difference. Deas recognized this when he wrote to the Admiralty in mid-February:

> We are infinitely better than we were. The guard and the male nurses are kept in order, and it is no longer the hopeless drag it was. Mrs Mackenzie and her staff are doing admirable service, smoothing the pillows and soothing the feelings as only a woman can do … and up to this time keeping in all respects within her proper province.[41]

Deas certainly appreciated how much better things were running since the nurses arrived, but he did not seem to understand the scope of their work and assumed it was simply a question of taking on housekeeping and women's supposed natural abilities, which men did not share, to soothe feelings. He was expressing the classic separate spheres evaluation of ladies' capacities. Henry Clifford also had no sense of the difference between what was to become professional nursing and femininity. He served on General Buller's staff, and when Buller became very ill and had to be sent home Clifford wrote to his family:

> What a blessing women are as nurses. It is not possible for a man to nurse as a woman can, and I always think how many poor fellows die out here, who if they had a mother, or a sister or a wife to take care of them, would live. I have tried very hard to do all I can for poor General Buller, but I am a rough, bad nurse, and I long for him to get into the hands of his sisters, or other kind friends at his home.[42]

213

Doctor-directed nursing

Mackenzie was obviously a good administrator for already in March when the Sanitary Commission visited the hospital they found it satisfactory. It then had a permanent agent and a clerk, allowing Davidson to spend more time on patient care, and Mackenzie had six working-class and two lady nurses. In June 1855 there was a serious outbreak of cholera that continued well into July, and 180 wounded sailors arrived after the 18 June assault, stretching the hospital's capacity and making the badly equipped and staffed transports for the sick and wounded especially overloaded. There was almost no medical or nursing help on the ships. Transport was the one area where the navy did badly. If a captain sent a surgeon to a transport, it was at the cost of leaving his own crew without medical aid. There had been little improvement in the naval transports since the Alma when two naval surgeons on the *Britannia*, which was carrying 200 wounded men to Scutari, reported there were no naval officers on board to prevent men being robbed by others or to superintend the messing and there were no nurses or orderlies. Nor was there an executive officer to look after the men's papers or sort out the constant confusion. It was simply a case of 200 men laid out on hay or bare decks with little hope of any care. Fifty-two of the 200 men on that voyage died.[43]

Wood was one of the 180 wounded men that the understaffed transports brought to Therapia. He had been severely ill with low fever and intestinal complaints for a week before the Waterloo Day assault and had been living on a diet of rice, tinned milk, laudanum, and other sedatives but somehow had managed to evade being put on the sick list.[44] After he was wounded he was taken to his uncle's ship to recuperate, but when his broken arm failed to heal he was transferred to Therapia on 18 July. There what he described as 'two resident ladies,' the Misses Baltazzi, nursed him.[45] Wood was pleased with the hospital and said he would have been very happy there if only he had not had to go through the excruciating probings of his wound. He was in Therapia for a week and then sent to England to recuperate in his parents' home. He arrived home early in August, desperate to return to the Crimea so he could continue fighting. Because the Naval Brigade was soon to be broken up, he decided to transfer to the army, which everyone anticipated would be embarking on a major campaign in the spring of 1856.

214

The naval hospital at Therapia

Wood returned to Scutari in January 1856 as a newly commissioned army officer. At the beginning of March he contracted typhoid fever and was sent to the Scutari General Hospital. His experience there gives us insight into the way the doctors and nurses saw motherly patient care. Their view contrasted strongly with the generally held belief expressed by Deas and Clifford. Wood developed pneumonia on top of the typhus and was aggressively treated with leeches, blisters, and mustard poultices. His doctors feared he was dying and urged his parents to come to Scutari to see him one last time. In the meantime the senior doctor discontinued his treatments so he could die in peace. Nightingale assigned Susan Cator and Ruth Dawson, two of her very best nurses, to tend him. Wood liked Cator but detested Dawson who, he said, was very rough and brutal. When she changed his dressings, instead of wetting them first, she just tore off the lint, bringing flesh away with it.[46] It was quite common for delirious patients to develop a paranoid view of their nurses or other individuals. Nightingale cited the case of Miss Wear as an example. Delirious with fever, Wear believed her nurse was trying to poison her. Her doctor changed the nurse, hoping a different nurse would be more acceptable, but the replacement nurse, Elizabeth Woodward, did no better. Woodward was a St. John's House trained nurse and another one of Nightingale's best nurses. When Wear's delusions continued, Nightingale changed the nurse yet again, sending Woodward to accompany the convalescent assistant surgeon George Lawson home. Lawson was suffering acutely from typhus and his doctors thought her nursing saved his life on the eight week and four day journey home.[47]

Wood's mother, Lady Emma Wood, reached Scutari on 20 March. Wood was delighted to see her; he very much admired her and believed that whatever good qualities he possessed he had inherited from her. Wood's head had been shaved, because it was believed hair prevented feverish heat from escaping, and he had developed a habit of rubbing his scalp until it bled. Dawson had been reprimanded for allowing him to do this so she sometimes held his arm to stop him. On the third day Lady Wood was in the hospital she opened the door to his room quietly and claimed she saw Dawson clenching her fist and punching Wood in the face. He himself had no memory of the incident because he said he was unconscious at the time. Lady

215

Doctor-directed nursing

Wood flew at Dawson and he never saw her again. His mother then personally took over his care. Wood asked if he could be transferred to the naval hospital in Therapia but they refused to receive him since he was now in the army. He thought his condition had improved after his mother's arrival, but the doctors disagreed. When his mother suggested taking him home to England they told her they thought he would die just from being moved to the ship, but Wood insisted he wanted to go home and on 15 April left the hospital for England.[48] Two months later, in June 1856, Lady Wood wrote to Lady Cranworth, one of the ladies responsible for recruiting nurses, charging Dawson with cruelty.

Nightingale was very angry because, as she wrote to Lady Cranworth, it was against all the rules of common sense and fairness to make such an accusation months later, when Lady Wood had never said a word to her or her deputies at the time. Nightingale left Scutari for the Crimea the very day that Lady Wood arrived so she could not speak personally about the care Wood received when his mother was in charge. Now, in June 1856, the hospital had been broken up and most of the doctors and witnesses had gone home. However, Dawson had not left the East but had found a position in Constantinople, so Nightingale went into the city to interview her. Nightingale pointed out that Lady Wood claimed her son had been in the Barrack Hospital under Miss Terrot when he was allegedly mistreated. In fact he had been in the General Hospital where Miss Tebbutt was superintendent, so Nightingale also wrote to Tebbutt, asking her about Dawson. Sarah Anne Terrot did work in the General Hospital but was never superintendent, and she was sent home sick in April 1855, seven months before Wood was admitted. In July Nightingale reported her findings to Lady Cranworth. Tebbutt said that Lady Wood had, together with an orderly, taken on Wood's nursing herself and that she thought Lady Wood was very unfair to Dawson, and had told her so.[49] The chief medical officer of the General Hospital asked Tebbutt to keep Lady Wood out of her son's room as much as possible because he became worse 'under her fidgety attendance.' Those doctors who were still in Scutari and who knew Dawson's work said that if anything she was too attentive rather than the reverse.[50]

Nightingale's assessment of Dawson gives us a picture of another kind of first class hospital nurse, one who was very different from

The naval hospital at Therapia

Elizabeth Drake. She thought Dawson had probably not been respectful enough to Lady Wood but considered her an excellent nurse, though severely flawed by her lack of propriety. She called her a thorough humbug, 'full of fine words, much cry & little wool.'[51] 'My own opinion of Dawson is this,' she told Lady Cranworth:

> that she has somehow fallen from a higher position in the world by her own fault – that she is under a deep sense of injury from some cause unknown,– that her manner is bitter, disrespectful, provoking to all the female world,– that she flirts undeniably with Officers,– & that she would not be sorry to amend her position that way,– that she does not wish (for some unknown reason) to return home,– that she makes favourites among her Patients, & those who do not like her she does not like,– that she forgot that Lady Wood was the young man's mother, but otherwise did not behave improperly, i.e. in disobedience to Medical orders, to that Patient,– that she is one of the best nurses I ever had but that I would never engage her again for the above-mentioned reasons – & because, at the Palace Hospital, she was used to be a kind of companion to the sick Officers.[52]

Lady Wood claimed Dawson dressed Wood's bedsores in a crude way, slapped his hands, and treated him roughly when he was delirious. Dawson told Nightingale she had been instructed to keep Wood in bed when he was delirious but he was never delirious after his mother arrived. Dawson had often sponged his hands but never struck him, either on the hand or anywhere else. She had often put his hands under the bed covers but never in an impatient way. She did his dressings infrequently (because after December 1854 the dressers were supposed to do the dressings) but when she occasionally had to, he never complained that she was doing so in an unpleasant way. Furthermore, Dawson said, he did not have bedsores but rather boils.[53] Lady Wood's motherly care of her son, in the eyes of his doctors and nurses, did not bear out Deas's and Clifford's belief that only women, and especially relatives, could really nurse. However, Deas was certainly correct in noting the better discipline of the nursing team that Mackenzie established, as well as the way she kept 'within her proper province.' She would undoubtedly have agreed with the better discipline and confining herself to housekeeping and nursing care, but she never mentioned smoothing pillows or mollifying the patients' feelings although she certainly thought Dr Davidson needed tactful, if not mollifying, handling. It is noteworthy that the

Doctor-directed nursing

Daughters of Charity who cared for the French and Piedmontese officers reminded them of their mothers and sisters in France, but the officers never characterized the Sisters as motherly. British officers did sometimes portray the working-class nurses as motherly. For example, when Langston's team arrived in Balaclava in January 1854 Calthorpe said that none of the nurses were young, 'all rather fat and motherly-looking women, and [they] quite come up to one's idea of orthodox nurses.'[54]

By mid-October Mackenzie had sixteen competent male orderlies as well as her female nurses. Four seamen did the cooking and she had marines doing the washing and ironing.[55] Nightingale imported washing machines and set up a separate paid laundry service in a Turkish washing-house in Scutari; she later established the same system in Koulali and Balaclava.[56] Mackenzie, however, used what was at hand. The greater resourcefulness the sailors developed as a result of living in their all-male wooden world also forced them to cross traditional gendered boundaries. Sailors and marines had to do their own sewing and laundry on shipboard, so when Mackenzie asked them to take over the laundry it was something they were used to doing. When in May two nurses went home sick their absence made Davidson realize how much the hospital had come to depend on them.[57]

Who were the nurses who helped Mackenzie achieve such excellent results? We have almost no information about the working-class nurses other than that there were three Devonshire Square Sisters among them,[58] and Mackenzie said they were respectable but indulged in violent rows and absurdities. However, we do know a little about three lady nurses who worked with Mackenzie: Miss Gertrude Vesey,[59] Miss Bartlett, and the Honorable Harriet Erskine. Vesey and Bartlett arrived together with Mackenzie on 10 January 1855. Erskine was one of the Anglican Sisters who went to Scutari with Nightingale in October 1854 and who accompanied Langston home in April. Nightingale commented later that Erskine was 'one of the best of the Lady Nurses. She was at Therapia with Dr & Mrs Mackenzie all good people. The naval hospital having been always well managed,' but Nightingale realistically added, 'The trial there was less.'[60] Erskine left the East with Langston on 27 April 1855, so she could not have joined Mackenzie's team any earlier than May 1855. Bartlett was a St. John's

The naval hospital at Therapia

House Sister, not one of their working-class nurses, and the Sister to whom Elizabeth Drake bequeathed a jar for flowers. She joined St. John's House on 28 March 1855 and was made a Sister on 8 May. She then worked at the Westminster Hospital until she went to Therapia. She volunteered for the navy in December as did Vesey, a volunteer lady who was at St. John's House for the required brief training.[61] Bartlett left Therapia and returned to St. John's House on 15 May, probably one of the two nurses who were invalided home making Davidson realize how much they contributed. On 24 July 1855 she asked, and was given permission, to return to the East.[62]

We know nothing about what Vesey had done before volunteering for the East but she apparently worked out well because she later wrote to Nightingale saying that Erskine had told her Nightingale would like her to become a Sister at St. John's House. Vesey was very flattered that Nightingale remembered her work in the East, but she had an older sister whom she could not leave on a permanent basis. She had spoken with Lady Superintendent Mary Jones, who suggested that she come as an associate sister, which she had agreed to do because associate sisters were only required to work at King's College Hospital occasionally and then only for a few weeks at a time.[63] Eliza Mackenzie was invalided home utterly exhausted and unwell in November 1855. The officers, seamen, and marines gave her a silver tea service 'in token of their Gratitude for her unwearied attention to their sick and wounded Comrades in Therapia.'[64] Erskine then took Mackenzie's place as lady superintendent. Unlike Florence Nightingale, these three ladies were never lionized. The British press said almost nothing about the successes of the ladies in the other hospitals, while its coverage of naval affairs tended to concentrate on the Baltic naval campaigns rather than the Black Sea fleet. Undoubtedly it was also partly because Nightingale was especially interesting since she came from the top ranks of society while the other lady nurses, with the exception of Jane Shaw Stewart, did not.

At the same time, although she was eminently successful, as Nightingale pointed out, Mackenzie had a far less complex challenge and she was also fortunate in her lady assistants. Vesey worked out well and both Erskine and Bartlett were trained, clinically experienced nurses. Bartlett was trained in the modern style and had eight months' experience at a distinguished teaching hospital and

Doctor-directed nursing

Erskine had the advantage of almost six months of military nursing experience when she arrived in Therapia. Both were also religiously committed to nursing. Mackenzie never had to face problems such as the incompetence or insubordination of Salisbury, Clough, Wear, Stanley, or Mother Francis Bridgeman. She also benefitted from arriving in the East two months after Nightingale, when the supply system was rapidly improving. Furthermore, Deas and Davidson had sought better nurses so she did not meet the kind of stubborn resistance that Sir John Hall and some of his doctors exhibited. Rater Deas and Davidson welcomed her, and Davidson praised the female nurses for the way they never shirked from any duty.[65] Mackenzie was in charge of one hospital with a capacity at its peak of only 159 beds (although at one point they had to accept more patients) while Nightingale had to deal with thousands of patients in hospitals some of which were hundreds of miles apart.

These were all significant advantages, but the greatest advantage Mackenzie enjoyed was the superior underlying health status of the navy's men. Now called the social determinants of health, these are currently thought to be responsible for 85 percent of good health. In proportion to its numbers the Naval Brigade suffered more wounds than the soldiers and, with the important exception of scurvy, were smitten by all the same diseases, but they recovered more quickly because the navy provided better determinants of health: the superior diet, accommodation, workloads, and the general support that their officers gave them. Even so, introducing a new, modern nursing service into an old dilapidated building served by a dismal naval transport service was not an easy job; Mackenzie worked so hard that she was forced to retire before the end of the war because her health broke down.

The sailors who survived the 18 June assault recovered quickly. By the end of July only thirty-nine of the Naval Brigade's 1,295 men were on the sick list but in August the hospital began filling again with bowel disease, fevers, and rheumatism. A week after the fall of Sevastopol, on 15 September 1855, the Naval Brigade was broken up.[66] The Therapia hospital continued for another nine months, closing in June 1856, about the same time as the army hospitals. It had served its purpose well. Mackenzie and Erskine provided good nursing, and of 230 operations performed, all using chloroform although sometimes

The supply ran out during longer operations, only twenty-two proved fatal.[67] In comparison with the Ottoman hospitals the naval hospital demonstrates clearly the complex components required for better patient outcomes: adequate funding, training and experience for the nurses and doctors, and good determinants of health for the patients. The horrible fate of the Ottoman soldiers was a direct result of an incompetent and bankrupt government which tolerated graft and peculation and provided almost nothing in terms of support for its soldiers.

Notes

1 Lambert, *Grand Strategy*, p. 12; Duckers, *Crimean War at Sea*, pp. xiv–xv.
2 Rodger, *Wooden World*, p. 486.
3 Ibid, pp. 35–6, 86–7, 99, 105; McLean, *Surgeons*, pp. xii, 1, 3, 10–11.
4 Lloyd and Coulter, *Medicine and the Navy*, vol. 4, p. 61; Lewis, *Navy in Transition*, pp. 259–60.
5 Shepherd, *Crimean Doctors*, vol. 1, pp. 21–2.
6 Brooks, *Long Arm*, pp. 3–4; *Medical Chronicle* (1855) Vol. 1, No. 9, pp. 372–3.
7 Taylor, *Journal*, vol. 1, pp. 133–4.
8 Robinson, *Diary*, pp. 109–10, 173–5, 196–7, 232, 242–4.
9 Brooks, *Long Arm*, pp. 3–4, 10–11; Lloyd and Coulter, *Medicine and the Navy*, vol. 4, pp. 144–5.
10 Calthorpe, *Letters from Headquarters*, pp. 100, 113–17; Lloyd and Coulter, *Medicine and the Navy*, vol. 4, pp. 144–5.
11 Bushby, *Camp Before Sebastopol*, p. 107.
12 Wood, *Crimea in 1854*, pp. 78–81; Beckett, 'Wood, Sir (Henry) Evelyn.'
13 There were four major bombardments of Sevastopol: the first beginning on 17 October 1854, the second on 10 April 1855, the third on 6 June, and the fourth on 6 September 1855.
14 Clifford, *Letters*, p. 201.
15 Brooks, *Long Arm*, p. 21; Wood, *Crimea in 1854*, pp. 252–3; Calthorpe, *Letters from Headquarters*, pp. 258, 285–6.
16 Hodasevich, *Within Sevastopol*, p. 87.
17 Wood, *Crimea in 1854*, pp. 88, 173, 193.
18 Clifford, *Letters*, pp. 234, 243.
19 Montaudon, *Souvenirs*, pp. 63–5, 230.
20 Clifford, *Letters*, pp. 132, 253–4, 257–8.
21 Wood, *Crimea in 1854*, pp. 187–8.
22 Ibid, pp. 78–81, 187–8, 217–21; Steevens, *Crimean Campaign*, pp. 153–4;

Doctor-directed nursing

Calthorpe, *Letters from Headquarters*, p. 235; Stuart, *Beloved Little Admiral*, p. 158.

23 Wood, *Crimea in 1854*, pp. 202–3.

24 Brooks, *Long Arm*, pp. 22–3, 26.

25 Wood, *Crimea in 1854*, pp. 217–21. These figures are cited in numerous secondary sources and seem to have originated with Wood. He does not give his source.

26 Baumgart, *Crimean War*, pp. 215–16.

27 Lloyd and Coulter, *Medicine and the Navy*, vol. 4, pp. 147–9.

28 McLean, *Surgeons*, p. 173.

29 Lloyd and Coulter, *Medicine and the Navy*, vol. 4, pp. 147–9; Penney, 'Letters from Therapia,' p. 414; McLean, *Surgeons*, pp. 161–3; Shepherd, *Crimean Doctors*, vol. 2, pp. 492–3.

30 McLean, *Surgeons*, 161–4, 168–73.

31 Laughton, 'Boxer.'

32 Duberly, *Mrs Duberly's War*, pp. 144, 147, 175, 188.

33 McLean, *Surgeons*, pp. 161–4, 186–7.

34 Different sources give different figures. Shepherd and Penney say that there were twenty-three naval ratings (Shepherd, *Crimean Doctors*, vol. 2, pp. 494–5; Penney, 'Letters from Therapia,' p. 414). Penney says fourteen Maltese arrived. It is probable that they counted people under different headings – that twenty-three sailors staffed the hospital, six of whom were nurses and the others were guards, clerks etc.

35 McLean, *Surgeons*, pp. 161–5.

36 Lloyd and Coulter, *Medicine and the Navy*, vol. 4, pp. 148–9.

37 Penney, 'Letters from Therapia,' pp. 415–16; Taylor, *Sea Chaplains*, p. 384; Taylor, *Eastern Hospitals*, vol. 1, pp. 9–10.

38 Lloyd and Coulter, *Medicine and the Navy*, vol. 4, pp. 148–9.

39 Penney, 'Letters from Therapia,' pp. 415–17, 420.

40 McLean, *Surgeons*, p. 173.

41 Penney, 'Letters from Therapia,' p. 418.

42 Clifford, *Letters*, p. 217.

43 McLean, *Surgeons*, pp. 165, 171–4, 186–7.

44 Wood, *Crimea in 1854*, pp. 290, 295, 318.

45 I have not found any information about these ladies. It is not clear whether 'resident' means the two sisters were residents of the town of Therapia or that they were residing in the hospital. The former seems more likely.

46 Wood, *Midshipman*, pp. 99–101, 107–9.

47 BL 43397, Nightingale to LeFroy, 11 January 1856, fol. 209; Lawson, *Surgeon in the Crimea*, pp. 179–80.

48 Wood, *Midshipman*, pp. 2, 107–9.

49 BL 43397, Nightingale to Lady Cranworth, 26 June 1856, fols 27–9.

50 BL 43404, Nightingale to Lady Cranworth, 17 July, fols 133–4.

The naval hospital at Therapia

51 BL 43404, Nightingale Report No. I, May 1856, fols 6–7.
52 BL 43404, Nightingale to Lady Cranworth, 17 July, fol. 134. Dawson had originally been a nurse at the Palace Hospital for officers. It closed in November 1855 and she then transferred to Scutari.
53 BL 43397, Dawson's statement, 15 July 1856, fol. 29.
54 Calthorpe, *Letters from Headquarters*, p. 235.
55 McLean, *Surgeons*, p. 191; Penney, 'Letters from Therapia,' p. 419.
56 BL 43393, Nightingale to Herbert, 28 December 1854, fol. 57; 19 February 1855, fol. 170; 22 February 1855, fol. 174.
57 McLean, *Surgeons*, pp. 189–91.
58 WI/SA/QNI/W2/4, Minutes of Committee, 20 October 1854, 9 February 1855, 25 April, 29 August 1856.
59 Vesey is alternatively spelled Vesie.
60 WI Ms 9030, Nightingale note on letter from Erskine, 29 May 1857, Letter 5.
61 LMA/H01/ST/SJ/A20/3, Lady Superintendent's Diary 1854–57, 28 March, 8 May, 5 and 25 November, 5 and 21 December 1854.
62 LMA/H01/ST/SJ/A20/3, Lady Superintendent's Diary 1854–57, 15 May and 24 July 1855.
63 LMA/H01/ST/NC2/V17/57, Vesey to Nightingale, 10 March 1857.
64 Penney, 'Letters from Therapia', p. 421.
65 Lloyd and Coulter, *Medicine and the Navy*, vol. 4, pp. 148–9.
66 McLean, *Surgeons*, pp. 189–90, 192–3.
67 Lloyd and Coulter, *Medicine and the Navy*, vol. 4, pp. 148–9.

11

The civilian hospitals

Introduction

Anticipating a campaign in the spring and summer of 1855 and hence many more casualties, the War Department realized the medical department needed more doctors. Given the outcry over poor medical care, the government decided to recruit experienced civilian doctors rather than commissioning newly graduated surgeons. The civilian doctors would run their own hospitals and have complete control over the female nurses. Two civilian hospitals were established in Turkey, the first in Smyrna and the second in Renkioi. Unfortunately, we do not have as many sources for these two hospitals as we do for the military hospitals. The Register of Nurses refers us to reports from the lady superintendents in Smyrna and Renkioi but those reports have not survived. George Macleod, who worked in the Smyrna hospital, wrote a book on the surgery of the war; we have a few letters from Henrietta LeMesurier, the second lady superintendent; and one of the lady nurses, Martha Nicol, wrote a book describing her experiences there. For Renkioi Edward A. Parkes, the doctor in charge, wrote a short account of its establishment and management, but otherwise there are only brief references here and there making up the primary sources for these two hospitals. Nevertheless, if more incomplete than the sources for the other hospitals, these documents do contain considerable and important information about the nursing there.

The War Department sent requests to hospitals throughout Britain asking for volunteer doctors. In order to attract more senior men it paid the civilians at a much higher rate than the army doctors, causing much discontent among them. More than 500 surgeons

The civilian hospitals

applied. Herbert and the Duke of Newcastle were well aware of the resistance that the proposed civilian hospital would incite among the army doctors. 'It will be necessary in spite of all opposition and all professional feeling to the contrary,' Newcastle told the House of Lords, 'to introduce into the army hospitals the civil element.' Andrew Smith and Hall had to accept this political decision despite the angry outcry from their staff. Hall took the introduction of civilians to mean that the War Department considered the military doctors incompetent and was therefore antagonistic to the project, later making many bitter comments about it. He pointed out that he himself, as chief doctor of the field army with forty years of service in every quarter of the globe, made only £1,200 a year while the top civilian doctors made up to £1,000 with a bonus to cover the loss from private practice fees. He also deeply resented the generous resources the government provided for the civilian hospitals which he felt, with some justification, it denied to the military hospitals.[1]

The hospital in Smyrna

The Smyrna hospital opened at the beginning of 1855 in a former Turkish army barrack. It suffered from all the same problems as the Barrack Hospital in Scutari – poor and usually blocked drains, little ventilation, inadequate and contaminated water supply, and hideous infestations of rats and fleas. It was situated on the waterfront, below the hill on which the town was built; the municipal open sewers flowed down the slope towards and sometimes through the building's ground floor. Worse still, Smyrna was some 600 miles as the crow flies from Sevastopol, and further by the sea route. However, it was the only building the Ottoman government had to offer. It did have one advantage over the Barrack Hospital: it was not used as a depot for soldiers as well as a hospital. In early March Hall sent a small staff of military doctors to open the hospital. The government placed Dr Meyer in charge who, having chaperoned Mary Stanley's group of nurses to the East, was in Scutari. Macleod acted as chief doctor until Meyer arrived; then he became head surgeon in Martha Nicol's division. She found his way of working prompt and businesslike and regretted his absence when he was sick with typhus. Macleod and the civilian doctors took charge in the second week of March 1855. The hospital was packed with about 800 patients in grossly overcrowded and chaotic conditions. There were relatively few wounded; rather, most had fever of the worst kind – spotted typhus – and some had frostbite, bedsores, dysentery, and chest complaints; many were dying, and of course all were alive with vermin.[2]

A party of twenty lady nurses and twenty-two paid nurses[3] left England for Smyrna on 3 March 1855 and started work in the hospital on 20 March.[4] Of the twenty ladies, only nine stayed for the whole time – four were fired, two invalided home, one died, and four left for other reasons. The working-class nurses did better. Of twenty-two, sixteen remained at the end of the war, four were invalided home, one was fired, and one died. On 31 March the hospital had admitted 993 patients of whom 127 died, a mortality rate almost as high as that at Scutari in its worst days. However, the new medical staff immediately began establishing order. They evacuated the unhealthy ground floor and began segregating contagious cases.[5] As in Scutari, many doctors at first resisted the new female nurses but all the doctors soon found them extremely useful. In winning the doctors' trust the ladies in the civilian hospitals had two major advantages over Nightingale: namely that they were not there trying to establish a permanent female nursing service in the army, one of Nightingale's overall goals; and civilian doctors were used to working with female, although not lady nurses in the hospitals at home. It may also be that because these ladies did not come from such an elevated level of society as Nightingale, the doctors found them less intimidating. Also the ladies did not have direct access to the War Department as Nightingale did, so they presented no threat to the doctors.

As in all the Crimean War armies, nurses, doctors, and orderlies all contracted the fevers the patients suffered. Illness among the staff was so prevalent in large part because public hygiene in Turkey was abominable. The Turks made absolutely no effort to bury dead horses, oxen, donkeys, or dogs; they left them where they died either to decay or be eaten by dogs and jackals. There were stagnant pools of refuse and carrion of all descriptions everywhere in the town. The drains were never cleaned. Fleas were omnipresent; every room in the house in Smyrna where the lady nurses eventually moved was infested with them, including the dining room, where they hopped about on the food and in the ladies' wine glasses.[6] Many of the ladies simply were

The civilian hospitals

not up to these unpleasant living conditions as well as the very hard physical work of nursing the soldiers. Typhus first broke out in one small room into which six working-class nurses had been packed, confirming the belief that overcrowding caused typhus. At one point six nurses were acutely ill, and when a nurse became ill another nurse had to be taken off the wards to care for her, resulting in even fewer nurses available for work. One working-class nurse, Mrs Payne, and one lady nurse, Drusilla Smythe, died of typhus, as did two orderlies. After contracting typhus Miss Aplin never regained her health and had to be sent home. Miss Osborne stayed until the hospital closed but was ill off and on the whole time.[7]

Nurse Payne was a 34 year old woman who had been a servant of Mrs Coote, the first lady superintendent at Smyrna. Payne had no hospital experience; she had worked for Mrs Coote's mother from the time she was 20 years old. When Mrs Coote was married, her mother sent Payne to the newlyweds' household as the cook and housekeeper. In Smyrna Payne worked as a nurse, another illustration of Dr Steele's point that people did not distinguish between nurses and domestic servants until after the Crimean War. Mrs Coote and her husband, Holmes Coote, a St. Bartholomew's Hospital surgeon, were living in a hotel when Coote was smitten with cholera. Dr Meyer sent Payne to nurse him. She had been feeling unwell for several days but had not mentioned this to anyone. At the hotel she was struck by cholera at 3 a.m. and died twelve hours later. At 7:30 a.m. when they heard Payne was ill, lady nurse Charlotte LeMesurier and Mrs Hely, one of the best working-class nurses, went to attend her. They spent their whole time with her constantly rubbing her in a vain effort to relieve the horrible muscle spasms of cholera. They were utterly exhausted from the continuous massaging when they returned to the nurses' home later that afternoon.[8] Payne was a stout, hearty woman, whose sudden death brought home to both lady and hospital nurses the deadly risks of their work.

After the first influx of patients in March it became clear that Hall had no intention of making good use of the new civilian hospital. He sent fewer and fewer patients, so that by the summer there was very little work for the staff. At the end of June four of the hospital's eight divisions were closed and the remaining four were only half filled through the early fall. Many nurses were almost unemployed. Seven

227

Doctor-directed nursing

ladies applied to Nightingale asking to be transferred to Scutari, Koulali, or anywhere they could be used, but Nightingale said she had no openings for ladies. Some ladies then thought of going home but decided to stay when they were told more sick would be coming. When Mr Coote went to Renkioi in June Mrs Coote went with him, so only eight of the original twenty ladies were left and all eight felt rather useless. The doctors felt the same way. Three doctors transferred to Balaclava; two went home in charge of invalids, and one did not return while the other came back but went to Balaclava.[9] Other doctors accepted local patients. Still others entertained themselves by going on excursions about the countryside, and forming the Smyrna Medico-Chirurgical Society, where they gave weekly papers. Interestingly, at a paper discussing whether Smyrna was a healthy site for a hospital, Mr Holmes Coote argued that it compared very favorably with the average London hospital.[10]

When Mrs Coote left, the elder of the two LeMesurier sisters, Henrietta, took over as lady superintendent.[11] The two LeMesuriers may well have been sisters or otherwise related to the Dr LeMesurier who was attached to the Turkish Contingent in Balaclava,[12] and that may be why Henrietta was chosen to succeed Coote. Coming from a professional family, and especially a medical one, was considered a good qualification for a nurse,[13] which is probably also why Elizabeth Herbert chose Mrs Coote as lady superintendent. On taking up her new position Henrietta LeMesurier feared she would have no easy job. When Mary Stanley's party left for the East Sidney Herbert had addressed them, telling them that they were all to be treated equally as hospital nurses.[14] The 'equality system,' as the ladies called it, caused problems of insubordination as well as social pretensions: some of the nurses thought it meant that in the East as well as all being treated as hospital nurses, they would also all have the social status of ladies.[15] The problem started as soon as Stanley's party landed in Turkey. When the ladies asked the nurses to do the housework in Therapia they responded by saying they had come out to nurse the soldiers, not to sweep, wash, and cook. One nurse refused to do any housework at all, and those who did, did so with an air of condescension. The problem continued at Koulali. We soon discontinued the hospital uniform, Fanny Taylor, a lady nurse, explained, because it was impossible to wear the same dress as the working-class nurses.

The civilian hospitals

'The ladies soon found,' she wrote, 'it was necessary for their own comfort and for the good of their work that in every possible way the distinction [between the social classes] should be drawn.' Taylor then went on to explain, no doubt influenced by Bridgeman whom she very much admired, 'None but those who knew it can imagine the wearing anxiety and the bitter humiliation the charge of the hired nurses brought upon us.'[16]

When the ladies in Smyrna moved from their cramped quarters in the hospital to their own house in May, they asked the nurses for volunteers to come and do their housework. With the exception of Mrs Gunning and Mrs Suter, all the working-class nurses refused, saying they came out as nurses, not as domestic servants. Working-class nurses were beginning to appreciate their own professional expertise and demanding recognition of it, but the ladies still considered them domestic servants. Suter was an excellent cook who 'thoroughly knew her place' while Gunning worked as the household servant. Furthermore, both Gunning and Suter infinitely preferred doing domestic work because they enjoyed the peace and quiet in the ladies' house as opposed to what Nicol called the brawling, quarrelling, and petty jealousies of the paid nurses who remained in the overcrowded hospital quarters. Later some working-class nurses changed their minds about doing housework because they realized that it was better for their health to get away for short periods from the noxious air of the hospital. In addition to Suter and Gunning, the ladies had an orderly who worked as a manservant and a Greek girl to help Gunning with the housework.

Despite these social problems, the ladies in Smyrna generally had better relationships with the working-class nurses than did the ladies in Nightingale's hospitals. Some of the paid nurses did behave very badly – so much so that Dr Meyer ordered that they were not to go out unless they were under the care of the matron. Still, Nicol said there were many nurses who were too sensible to think they were ladies, and many worked very hard and supported the ladies in every way they could. The Smyrna ladies did not completely do away with the uniform because they thought it helped differentiate the nurses from other women, but they deplored ladies wearing the same uniform as the nurses and washerwomen. The regulation uniform consisted of a dress with a sash embroidered with the name of the hospital worn across the shoulder.

Doctor-directed nursing

To distinguish themselves from the paid nurses, the ladies wore the regulation dress but without the sash.[17] When LeMesurier took over as superintendent there was so little work to do that all the nurses, both lady and working-class, were restless and full of complaints. Nevertheless, LeMesurier thought there was 'sterling principle' among both classes of nurses. She thought if there were more work they would all soon be doing much better, which indeed turned out to be the case.

Henrietta LeMesurier also believed that Nightingale's friend Elizabeth Herbert, who selected all the nurses for Smyrna, had absolutely no business sense. First of all, she sent as many ladies as working-class nurses when it was obvious that only women used to hard work were suitable for what is now called direct nursing care, the physical care of the patients. Second, like Nightingale, LeMesurier thought it very difficult to determine the character and capabilities of a nurse in one interview, but she said Herbert had made no greater mistake than appointing Mrs Coote as lady superintendent. No one could look at her twice without seeing that she would be incompetent. There had been all kinds of disorder and difficulties under her direction and LeMesurier thought it a wonder that there had not been seven times more.[18] It is notable that Coote did not dismiss any nurses in the three months she was in charge, while LeMesurier dismissed five, four of whom were ladies. Nightingale, as we have seen, found it difficult to dismiss ladies and would write two years after the war that one of the reasons she hesitated to include ladies in an ideal nursing workforce was that 'Their dismissal (like those of [religious] Sisters must always be more troublesome, if not more difficult than that of the other nurses.'[19] However, LeMesurier had no qualms about firing troublesome ladies. Miss Tomlinson was insane, Miss Jackson was 'perfectly unsuitable,' and Miss Winthrop was a mischievous person who spread evil reports. The ladies in London must have had high hopes for the fourth dismissed lady, Mrs Brereton, who was an officer's widow and the daughter of a doctor, because she was paid a full pound a week rather than the standard eighteen shillings for ladies. However, LeMesurier found 'a great want of discretion and most discreditable disorder in her preliminary transactions,' whatever that might mean, and fired her in September. The fifth nurse, Mrs Butler, an experienced working-class nurse from St. Bartholomew's Hospital Accident Ward, LeMesurier dismissed for misconduct.[20]

The civilian hospitals

The eight divisions of the Smyrna hospital ranged in size from 60 to 125 patients depending on how busy the hospital was. A head doctor and two assistant physicians or surgeons, two lady nurses, two working-class nurses, and a ward master were assigned to each division. There was one orderly for every ten to twelve patients and also two Greeks who came in to do the scrubbing.[21] Army regulations prescribed one orderly for every ten patients in the hospitals and one for every twenty-five on the transports but there were frequently fewer, and of those few Macleod considered many utterly unfit for their jobs. Nor did he like the civilian orderlies he met. He thought that, unlike the French soldier nurses, they lacked military spirit and discipline and the soldiers despised them. Macleod used a higher proportion of orderlies in his division, two orderlies to sixteen beds. Each was responsible for eight patients; one was designated the diet orderly and the other the medicine orderly. The diet orderly brought the food from the kitchen and distributed it to the sixteen men while the medicine orderly collected the medicines from the apothecary, distributed them, and had charge of the dressings.[22] The chief of the two lady nurses in each division was responsible for supervising the nurses, orderlies, and ward masters, and for the linen and utensils. She was to notify the medical officer of any sudden change in a patient, see that meals were served on time, and she always supervised the orderlies when they apportioned the food. As in Scutari and Koulali, the ladies gave no extras without a doctor's order. They also ensured that the ticket at the head of each patient's bed was up-to-date and formed an accurate record of the treatment given. The first lady only left her wards when the second lady nurse was there. The second lady nurse cared personally for the critically ill men and she, rather than the orderlies, gave them their medicines and drinks. The working-class nurses monitored the less acutely ill patients for changes for the worse and gave them their medicines, wine, and drinks.[23] Nicol gave some examples of the orders she received from the doctors that illustrate how dependent on clothing, feeding, and fluids medical treatment and nursing care were in the mid-1850s. They also indicate how little authority of their own these lady nurses had as compared to the Daughters of Charity and Sisters of Mercy. For example, 'Walker: shirt and sheets; Graney: shirt and flannel; Curran: shirt and flannel; McKane: flannel and socks; Smith: boiled rice for dinner; Fletcher:

Doctor-directed nursing

two eggs at different times; Cermody: discontinue medicine; Barber: egg flip.'[24]

As in all the hospitals, the Smyrna nurses' most difficult task was managing the frostbite cases. Giving stimulants and nourishment to utterly prostrated fever patients was also especially trying. These patients were always unwilling to be roused from their semi-comatose state to eat or drink. But without intravenous therapy the only way to rehydrate the low fever patients was to pour 'restoratives,' down their throats every five to ten minutes. When one of Nicol's best orderlies fell ill and was in this stage of fever he was just barely able to swallow and groaned each time he did. Nevertheless, the night nurse and her orderly succeeded in getting him to take almost a whole bottle of brandy by morning. Somewhat surprisingly, despite what would seem to us this counter-productive treatment, he recovered.[25]

We tend to forget in our day of antibiotics how much higher and longer lasting fevers were and how much lengthier the convalescence was. Robert James Graves, the great Irish clinician, told his students that they must expect fevers to last fifteen or twenty-one days or even more. The fevers were so high that nearly all patients became delirious, or as Graves put it, 'in a state analogous to insanity.' He emphasized the importance of a highly qualified nurse for these patients. He himself refused to attend any private case of dangerous, protracted fever unless the family was prepared to hire such a nurse.[26] Nightingale herself provides an illustration of how lengthy recovery from fever was at that time. On her first visit to Balaclava she was stricken with Crimean Fever on 13 May 1855. As was typical, she became delirious and hallucinated. Twelve days later, on 25 May, she was pronounced out of danger but remained unable to feed herself or to speak above a whisper. She returned to Scutari on 5 June, twenty-three days after collapsing, but was so weak she had to be carried from the ship to the house on a stretcher. Together with Mrs Roberts she went, still by stretcher, to convalesce in the naval hospital in Therapia, where she and Roberts had a whole ward to themselves. She returned to Scutari on 5 July, feeling much stronger but looking much older and unable to stand for any length of time. Nightingale believed, with good reason, it was Roberts's nursing which had saved her life.[27]

The Smyrna ladies worked just as well with their orderlies as they did with the working-class nurses. Nicol had complete confidence in

The civilian hospitals

her hospital nurses and reported that she had a good ward master and four of her orderlies were excellent, steady, hard-working men whom she called 'capital assistants.' The ladies also used convalescents as orderlies. As Nightingale had petitioned Raglan, they petitioned General Storks to let them keep the men who were especially good at this job rather than sending them back to the front. Storks and Dr Meyer got on well and Storks was always helpful.[28] Friendlier relations with the military authorities made it much easier to deliver good nursing care, as did basic resources such as adequate staffing, food, clothing, bedding and so on, but successful nursing care required knowledge and experience as Graves indicated.

After the fall of Sevastopol in September some of the ladies again thought of returning home. One lady, Miss Écuyer, applied a second time to Nightingale who this time accepted her, appointing her matron of the Scutari General Hospital. In October sixty-one patients arrived and at the end of the month another 161 were landed with no advance notice. All the men were received, bathed, clothed, and fed within two hours. Shortly after that 215 more men landed.[29] The nurses' efficiency was partly due to the fact that the hospital was now well organized and had a much higher ratio of staff to patients than in the spring. The Smyrna doctors and lady nurses thought of nursing holistically and now established a small library, which was heavily used. Some of the chaplains, doctors, and lady nurses were good musicians and there was a piano in the chapel. Appreciating how helpful music and games were for the morale of the men, they held regular practising days for the choir and gave the men singing lessons. The hospital was finally running admirably, but just at this point the staff learned that it was to be broken up and turned over to the Swiss Legion for their barracks. All the patients and seven nurses were sent to Renkioi; the last man left on 26 November 1855. The lady nurses all regretted the hospital closing just when it was functioning so well. Col. LeFroy, whom the War Department sent to investigate conditions in the Eastern hospitals, came a second time and said he could hardly believe it was the same hospital he had visited some months previously.[30]

Although at first he had been one of the most outspoken in opposing female nurses, Macleod became a strong proponent of them. Some were injudiciously chosen, he later avowed, but every unprejudiced observer acknowledged that when they were carefully chosen and properly organized the female nurses did vast amounts of good. Like Nightingale, Macleod thought ladies out of place except as superintendents of nurses but he came to consider lady superintendents indispensable. For the ordinary nurses he believed only 'strong, active, respectable *paid* [working-class] nurses' with preliminary training in civilian hospitals at home should be used. There should always be female nurses in the base hospitals, Macleod said, with orderlies doing all the cleaning. The ward master should be responsible to her as well as to the doctors, but in the field hospitals only men should do the nursing. Like Chenu, Macleod considered religious commitment an almost essential qualification for all grades of nurses but thought it could not be relied on alone as the motivation for such an arduous service; hospital nurses must be well paid.[31]

Martha Nicol described her motivation somewhat differently. She was not a paid nurse so the high wage was not an incentive for her as it became for some ladies later in the war. Nor was she religiously motivated; she said she never thought of herself as a kind of Sister of Mercy. Rather she volunteered as a woman 'who had little to do at home, and wished to help our poor soldiers.' She did not think the work the ladies did in the East was any more praiseworthy than the work they did every day at home, but it was easier because it was new and exciting rather than 'the uneventful monotony of daily doing good at home.'[32] This may well have been the case for a number of other unpaid lady volunteers. It was obvious that the ladies who were able to stick it really enjoyed the work and the greater responsibility it placed on their shoulders, as well as the many friends they made. Nicol referred to 'dear old Smyrna' and said it was with great regret that she left it on 1 December 1855. 'We had all spent so many pleasant days there,' she said, and 'from being strangers to each other, we had become interested in one another, and some of us formed friendships which, we hope, will last all our lives, while from the medical men with whom we worked we had always experienced the most gentlemanly courtesy and friendliness.'[33]

The hospital in Renkioi

The sick rate in the army reached its height in February and March 1855, leading the War Department to open a second civilian hospital

The civilian hospitals

to relieve the pressure on Scutari and Smyrna. This second hospital was a great contrast to the Smyrna hospital: it was a purpose-built, state of the art building. Using all the latest sanitary knowledge and equipment Isambard Brunel, most famous for his railways, bridges, and iron ships, drew up the plans in eight days.[34] The War Department placed Dr Edmund Alexander Parkes in complete charge of the hospital. Parkes had had an interesting career and was very distinguished. Immediately after graduating from University College Hospital Medical School in 1841 he enlisted in the army and served three years in India and Burma. He then returned to University College where, at the age of 30, he was made chair of clinical medicine. After the Crimean War he went on to become a founder of the Army Medical School in 1860. He was an expert on public hygiene, and later became famous for his *Manual of Practical Hygiene* written for the army medical department. He was also a skilled administrator, extremely popular, and noted for his gentle character.[35] At Renkioi he never seemed to have any of the disciplinary problems which dogged some of the other hospitals. Brunel consulted closely with Parkes as he drew up his plans. Because the public now appreciated the hardships the soldiers faced and believed they should have good medical care, the two men were able to design a hospital with all the latest comforts. Parkes's primary concerns were a good water supply, ventilation, and proper cooking and laundry facilities.

Parkes arrived in Constantinople on 18 April 1855 and immediately began searching for a suitable location for the hospital. There was not enough space for another hospital in Scutari and he did not have time to personally inspect Sir John Hall's choice of Sinope because Brunel's unassembled prefabricated huts were already at sea on their way to the East. Sinope, though closer to Balaclava, was 350 miles away from Constantinople. Hall became even more cross and bitter when Parkes rejected his choice for the site,[36] but Renkioi met all the requirements of the latest sanitary science. Now called Canakkale, Renkioi was approximately 100 miles[37] west of Scutari but the healthy location seemed more important to Parkes than the inconvenient distance from the other base hospitals. It was also an exceptionally beautiful part of the Dardanelles, overlooking the Sea of Marmara. The prefabricated wooden huts were to be built on a hill where sea breezes would cool them in the hot Turkish summer.

Doctor-directed nursing

There was a pure water supply with excellent drainage which could provide the 25,000 gallons of water per day required by the modern water closets, laundry, bathing facilities, and sewers. *The Times* correspondent was amazed by the water's freshness and abundance. 'In this climate,' he wrote, 'there is really no luxury more highly prized.'[38] The hospital was to consist of 1,000 beds with fifty in each hut. Bed capacity was subsequently expanded to 2,250. The huts provided good cubic footage of air for each patient,[39] and each had a lavatory, water closets with instructions posted on the wall explaining how to use them, bathrooms, and a constant water supply, with sewage carried off down the hill in wooden pipes. The laundry was another state of the art facility. Using Greek washerwomen, a superintendent from one of the London bath houses ran it. The drying closets had a temperature of 400°F which (to use an anachronistic concept) sterilized the bedding and clothing, killing bugs as well as bacteria.[40] Work began on 21 May 1855 and by 12 July six huts were ready to receive patients; when in March 1856 the work was discontinued, the hospital could have accommodated 2,200.[41]

The Renkioi hospital was always underused, partly because of Hall's attitude, but more importantly because by July 1855 the health of the British soldiers was so much better that fewer needed hospitalization. In addition, with the opening of the Castle Hospital in Balaclava there were more beds in the Crimea. Only eleven shiploads of patients arrived in Renkioi, the first not until 2 October 1855 and the last on 11 February 1856. The men were largely casualties from the final assault on 8 September, some convalescent cases from Smyrna when it closed, and some from Scutari.[42] In Scutari, although it was only a five-minute walk from the dock to the Barrack Hospital, it had taken four to five hours to unload the men. This was partly because there were not enough stretchers and the dock was in very poor repair. At least two soldiers drowned trying to get off the ship onto the dock when the sea was rough. Struggling along unaided, many men made their own way up to the hospital. For example, one night as they were returning from their wards Sisters Sarah Anne Terrot and Elizabeth Wheeler met a tall soldier staggering about through the wards crying like a child. He told them he had landed with a number of other patients but could not keep up with them as they walked from the pier to the hospital. He fell behind, lost his way, and when he finally found

The civilian hospitals

the hospital, could not find a bed. The two Sisters took him from ward to ward until they finally located an empty bed.[43] Matters were much better organized in Renkioi. A quarter mile-long railway was built from the pier to the hospital so that when the patients disembarked they were whisked comfortably from the ship to the hospital.

The medical staff visited the wards every morning and evening, and at night a doctor known as the orderly officer went through every ward twice.[44] Four orderlies were assigned to each hut of fifty sick men, slightly fewer than the army regulation proportion of 1:10 but there were now nurses who more than made up the difference. Parkes was very satisfied with his orderly corps. They were not commandeered from the soldiers but consisted of civilians, some men sent from the naval hospital at home in Chatham, and some convalescents. He thought the civilian orderlies well chosen and some of the convalescents proved excellent. Three or four of the convalescent soldiers had a real aptitude for nursing, which Parkes described as feminine sympathy, kindness, and consideration. 'But generally the orderlies,' Parkes wrote, 'no matter how attentive and kind they might be to the sick, were better adapted for the rough work of the wards rather than nursing the patients.' He chose the ward masters and assistant stewards from the civilian orderlies, not the experienced Chatham orderlies. The orderlies took charge of the stores and linen in the wards and did all the cleaning and outdoor work so that the ladies could concentrate entirely on the critical cases and superintendence.[45] Parkes had a total staff of forty-two orderlies, of whom thirty-three were engaged in nursing while nine combined nursing with other duties such as dispensing drugs.[46]

On 23 July 1855 twenty-two working-class women and five lady nurses arrived in Renkioi. These nurses differed from all the other nurses the government sent, in that the doctors, not the ladies in London, recruited them. Lady Superintendent Maria Parkes was Dr Parkes's sister. As in the military hospitals and at Smyrna, there was the same initial resistance to the female nurses among some of the doctors. One young assistant surgeon thought the lady nurses rather a farce. 'The chief thing they have to do,' he said, 'is to look after the wine etc [sic] and prevent the nurses drinking it … I look upon them as a failure for any practical use beside looking after the stock of clothes, wine etc in the ward – call them storekeepers and it would

Doctor-directed nursing

come nearer the mark.'[47] He had a certain point in that storekeeping and maintaining sobriety among the nurses were important parts of the ladies' duties but in fact the lady nurses did a great deal more. Miss Parkes and the matron, Mrs Newman, superintended the nursing department as a whole. The sub-matron, Miss Raynes, and the storekeeper, Miss Griesdale, helped Mrs Newman while Miss Parkes and Miss Frodsham supervised the paid nurses in the various huts. These two ladies spent their whole day moving from one ward to another (each hut of fifty beds was called a ward) seeing that the nurses and orderlies carried out the doctors' orders precisely. Only Parkes and Frodsham administered wine and medical comforts, thus saving, they believed, many lives. They followed doctors' orders accurately and the results, Dr Parkes declared, were excellent.[48] The young surgeon who considered the ladies a farce reported they were neither young nor pretty with the one exception of Maria Parkes whom he considered a lady-like, quick kind of girl but she also was not very young.[49] The ladies in London described her as a pleasant and sensible woman,[50] but apart from this, we know almost nothing personally about this exceptionally able woman who managed her nurses so well. Of the total of thirty-five nurses whom she supervised, the twenty-eight originally sent to Renkioi and the seven who later transferred from Smyrna, she dismissed only three. Only Henrietta LeMesurier, who fired five out of forty-two nurses, seemed able to keep so many of her original staff. Parkes dismissed M. Wilson on 18 September 1855 for disorderly conduct and bad character, and Mary Grey and Marion Hepburn on 29 January 1856 for drunkenness and disorderly conduct. Like Dickens's fictional Sarah Gamp, Mary Grey was a domiciliary nurse, another evidence of the validity of the gamp icon. Only two nurses had to be invalided home, an indication of the superior hygiene in the hospital. Two nurses who had gone to Renkioi when the hospital in Smyrna closed were on contract and went home early when their contracts expired.[51]

Miss Parkes used eight of the twenty-two hospital nurses as needlewomen, servants, or laundresses, a proportionately larger domestic staff than that in Nightingale's hospitals. This suggests that Parkes, like St. John's House, used the remaining nurses exclusively for nursing care. Two of the eight women who did not work with patients had teaching hospital experience. Sarah James was clever

The civilian hospitals

and sober but had a bad temper so Parkes apparently thought she would be better used as a laundress. Mary Viney had some training at the Middlesex Hospital but apparently was not adequately proficient as a nurse so Parkes placed her in the laundry as well. Of the nine who worked as nurses in the wards, two were good nurses but not of sober habits. Both came from prestigious London teaching hospitals, Elizabeth Clarke from University College Hospital where Dr Parkes taught and Mary Ann Reid from St. Bartholomew's. Clarke was a good nurse who understood her job and was attentive in her wards. Reid, whom Dr Parkes had personally recommended, was also industrious in her wards. It is curious that many of the intemperate nurses were recommended by doctors. Were doctors more willing to put up with intemperance, was it simply a case of the nurses' merits outweighing their weakness, or were the doctors unaware of the drinking? Given the paucity of information, it is impossible to know. Of the strictly sober nurses one, Agnes Miller, had been at the Edinburgh Lunatic Asylum for five years and was very sober but 'very slow, almost deficient.' Five of the nine nurses were excellent, sober, industrious, honest, respectable, and trustworthy women.

Miss Parkes also seems to have been more supportive of her staff than some lady superintendents for she reported three, one of whom was a lady nurse, as having made a shaky start but became very good nurses. Anne Newman, also an experienced nurse from the London teaching hospitals, was not quite satisfactory at first because, like Eliza Roberts, she had a quick temper, but she improved, becoming one of the best medical nurses. Caroline Brown, a St. Bartholomew's nurse who was invalided home in April 1856, was another nurse who was not entirely satisfactory at first but changed entirely for the better. The lady nurse, Miss Frodsham, was not steady when she started but became a very good nurse – clever, very kind, and she had good presence of mind. Parkes kept three Scottish nurses, Janet Duncan, Margaret Elmslie, and Agnes Miller, until all the patients had left in July 1856. Margaret Elmslie was an excellent nurse from the Edinburgh Royal Infirmary, sober, honest, industrious, and trustworthy. Janet Duncan and Agnes Miller both came from lunatic asylums and were also excellent nurses.[52] It is a curiosity that a number of first class nurses came from lunatic asylums, because they could not have had the kind of clinical experience in surgical dressings or dealing with all the fever and bowel disease which the general hospital nurses had and yet they did well in the Eastern hospitals.

One of the most striking differences between Nightingale's nurses and the Renkioi nurses was that, of the five lady nurses, Parkes was the only unpaid person. All the ladies in Mary Stanley's party were unpaid, but gradually more ladies who came to the East were paid, and increasingly paid more highly. Mother Francis Bridgeman reported that Amy Hutton, the second superintendent at Koulali, told her Lady Canning said that ladies were no longer volunteering unless they were paid.[53] Nightingale believed the excitement over the nursing mission which the press encouraged was responsible for raising the wages, which she considered too high in some cases. She thought some of the hospital nurses from the original party who started at ten shillings a week were superior to those who were later paid eighteen as a starting salary. She did not express her opinion on the paid lady nurses[54] but one imagines she may have disapproved of them. The Renkioi ladies were paid even better. Miss Frodsham earned the standard lady's wage of eighteen shillings a week or £46/16/- a year. This, with a few exceptions such as Eliza Roberts, was the highest wage that Nightingale paid either lady or hospital nurses. Miss Griesdale received twenty-one shillings a week or £54/12/- a year, and Miss Raynes £1/9/- a week or £75 a year.[55] Sarah Stickney Ellis's sense that ladies gave up their social status if they accepted a wage was losing ground, although obviously it was easier to accept a salary abroad in wartime than it would have been at home in peacetime.

Dr Parkes encouraged the convalescents to get up and start moving as soon as possible. In the winter he issued overcoats to the men so they could go out in the fresh air, and, as in Scutari and Smyrna, provided them with skittles, quoits, bat and ball, drafts and backgammon games. The government paid for most of these, as well as for books and newspapers.[56] Parkes was also very pleased with the female nurses. 'I am certain,' he wrote later, 'that many soldiers received as much anxious attention as the richest man in this metropolis [London] could have purchased, and owed their lives entirely to the devotedness and untiring sympathy of their female attendants.' The system of a small number of ladies superintending the ordinary paid nurses was most satisfactory.[57] There were a few working-class nurses

The civilian hospitals

who were inefficient and disorderly but Parkes attributed this to the fact that he and Sir James Clark[58] personally selected the nurses and had to do it very quickly. Although he remained in London, Clark was deeply involved in planning the hospital together with Parkes.[59]

Woman's mission and innovation in nursing

Nightingale thought placing nurses directly under the control of the doctors unacceptable in a military hospital because the army doctors had no experience with female nurses. 'Bind the *Superintendent* by every tie of signed agreement & of honor to strict obedience to her Medical Chief,' she wrote,

> But let all his orders to the Nurses go through her – I mean, of course, not with regard to the medical management of the Patients, but with regard to the placing & discipline of the Nurses – I have never had the slightest difficulty about this ... I would never have undertaken the Superintendency with that condition that the Nurses consider themselves 'under the direction of the Principal Medical Officer' – *I* am under his direction – *They* are under mine.[60]

But in all three of the British hospitals where doctors directed the nursing – Smyrna, Renkioi, and Therapia – doctor-directed nursing worked well. Nightingale did not hesitate to dismiss hospital nurses but was wary of dismissing ladies, while four of the five nurses LeMesurier dismissed were ladies. Was she less guided by social status than Nightingale, or did the doctors demand their dismissal? There is no way of knowing. Parkes and Meyer did officially report to General Storks but he was usually very helpful and did not interfere with their staffing, budgets, and supplies. Hence they had none of the difficulties with red tape which so impeded Nightingale and the military doctors. In addition, especially at Renkioi, the civilian hospitals were amply supplied and had a larger medical staff with experienced surgeons.

Nicol and her colleagues were quite prepared to accept the hospital nurses' brawling and fighting as a fact of life; they did not feel an obligation to raise their characters. Maria Parkes mentioned the way several nurses had improved in character but she was thinking in terms of a better work ethic and approach to the patients, not in Nightingale's sense of religious and moral character. The lady

Doctor-directed nursing

superintendents in Smyrna and Renkioi saw the advantage of assigning nurses to patient care only, and working-class nurses recognized their professional expertise and defined themselves by their nursing duties; they wanted to leave their origins in domestic service behind. This was true of nurses who had never had anything to do with St. John's House, which originally made a principle of removing all household work from nurses.

These were all innovations but the ideology of woman's mission, which was to so impede the development of nursing, remained very much alive in the British hospitals. British doctors seemed less open to transnational ideas of using soldiers as nurses. Macleod thought that only women could provide the patients with what Kinglake called kindly sympathy. Macleod believed that attention to trivial, apparently insignificant detail and the patience and gentleness which women brought to the sick bed were not to be found in vigorous young soldiers. Although Parkes observed that four of his orderlies had a wonderful aptitude for nursing, he continued to think of devotion, untiring sympathy, and consideration as feminine qualities. By contrast, the French doctors, who worked with both male and female nurses, found both necessary. They were not concerned with the issue of gendered characteristics but rather with who could do the work the best. Scrive spoke of the energy and devotion to their patients of his soldier nurses, and French doctors wanted trained male soldier nurses for the battlefield as well as in the hospitals because of their greater physical strength and their familiarity with the mayhem of battle.

Notes

1 Shepherd, 'Civil Hospitals,' pp. 199–201; Stanmore, *Sidney Herbert*, vol. 1, pp. 367–8; Silver, *Renkioi*, p. 181.
2 Shepherd, 'Civil Hospitals,' p. 201; Nicol, *Ismeer*, p. 33.
3 The Register states twenty-one paid nurses but actually lists twenty-two.
4 LMA/H01/ST/NC8/1, Register of Nurses, pp. 12–18; Shepherd, 'Civil Hospitals,' p. 201; Nicol, *Ismeer*, p. 86.
5 Shepherd, 'Civil Hospitals,' p. 201.
6 Nicol, *Ismeer*, pp. 88, 208–9.
7 Ibid, pp. 45–6, 53–4, 83, 308–9.
8 BU, LeMesurier Papers, H. LeMesurier to M. LeMesurier, 6 July 1855.

The civilian hospitals

9 Nicol, *Ismeer*, pp. 176–7, 210, 261–3.
10 Shepherd, 'Civil Hospitals,' p. 202.
11 Nicol, *Ismeer*, p. 171.
12 Buzzard, *With the Turkish Army*, p. 35; Shepherd, *Crimean Doctors*, vol. 2, p. 432.
13 See for example LMA/H01/ST/NC8/1, pp. 12, 15, 20.
14 Taylor, *Eastern Hospitals*, vol. 2, pp. 12–13.
15 BU, LeMesurier Papers, H. LeMesurier to M. LeMesurier, 6 July 1855.
16 Taylor, *Eastern Hospitals*, vol. 2, pp. 13–14, 36–9.
17 Nicol, *Ismeer*, pp. 85–6, 89–90, 307–11.
18 BU, LeMesurier Papers, Henrietta LeMesurier to her sister Martha, 6 July 1855.
19 Nightingale, 'Introduction of Female Nursing,' p. 8.
20 LMA/H01/ST/NC8/1, Register of Nurses, pp. 12–15.
21 Nicol, *Ismeer*, p. 44.
22 Macleod, *Surgery in the Crimea*, pp. 48, 54fn.
23 Nicol, *Ismeer*, pp. 93–6.
24 Ibid, p. 37. Egg flip was egg, beaten, with water and brandy or rum added.
25 Ibid, pp. 33–5, 61–5.
26 Graves, *Clinical Lectures*, pp. 114–15, 117.
27 WI Ms 8895, Nightingale to Dearest People [her family], 18 June and 5 July 1855, Letters 17 and 21; Bostridge, *Florence Nightingale*, pp. 277–80.
28 Nicol, *Ismeer*, pp. 125, 255, 309, 325.
29 Ibid, pp. 311–12.
30 Ibid, pp. 117, 164–5, 184–5, 336–7.
31 Macleod, *Surgery in the Crimea*, pp. 49–54.
32 Nicol, *Ismeer*, pp. 9–10.
33 Ibid, pp. 339–40.
34 Shepherd, 'Civil Hospitals,' p. 202.
35 Harrison, 'Parkes, Edmund Alexander.'
36 Silver, *Renkioi*, pp. 61, 68–70, 95.
37 On the map Renkioi looks a bit further than 100 miles from Scutari.
38 Silver, *Renkioi*, pp. 68–9, 97, 130.
39 1,000 cubic feet of air per bed was the rule of thumb, but few hospitals in London met this standard.
40 Silver, *Renkioi*, p. 98.
41 Parkes, *Report*, pp. 17–18.
42 Silver, *Renkioi*, pp. 108, 110.
43 *PP* 1854–55, vol. 9, Part I, pp. 283–4, 572; Terrot, *Reminiscences*, pp. 33–4.
44 Silver, *Renkioi*, pp. 92–3, 111.
45 Parkes, *Report*, pp. 31–3.
46 Silver, *Renkioi*, p. 200.
47 Ibid, p. 93.

Doctor-directed nursing

48 Parkes, *Report*, pp. 31–2.
49 Silver, *Renkioi*, p. 132.
50 LMA/H01/ST/NC8/1, Register of Nurses, p. 27.
51 BL 43402, Miss Parkes's Report, fol. 2.
52 LMA/H01/ST/NC8/1, Register of Nurses, pp. 27–30.
53 Bridgeman, 'Account,' p. 220.
54 Leeds Record Office, Canning Papers/177/2/2, Nightingale to Lady Canning, 9 September 1855.
55 LMA/H01/ST/NC8/1, Register of Nurses, p. 27.
56 Silver, *Renkioi*, p. 121.
57 Parkes, *Report*, pp. 31–2.
58 One of London's most distinguished doctors, Physician to the Prince Consort and later to the Queen.
59 Silver, *Renkioi*, pp. 92–3.
60 Leeds Record Office, Canning Papers/177/2/2, Nightingale to Lady Canning, 9 September 1855.

12

Russian nursing:
Pirogov and the Grand Duchess

The Russian army and its medical department

The Russian army as a whole was the largest in the world and enjoyed an international reputation of invincibility. However, many major problems invalidated this perception. First of all, the Russians had no universal draft in the Western European sense of the word because such a system would have destroyed the Russian agrarian economy which was based on serfdom. As soon as they joined the army, serfs became free men and, if they survived the long term of service, they remained free men. When the war forced the government to recruit more serfs it proved a tremendous drain on the agricultural workforce. In January 1856, when negotiating peace terms, the Russians knew that continuing the war would incur national bankruptcy. The four allies had a combined population of 108 million compared with Russia's 65 million, and their combined revenues amounted to three times that of the Russian government. The 800,000-man army that the Russians were maintaining in 1853, even before they began increasing the numbers for the war effort, almost bankrupted the state. 'The military burden,' John Shelton Curtiss wrote, 'was more than the country could afford.'[1]

In Russia's pre-industrial society each regiment had to be economically self-sufficient with its own shoemakers, tailors, blacksmiths, carpenters, metal workers, etc. Nearly all the serfs were illiterate and few knew any skilled trades so the army had to give them time to learn the necessary trades. It was a costly and inefficient system, and meant there was less time for basic military training. However, without skilled craftsmen the army could not have functioned.[2] During the winter the men were not under army discipline. The government gave

245

Doctor-directed nursing

the commandant of each regiment funds and a certain amount of supplies, which he distributed as he wished, but there was a constant shortage and the soldiers usually had to supplement them from what was available in the local countryside. The soldiers were so badly paid and supplied that, to make ends meet, they were allowed to take on outside work, a practice which was open to widespread abuse.[3] Also, Russian commanders accepted a higher rate of loss than any other armed force and the humanizing trends noted in the British and French armies had not yet reached the Russian army. Foreign observers were amazed by the way senior officers struck and publicly threatened junior officers.[4] Discipline was brutal; floggings were a daily event and it was said that there were whole regiments made up of men with wounds inflicted by their own officers.[5] Curtiss devotes a whole chapter in his book on Nicholas I's army to the incredibly brutal way officers treated their men. Flogging, which was far more severe than in the British army, and running the gauntlet were standard punishments. The death rate in Russia was not much higher than in other European countries, thirty-five or thirty-six per thousand, but it was three times as great in the army as for civilians of similar age, a result of the army's organization, economy, and cruel system of training.[6]

'The most modern part of the army was the officer corps,' Geoffrey Best noted, but, he said, foreign observers repeatedly remarked on the contrasts in the officers corps – 'sharper and starker by far than anywhere else: lethargy, ignorance, corruption and incapacity in depressingly large quantity at one end, intelligence, energy and polished cosmopolitan professionalism at the other.' The top military colleges were equal to those in Western countries, but only a minority of officers went through them. About five-sixths of the officer corps was noble, but most came from the minor nobility and many were what J. N. Westwood, one of the classical historians of modern Russia, called dull, spoiled children for whom the army seemed the only suitable employment.[7] Also many officers were promoted from the ranks. Captain Hodasevich, a Russian army officer who was Polish by birth and later deserted to the allies in order to enlist in the Polish Legion, joined his regiment in 1851 when he finished his training as a cadet. To his great disappointment he found all the officers in his company were men promoted from the ranks. They assured him that unless he swore at his men and used his fists he would never be able to establish discipline. Because Hodasevich did not adopt this policy the other officers called him 'the young lady with white hands.'[8]

The infantry was poorly trained and badly equipped while the cavalry was trained for glittering parades and reviews rather than scouting and outpost duties.[9] By contrast, the Russian engineers and artillery were second to none. The artillerists had inferior guns compared to those of the allies but they were very inventive with their poorer equipment. However, artillery and engineering officers had a low social status; they were considered technicians.[10] Tolstoy arrived in the Crimea as a 25 year old artillery officer two days after the Battle of Inkerman, and was one of the last to leave the city when it fell. He visited the hospitals frequently, where he spoke with French as well as Russian patients. He took a dim view of the army and its training. He believed the enemy soldiers were proud of their positions as professional soldiers, had good weapons and the skills to use them, while the Russian soldiers had to undergo 'stupid foot and arm drills, useless weapons, oppression, lack of education, and bad food and maintenance, all of which destroyed the men's last spark of pride, and even gave them too high an opinion of the enemy.'[11]

Historians find it difficult to explain how the Russian soldiers maintained such excellent fighting spirit and élan when they were so brutally trained, so appallingly treated, and so badly officered.[12] Sevastopol was a naval base, and sailors and engineers led the brilliant defence. It may have been partly because the three outstanding leaders were Captain Édouard Totleben, an engineer, Admiral Vladimir Kornilov, and Vice-Admiral Pavel Nakhimov. They used the soldiers and sailors interchangeably and naval officers commanded all but one of the bastions and batteries. These three men were professional military men of the new type, who contrasted strongly with the courtier Prince Menshikov, the supreme commander of the Crimean armed forces.[13]

Pirogov thought the navy did better by its men than did the army[14] and Tolstoy deemed the sailors superior fighters. Tolstoy's three Sevastopol stories, depicting the defenders in December, May, and August, the first two written during the siege and the third immediately afterwards, have fictionalized heroes but Tolstoy's superb observational skills give us a wonderfully accurate and detailed

Doctor-directed nursing

picture of Sevastopol under siege. The narrator of 'Sevastopol in December' notes on his first day in the city that everyone has more respect for the men who work in the Fourth Bastion. More men were killed there and most of the stretcher parties who constantly pass him on the streets are carrying wounded men from this fearsome bastion. The narrator goes to see the bastion for himself and is filled with admiration for the naval men who man it. The officer in command 'walks from one embrasure to another so quietly,' Tolstoy wrote, 'talks to you so calmly and without affectation, that in spite of the bullets whizzing around you oftener than before, you yourself grow cooler, question him carefully, and listen to his stories.' He shows you some firing. 'Gunner and crew to the cannon,' he orders, and fourteen sailors man a gun. The first shot goes home into the French embrasure and the sailors are thrilled to see two dead soldiers being carried out. The battery commander orders a second and third shot and the French respond, hitting a Russian sailor, tearing part of his chest away.

A stretcher party appears almost instantly. The Russians had first aid stations at every bastion, which explains why the stretcher-bearers got there so quickly. The wounded man lies down on the stretcher on his good side to be taken to the hospital and says with difficulty in a trembling voice, 'Sorry, lads.' One of his comrades puts a cap on his head and then calmly and indifferently returns to his gun. Seeing the narrator's horrified face, the naval officer tells him he gets seven or eight similar casualties every day; once he had eleven all at once from one shell.[15] This episode is another illustration of how different military patients are. The sailor, with what was sure to be a mortal wound, is more concerned about leaving his comrades with one less experienced man than about himself. It also shows how efficient the stretcher-bearing teams were, and how disciplined, rather than seemingly indifferent, the wounded man's team-mates were, very much like the British sailors who so impressed Clifford. Still, the sailors may have been even better fighters than the soldiers, but the fact remains that the Russian infantry was noted for its bravery, tenacity, and superb fighting spirit. 'The hardiness and team spirit of Russian soldiers,' Geoffrey Hosking wrote, 'remained as strong as ever under good leadership as the Crimean War demonstrated,' but, he added, 'inferior small arms, an inadequate supply system, and practically

Russian nursing: Pirogov and the Grand Duchess

no communication or industrial structure meant they could not maintain fighting capacity in the long siege.'[16]

The Russian army had many failings but its biggest problem was the widespread corruption that permeated it. It was not as severe as in the Ottoman army but it was crippling. Furthermore, the supply system made it extremely easy for dishonest officers to divert funds into their own pockets. Tolstoy commented in his *Diaries* that it was so easy to steal from the commissariat that 'it was impossible not to steal.'[17] The War Department gave the colonel of each regiment money to buy food and clothing for his men. They often bought the cheapest possible goods and kept the money saved for themselves. Cavalry officers inflated the price of remounts and especially of forage for their horses. The colonel of every regiment kept a special fund in which the soldiers could deposit cash. The Tsar often gave the soldiers money after an exceptionally fine parade or when they were wounded, and many had money they earned working privately. Officers could and did easily misappropriate this money. Even the engineering and artillery branches, the elite of the army, had corrupt officers.[18] 'The common soldier,' Elise Wirtschafter wrote, 'fought to scrape together the most simple necessities in the face of chronic shortages, corrupt or impecunious officers, and the hostility of overburdened civilians [on whom they were billeted in the winter]. The line between abuse and improvisation was permanently blurred.'[19]

The medical department was on a peacetime footing when 6,000 soldiers were wounded at the Alma. It had only 2,000 beds and enough supplies for 2,000 wounded, and a few weeks later the 12,000 casualties at Inkerman threw the department into total chaos.[20] In late October, as in the allied armies, sickness, largely bowel disease, began to increase. Making matters worse, the medical department was one of the worst centers of corruption in the army. Hospitals were usually very clean and gave the impression of being in excellent order, but behind this façade there were many problems. The head of the army medical department was Sir James Villiers, a Scot. He was also personal physician to Nicholas I, and president of the Medical-Surgical Academy in St. Petersburg where Pirogov worked, and where they had many fights. Although he had lived in Russia for over fifty years, Villiers never learned Russian, nor was he interested in military medicine. The chief doctors in the army's medical department were rarely

Doctor-directed nursing

chosen for their knowledge or expertise but obtained their positions by seniority or influence. Many did not even try to visit each of their 200 to 300 patients every day, and many supplemented their income by graft. Assistant doctors neglected their soldier patients to build up private practices. The apothecaries were perhaps the most corrupt of all. They stole drugs and wine or substituted cheaper products for the ones the doctors ordered, and there were also cases of straightforward embezzlement. Profiteering from buying provisions was one of the commonest forms of graft. Hospital administrators padded laundry and food bills and kept non-existent patients on their books so they could draw more money. In addition to all these problems, just as there were always too few military nurses in the French army, there was always an inadequate number of feldshers, the Russian equivalent of modern medics.[21] Baudens compared feldshers to the French dressing soldiers, and the Russian surgeons he spoke with praised their conduct, intelligence, and obedience.[22] There were some excellent feldshers, but they varied in quality and ability and a great many were not reliable. As with the orderlies in the British army, the feldshers would perform better when the Sisters were there to help and supervise them.

On top of all this, there were few experienced surgeons in Sevastopol in the fall of 1854. Recognizing the shortage of doctors, the government rapidly recruited 1,238 new doctors. It gave medical students their degrees one year before their training finished if they would enlist in the army: 824 of the 1,238 were students who had not finished their degrees. Retired men and physicians from the civilian bureaucracy volunteered,[23] while the government advertised for doctors through its diplomatic offices abroad, attracting 114 foreign doctors, mostly Germans and Americans. Hoping to get experienced surgeons, the government paid them better than the Russian army doctors, but the foreign doctors were only a limited success. There were exceptions, but they were mostly young people with little or no experience and, as in the Ottoman medical department, many had dubious qualifications. There was not a single qualified surgeon among them and only a small portion had any training in surgery. They could be useful as helpers in the operating room but, because few spoke Russian and they were unfamiliar with Russian hospital practice and pharmaceuticals, they were not much

Pirogov and the Grand Duchess Elena Pavlovna

The arrival of Pirogov, one of the great nineteenth-century European surgeons, was the beginning of a dramatic change in the dire hospital situation. This brilliant surgeon was born in 1810, the thirteenth of fourteen children of a major in the War Department's supply office. Pirogov's father's income was generous and, being a good accountant and lawyer, he earned additional money in private practice. The family had a spacious house with a small but beautiful garden. Pirogov was sent to private school when he was 11 or 12 but during his two years at school many disasters befell the family. Pirogov's father was completely honest and never took bribes but one of his commissars absconded with 30,000 roubles. Pirogov senior had to repay a significant part of this himself and his whole estate – house, furniture, even clothes – were distrained.[25] He resigned from his job, went into private practice, and withdrew Pirogov from the school he could no longer afford.[26] Soon after, he died unexpectedly of apoplexy. And within a month of his death Pirogov, his mother, and two sisters who were still living at home had to hand over their house and everything in it to the State Treasury and personal creditors. A second cousin of his father kindly took them in for more than a year. Then Pirogov's mother rented an apartment and rented out half of it, two rooms with meals and tea. Pirogov entered medical school at the University of Moscow when he was 14. It took him two hours each way to walk to school so he could not work to help support the family. His mother found it more acceptable to work herself rather than see Pirogov become a state-aided student, which she considered humiliating. After a year her circumstances improved a little and she was able to lease a house and rent rooms to students. She and her two daughters made ends meet, but only with what Pirogov described as a desperate struggle.

Pirogov thought the academic standards at Moscow University backward and superficial. He graduated having never held a lancet in his hand or seen a typhus patient, but he won a four-year scholarship to the University of Dorpat (now Tartu in Estonia) which was then

Doctor-directed nursing

the best university in Russia. While Pirogov was in Dorpat, living conditions for his mother and two sisters improved a bit more. One sister had found a job as a supervisor in a girls' orphanage and the other gave lessons at home.[27] Pirogov's subsequent medical education illustrates how international medicine was at the top levels.[28] After completing his degree in Dorpat, he spent three years in Germany where he visited the leading clinics and attached himself to the Charité Hospital in Berlin. He was not impressed with medical practice in Germany because, he said, it was not based on anatomy and physiology. He described the Charité as a graveyard, a reservoir of filth and putrid infection due to the Germans' lack of understanding of pyemia. 'It is difficult to imagine how little the German doctors and surgeons of those days knew,' he wrote later, 'and how little they were interested in understanding the basic pathological processes.' During his whole time in Berlin, he did not hear one word about purulent infection. It was from the books of the Frenchmen Cruveilhier[29] and Velpeau[30] that he first understood 'the principle of the mechanism of formation of metastatic abscesses after operation and damage to the bones.'[31] Although germ theory was not put forward for another generation, Pirogov had a strong sense that suppurating wounds could spread secondary abscesses throughout the body, that pus was not a necessary part of wound healing, and that healing by first intention was not freakish but desirable and achievable. Pirogov's advanced concept of purulent infection was a major reason why 65 percent of his amputations of the arm were successful. In the case of amputations at the hip, considered the most dangerous and difficult of all amputations, he had a survival rate of 25 percent while the British and French reported only 10 percent.[32]

Although he was only 26 in 1836, Pirogov was appointed Chair of Surgery at Dorpat, and five years later went to the St. Petersburg Military Medical-Surgical Academy as head of surgery. With the exception of three years with the army in the Caucasus, he taught there until he left for the Crimea in 1854. Ether was first used in Europe in London in December 1846; after first trying it on himself, Pirogov began using it on the battlefield in the Caucasus in 1847.[33] He was also the first to use plaster casts in the field. In 1851, while watching a sculptor using plaster on cloth, Pirogov immediately saw its application to surgery. He tried it on a compound fracture of the tibia and found the plaster dried in a few minutes and the wound healed by first intention. Plaster casts also had the advantage of making transportation of soldiers with broken limbs easier.[34] During the Crimean War Pirogov did some of his most brilliant work, including organizing a kind of assembly line surgery and devising an amputation of the foot which left some of the bone in place to provide more support for the leg. When he published his works on field surgery in 1864 they became standard textbooks, earning him an international reputation as the father of field surgery. The principles he set out were widely followed until World War II.[35]

This very distinguished surgeon was horrified by the graft he found in the army when he served in the Caucasus and equally appalled by the corruption in the Academy's 1,000-bed hospital in St. Petersburg. When he accepted the chair of surgery at the Medical-Surgical Academy he looked forward to transforming the hospital into 'a safe place for the sufferer and a Temple of Science,' but found that the staff were very mediocre, corrupt, and largely appointed through nepotism and graft. There were a few exceptions, one of whom was Karl Karlovich Seidlitz who became a close friend.[36] Pirogov's outspokenness about the corruption in the Medical-Surgical Academy made him extremely unpopular with his less honest colleagues. What use is a clever operation or any kind of treatment, he asked, if the patients are then placed in conditions which are not conducive to healing? Certainly Scrive, who had been placed in the same circumstances although for different reasons, would have whole-heartedly agreed with him. Pirogov believed it was the moral duty of the military physician to root out corruption because it caused more damage than epidemics or even medical mistakes. Vicious opposition met his efforts to improve the Academy. Corrupt doctors initiated smear campaigns, bribed patients to claim that he performed operations on them against their will, and there was even an attempt to have him declared insane. The fact that he had the largest and most successful surgical private practice in St. Petersburg increased his colleagues' jealousy. His position became so unpleasant that he finally decided to resign. He wrote to the Board of the Academy:

> I became convinced on many occasions that you rely on the opinion of ignoramuses; on those who are behind the times and hate everything that is beyond their limited understanding. You accept the opinion of those to

Doctor-directed nursing

whom the hospital is merely a soldiers' barracks, the patients annoying subjects, and chloroform and surgical instruments too expensive for hospital economy. Is it possible for one with sense, with honest intentions, with integrity, with devotion to science, to remain a consultant in a hospital degraded by the Physician-in-Chief [Villiers] ...[37]

However, he was convinced to stay.

When fighting on the Danube intensified in the summer of 1854, Pirogov asked for a commission in the army but his requests were repeatedly ignored.[38] A man who openly did his best to prevent illicit medical incomes and redirect the money to patient care, and who described the chief of the army medical department as an ignoramus who degraded the Medical-Surgical Academy, was the last person the many dishonest military doctors wanted in the service. They could not appreciate Pirogov's humanitarianism and integrity; to them he was an *enfant terrible*. Fortunately for the soldiers, Pirogov had a court connection, the Grand Duchess Elena Pavlovna, the widowed sister-in-law of the Tsar. She was a noted philanthropist who was renowned for her salons. Unhappily married and frustrated by the restrictions that her rank and gender imposed, in the 1830s she had begun a series of musical evenings at her home, the magnificent Mikhailovsky Palace. The musical evenings soon extended to scholars and statesmen who shared her interest in philosophy, literature, and politics. By the 1840s her salons had become a center of artistic and intellectual life in St. Petersburg.[39] Later, after the war, she would use her political influence to become instrumental in the emancipation of the serfs. Pirogov met Elena Pavlovna in 1848 when she invited him to her palace to tell her about using ether in the Caucasus. It was she who convinced him to withdraw his resignation from the Medical-Surgical Academy, which he was prepared to do when he knew he had her powerful backing. He helped in the charitable hospital for the poor that she ran, so they had known each other and worked together for six years when he asked for her help in obtaining an army commission.[40]

Inspired by the Russian Orthodox tradition of philanthropy as well as the work of the Daughters of Charity in the French military hospitals, in September 1854 the Grand Duchess began trying to organize a nursing sisterhood for the Russian army. There was a precedent for this kind of nursing in Russia. In 1803 the Dowager

Russian nursing: Pirogov and the Grand Duchess

Empress Maria Federovna, the mother of Alexander I, founded a home for impoverished widows of the nobility and their unmarried daughters. These ladies received some training as nurses and worked in hospitals but they were paid and did not form a religious sisterhood. In 1818 they were formally organized into the 'Compassionate Widows of the Empress'. There were several groups of these Widows in St. Petersburg and Moscow, and a number of them would work in the Crimean military hospitals. Then, in the 1840s a new kind of Russian Orthodox sisterhood appeared, lay Sisters of Mercy. These Sisters, very much like many of the Anglican Sisters, were looking less for a more intense religious life than for structured charitable work. In a similar way, they nursed the sick and helped abandoned children and 'fallen women.' The first two of these new communities gave one to three years of practical training in some medical procedures and in hygienic practice so the Sisters could look after patients both in their homes and in hospitals.[41] However, there was a very big difference between these new, more secular sisterhoods and the one that Elena Pavlovna envisioned. Her Sisters were to be lay Sisters, but they were to do entirely military nursing and would work not only in base hospitals as did the British nurses and the French Daughters of Charity, but they would also work in field hospitals which the Russians usually called bandaging or dressing stations.

When Pirogov met with the Grand Duchess in October 1854 she described her projected sisterhood to him, and Pirogov then explained his beliefs about military medicine, which meshed well with her plan. The chaotic accumulation of the wounded at the dressing stations caused many unnecessary deaths and complications that he believed could be avoided if there were immediate diagnosis rather than just treating patients in the order they came in. Diagnosis would enable the staff to identify the wounded who needed instant help, those who could wait, and those who were hopeless, and then send them to the most appropriate places. In order to do this, however, there had to be a larger number of personnel at the scene of the fighting. Because in war, as in great epidemics, the number of physicians is never sufficient, Pirogov believed one had to fill the gap with less qualified people.[42] He had seen female nurses only once in his life, the nuns in the Paris hospitals, and then only in passing, but he agreed with the Grand Duchess that women could be used to expand

Doctor-directed nursing

the triaging staff at the dressing stations. He later wrote that he had never seen the Grand Duchess in such an emotional state as she had been at that October meeting. She leapt from her chair and, striding around the room with a flushed face and tears in her eyes, she asked, 'Why didn't you come to me sooner? Your request would have been granted long ago and my plans would have been realized long ago ...'

Within twenty-four hours, Elena Pavlovna had spoken with the Tsar who immediately approved the project. Pirogov and Elena Pavlovna then worked out the details of how they would set up the nursing service. Pirogov would be the director of the whole enterprise and would take his own team of civilian doctors. In consultation with the military authorities, he would decide where the nurses should be placed.[43] Apart from meeting the desperate need for more paramedical help, the project appealed to Pirogov because the Sisters would be completely independent of the dishonest military administration and he hoped they would be able to neutralize some of the horrible abuses in the hospital system.[44] The new sisterhood, officially founded on 23 October/5 November 1854, was called the Sisters of the Exaltation of the Cross.[45] Just as the Daughters of Charity of St. Vincent de Paul were often called Sisters of Charity for short, the Russian Sisters were often called Sisters of Mercy, Sisters of Charity, or Sisters of the Cross.

One could place the Russian Sisters in the category of sisterhood nursing. They were professed in a religious service in the Mikhailovsky Palace chapel, at which point they were presented with a pectoral cross. They had a chaplain and their year-long vows incorporated the traditional vows of chastity and obedience, although not poverty. But there were major differences. They took one-year vows, not lifelong vows, and their uniform was not the traditional nun's habit but a forerunner of the classic nurse's uniform: a brown dress with a white apron and veil. The sisterhood was open to any denomination, Catholic, Orthodox, or Protestant,[46] making it different from any other sisterhood in Europe. The Tsar sent Pirogov to the Crimea not as an army doctor, but as a civilian 'Consultant Surgeon and Director of a Special Unit of Female Nurses.' The Sisters therefore reported directly to Pirogov rather than to a female religious superior, something no abbess would ever have permitted. The Sisters were created for the sole purpose of military nursing, and they did not observe any regular religious offices. They could also be placed

256

with the British nurses in the category of female nurses imposed on an unwilling medical service but, although most regular army doctors strongly opposed them, the Sisters had the strong support of Pirogov's team of doctors and he was the chief doctor in the Crimea, personally appointed by the Tsar. Pirogov believed the reason the Russian generals opposed the Sisters was because they did not want them to see 'the insatiable thievery of the hospital administrators.' There was considerable resistance to the new sisterhood at home too. Many thought it too dangerous for women to be working in the public sphere and especially on the battlefield, while some feared the public might associate them with sexually promiscuous camp followers and working-class women.[47]

The day after meeting with Pirogov and receiving the Tsar's approval, the Grand Duchess sent out a call for volunteers. Women from the lower nobility, wives, widows, and daughters of merchants and army and naval officers, a few semi-literate individuals, and at least one nun (who was actually a novice) came forward. To demonstrate that nursing was not beneath the dignity of a Russian noblewoman, Elena Pavlovna went with some of the new recruits to Pirogov's hospital clinic, attended an amputation, and bandaged a post-operative patient herself.[48] During the war, 236 Sisters of the Exaltation of the Cross would serve – almost exactly the same number of nurses the British War Department sent out to the East. Of these, 161 served in six Crimean hospitals and on the Crimean battlefields. The other seventy-five Sisters worked in the Black Sea ports of Odessa, Kherson, and Nikolaev and in Finland where they nursed sailors wounded in the Anglo-French naval raids.[49] During the course of the war seventeen of the Sisters working in the Crimea died, mostly from typhus. The first group of Sisters was quickly chosen, and were not used to the hard physical labor of nursing, or the kind of responsibility which they now had to shoulder. The first head of the Sisters, Aleksandra Petrovna Stakhovich, also proved a poor choice and Pirogov would later insist that she be replaced. But the most serious problem the new Sisters encountered was their lack of nursing knowledge: the first group had only a few days, or two weeks at most, of training at the St. Petersburg Military Hospital. This, however, was soon remedied: later groups were given two to three months of training,[50] which was a great deal at that time.

Doctor-directed nursing

On 25 October/5 November, twenty-eight Sisters were professed in the chapel of the Mikhailovsky Palace and left the next day for the Crimea. Pirogov, with a staff of ten doctors, his medical aide Kalashnikov, and feldsher Nikitin, both of whom had worked with him in the Caucasus, left St. Petersburg ahead of the Sisters, arriving in Sevastopol on 12/24 November after a thirteen-day journey.[51] Shortly afterwards Christian Hübbenet, a professor of surgery at the University of St. Vladimir in Kiev (now renamed the University of Kiev), arrived bringing some of his medical students with him. Like Pirogov, he would soon become heavily dependent on the Sisters. Up until this point the main primary sources for this chapter have been Pirogov's unfinished autobiography, *Questions of Life*, and Tolstoy's *Diaries* and Sevastopol stories. There are rich resources for the activities of the Sisters in Russian archives and at least two Sisters wrote memoirs, but these have not been translated into English. From here on, however, I use the writings of the two men who worked the most closely with the Sisters in the Crimea, Hübbenet and Tolstoy. Hübbenet's report on the medical care of the wounded (*Die Sanitäts-Verhältnisse der Russischen Verwundeten während des Krimkrieges*) has been translated from Russian into German. I am also fortunate in having a translation of Pirogov's letters to his wife (*Sevastopol'skiia pis'ma*), in which he expressed himself extremely frankly, and the pamphlet he wrote in 1856 (*Historical Survey of the Activities of the Sisters of the Community of the Holy Cross in Caring for the Wounded and the Ill in Military Hospitals*) in which he described the contributions of individual Sisters in great detail.

On arrival in Sevastopol, Pirogov first visited the hospital, where he found 4,000 wounded and what he described as rivers of blood. He then went to present his credentials to Menshikov to whom, as director of the medical department, he reported directly. Pirogov was not pleased with the commander-in-chief. Menshikov had no experience with line troops, was a poor leader, spoke of his troops and generals in disparaging terms, and distrusted his subordinates. The able Prince Viktor Vasilchikov, who became his chief of staff shortly after Inkerman, complained bitterly of his timidity and inertia.[52] On first meeting him Pirogov told his wife that he was puzzled by the peculiar Spartan lifestyle Menshikov affected. He wore a dirty kaftan and was living in a tiny hut. Menshikov asked him if he had seen the hospital,

Russian nursing: Pirogov and the Grand Duchess

to which Pirogov answered that he had indeed but conditions there were so horrendous that he wished he had not.[53] The hospitals were indeed in a shocking state. In early November an army surgeon visited the naval hospital. It was full of men wounded at the Alma two weeks previously who had never had their wounds dressed except by their own efforts, using their own shirts which they tore up for bandages. Soldiers came to bring them food but they had never seen a doctor. The men begged the surgeon for help and he attended to as many as he could with what instruments he could find in the hospital. When he tried to leave, those he had not been able to help begged him to stay and he was only able to get away by promising to come back.[54]

Menshikov replied to Pirogov's comment about the hospitals by saying that it had been even worse right after Inkerman: 'We didn't know where to start, they [the wounded] were lying on the bare ground under the pouring rain.' Pirogov thought to himself, 'And who, the devil take it, is to blame, if not you yourself ... as he [Menshikov] drily and dispassionately justified himself while at the same time admitting his own guilt.' Menshikov asked about the Sisters of Mercy, 'Will they be of any use? What if we should have to open yet a third syphilitic section to the hospital?' 'I don't know Your Grace,' Pirogov answered, 'Everything will depend on the character of the women who are chosen. The idea behind the undertaking is a good one and is already well on its way to being implemented.' Menshikov then went on to say that the army already had a nurse, Darya, a local woman who bandaged the wounded on the battlefield. 'They say that she has been a big help,' he explained, 'that she even did some bandaging of the wounded herself at the Alma.' Pirogov was disgusted. It was eighteen days after Inkerman and 2,000 wounded remained crowded together in the hospitals on dirty mattresses. He learned that Menshikov and the ranking staff doctor had not visited the hospital until a week after the battle, and that was to visit a general. While there, Menshikov did not even look at the crowded, mutilated, half-rotting wounded soldiers lying on their plank beds.

Pirogov took a very different approach to the soldiers. One of the Sisters later said of him, 'He cared for his patients as a father would care for his own children, and his example of love for one's fellow man and of self-sacrifice had a strong effect upon everyone. We all gained renewed enthusiasm at the sight of him; his patients were

Doctor-directed nursing

made easier by his very touch.' Another Sister said that he worked so tirelessly and was so full of life that he instilled new energy and the eagerness to do one's job in his co-workers. Above all, the soldiers knew that they could approach him with any complaint and the most naive requests, and that he would always listen to them and do everything he could to help them. 'Who will undertake to put up a good fight when he knows that when he is wounded he will be abandoned like a dog?' Pirogov asked himself as he wondered what lay beneath Menshikov's affected lifestyle.[55]

The day before Pirogov arrived in Sevastopol, Hodasevich went to the hospital in the barracks on the north side of the city to visit Masnikov, an old schoolfriendwho had been wounded at Inkerman. Hodasevich found him among the dead and dying who overflowed from the buildings into the courtyards. He lay in the dust and dirt surrounded by corpses whom no one was removing. Hodasevich said he then understood why a Russian soldier preferred death to a slight wound. Masnikov had been hit in the shoulder by a rifle ball and felt it sinking down deeper into his body. He begged Hodasevich to bind his shoulder with anything he could find. A feldsher would dress the slightly wounded but said it was useless to tend those for whom there was no hope. A slightly wounded officer told Hodasevich the feldshers would not help anyone unless they paid them, but a poor local woman named Maria came and brought the men tea and washed and dressed the wounds of some. Pirogov later examined Masnikov but said he was too weak to survive surgery. He died two days later. 'Had the operation been performed earlier, his life would have been saved,' Hodasevich wrote.[56]

Before the Sisters of the Exaltation of the Cross arrived there were a number of local women, who came from all social classes, who helped with dressings and gave out tea.[57] Pirogov described four of these women who worked at the Assembly of Nobles, which had been converted into the principal dressing station or field hospital for the western side of the city. This building consisted of what we would probably call assembly rooms, a kind of club with a ballroom, billiards room, and so forth. The local women consisted of a girl of 17 who was the daughter of an official, a soldier's wife, and the middle-aged wife of a sailor who did her hair in ringlets and always had a cigarette hanging from her mouth. The sailor's wife distributed

Russian nursing: Pirogov and the Grand Duchess

tea which she and friends paid for themselves. The fourth was Darya, whom Pirogov characterized as not unattractive and 'not the timid type.' She was a laundress, the 18 year old daughter of a sailor, who, with a cart and supplies which she purchased with her own money, dressed the wounded at the Alma and became famous as a heroine of Sevastopol. She went on to nurse in the Sevastopol hospitals, helping in the operating room.[58] When the Tsar's sons visited Sevastopol, he ordered them to kiss her and give her 500 roubles, and he promised her another thousand when she married.[59] Darya later asked to join the sisterhood but she had what Pirogov tactfully called a problematic lifestyle. When he explained the sisterhood's rules to her, pointing out that she would have to remain celibate for a year, she answered 'Why not, can do,' but never came back.[60] Once the more reliable, trained Sisters arrived these untrained local women were pushed into minor roles. The local women did give the patients tea but not accurately, Pirogov said, and they did everything with an eye to future rewards, even Darya with her 500 roubles and the Tsar's gold medal pinned to her bosom. By contrast, the Sisters carried out doctors' orders reliably and precisely, giving the correct amounts of medicine, food, and fluids. 'The Grand Duchess has truly done a great service to humanity and has created a revolution in military hospitals,' he declared.[61]

In the twelve days that Pirogov spent in Sevastopol before he left for Simferopol, he was able to sort the patients into appropriate groups, separate those with clean wounds from those with suppurating wounds, and operate on almost all those who needed surgery. In early December Pirogov received notice that sixty Compassionate Widows from St. Petersburg, who would be under his sole direction, were on their way to the Crimea. A total of ninety-one Compassionate Widows served, but he did not think them efficient nurses.[62] Pirogov spent a full week in Simferopol visiting more than 1,000 wounded who were housed in about twenty makeshift hospitals, and then he returned to Sevastopol.[63] Map 4 indicates why Pirogov had such freedom of movement in and out of Sevastopol and Simferopol, and why the allies had to make a frontal assault rather than starving the city out. The allies were encamped on the south side of the city and controlled only the small strip of land from the Tchernaya River to Balaclava. The Russians held all the rest of the Crimean peninsula and could move troops and supplies in from the north side by both

261

Doctor-directed nursing

land and sea. On returning to Sevastopol Pirogov reorganized the hospitals, placing the Sisters in charge of hospital administration.

Notes

1 Curtiss, *Russian Army*, pp. 99–101, 110–11, 367.
2 Wirtschafter, *Russian Soldier*, pp. 75, 83, 85–7.
3 Ibid, pp. 75, 77, 83, 85–9; Kagan, *Military Reforms*, pp. 241–2; Curtiss, *Russian Army*, pp. 215–17.
4 Best, *War and Society*, pp. 186.
5 Figes, *Crimean War*, p. 119.
6 Curtiss, *Russian Army*, p. 250, 273–94.
7 Best, *War and Society*, pp. 224–5; Westwood, *Endurance and Endeavour*, pp. 63–6.
8 Hodasevich, *Within Sebastopol*, p. 42.
9 Curtiss, *Crimean War*, pp. 333–4; Curtiss, *Russian Army*, pp. 120–6.
10 Curtiss, *Russian Army*, pp. 144–9; Best, *War and Society*, pp. 224–5.
11 Tolstoy, *Diaries*, vol. 1, p. 97.
12 Tolstoy, 'Sevastopol in August,' pp. 282–3.
13 Figes, *Crimean War*, pp. 233–4.
14 Pirogov, *Sevastopol Letters*, p. 137.
15 Tolstoy, 'Sevastopol in December,' pp. 197–200; Tolstoy, *Diaries*, vol. 1, p. 98.
16 Hosking, *Russia*, p. 285.
17 Tolstoy, *Diaries*, vol. 1, p. 104.
18 Curtiss, *Russian Army*, pp. 212–20.
19 Wirtschafter, *Russian Soldier*, pp. 94–5.
20 Curtiss, 'Russian Sisters,' pp. 87–8.
21 Curtiss, *Russian Army*, pp. 220–6.
22 Baudens, *Guerre de Crimée*, pp. 109–10; Pirogov, 'Historical Survey,' p. 32.
23 Frieden, *Russian Physicians*, p. 37; Hodasevich, *Within Sebastopol*, pp. 101–2.
24 Hübbenet, *Russian Wounded*, pp. 7–9; Fried, 'Pirogoff in the Crimean Campaign,' p. 520fn; Pirogov, *Questions of Life*, p. xix. Hübbenet is now more often transliterated Giübbenet. I use Hübbenet because that is how it is spelled in the title of this edition.
25 A legal process whereby, when a debtor cannot repay with money, the creditor seizes his property instead.
26 Pirogov, *Questions of Life*, pp. 82, 84, 111, 156, 164.
27 Ibid, pp. 259–65, 275–9, 329.
28 Pirogov belonged to five European scientific academies. Rappaport, *No Place for Ladies*, p. 116.
29 Jean Cruveilhier (1791–1874), Chair of Pathological Anatomy at the University of Paris.

Russian nursing: Pirogov and the Grand Duchess

30 Alfred-Armand-Louis-Marie Velpeau (1795–1867), Chair of Clinical Surgery at the University of Paris.

31 Pirogov, *Questions of Life*, p. 369.

32 Figes, *Crimean War*, pp. 298–9.

33 Mikulinsky, 'Pirogov, Nikolay Ivanovich'; Pirogov, *Questions of Life*, p. xiv.

34 Fried, 'Pirogoff in the Crimean Campaign,' p. 533.

35 Pirogov, *Questions of Life*, p. xvi. There is not space here to mention all his most important publications or his numerous honors.

36 Seidlitz is often transliterated Zeidlitz and sometimes Heidlitz.

37 Fried, 'Pirogoff in the Crimean Campaign,' pp. 523–4, 528–9.

38 Soroka and Ruud, *Grand Duchess*, p. 199.

39 Ibid, pp. 142, 145–6.

40 Ibid, pp. 199, 241–81.

41 Meehan, *Holy Women*, pp. 75–7; Stoff, *Russia's Sisters of Mercy*, pp. 18–24; Murray, 'Russian Nurses,' p. 131.

42 Soroka and Ruud, *Grand Duchess*, p. 199; Fried, 'Pirogoff in the Crimean Campaign,' p. 529.

43 Soroka and Ruud, *Grand Duchess*, pp. 199–202.

44 Malis, 'Editor's Introduction,' p. 6.

45 Pirogov, *Sevastopol Letters*, p. 31; Soroka and Ruud, *Grand Duchess*, pp. 219–22.

46 Soroka and Ruud, *Grand Duchess*, p. 310.

47 Curtiss, 'Russian Sisters,' p. 85; Stoff, *Russia's Sisters of Mercy*, pp. 20–1, 23–4.

48 Malis, 'Editor's Introduction,' p. 5; Pirogov, 'Historical Survey,' p. 31.

49 Soroka and Ruud, *Grand Duchess*, p. 205; Sorokina, 'Russian Nursing,' pp. 57–8, 61.

50 Rappaport, *No Place for Ladies*, pp. 117–18.

51 Pirogov, *Sevastopol Letters*, p. 59.

52 Curtiss, *Russian Army*, pp. 328–9, 337; Curtiss, *Crimean War*, pp. 305, 307.

53 Pirogov, *Sevastopol Letters*, p. 72.

54 Hodasevich, *Within Sebastopol*, pp. 89–90.

55 Malis, 'Editor's Introduction,' pp. 12–13, 21–2; Pirogov, *Sevastopol Letters*, pp. 72–3.

56 Hodasevich, *Within Sebastopol*, pp. 138–9.

57 Hübbenet, *Russian Wounded*, p. 7.

58 Figes, *Crimean War*, p. 220fn.

59 Pirogov, *Sevastopol Letters*, p. 59.

60 Soroka and Ruud, *Grand Duchess*, p. 202.

61 Hübbenet, *Russian Wounded*, p. 7; Pirogov, *Sevastopol Letters*, pp. 77, 88, 90, 100.

62 Murray, 'Russian Nurses,' p. 131.

63 Pirogov, *Sevastopol Letters*, pp. 59, 76–80.

13

The Sisters take over

The Sisters at work

The new Sisters would make an enormous difference in the care of the soldiers. Four parties arrived before the fall of Sevastopol and a fifth after. The first group of twenty-eight Sisters reached Simferopol at the end of November 1854. The second group of thirteen Sisters arrived on 13/25 January 1855, a group of six under the direction of the famous Sister Ekaterina Mikhailovna Bakunina four days later, and the fourth party of nineteen two months later on 28 March/9 April. The new Sisters, like the first party, were directly responsible to Pirogov and his doctors, not to Head Directress Stakhovich. Her job was to visit the Sisters in the various hospitals to see that they were doing well. For example, when Darya wanted to join the sisterhood, it was Pirogov she spoke to and who explained the rules to her. The first Sisters started work in Simferopol on 1/13 December 1854. They worked in 'day and night shifts, assisted with dressings and operations, distributed tea and wine, and watched over the servants, orderlies, and,' Pirogov wrote to his wife, 'even the doctors.' He thought 'the presence of a woman, neatly dressed and providing sympathetic care, brought life to the pitiful vale of suffering and misfortune.' At first he was favorably impressed by Stakhovich, 'a woman in spectacles but not yet old, who has managed to keep them [her Sisters] quite well up to now; she carries herself energetically.' Pirogov noted that some Sisters were well educated; there was a nun, and an officer's widow who spoke five languages.

He was absolutely delighted with the Sisters' work and quickly became highly dependent on them. 'They have turned the hospitals upside down,' he told his wife, 'they see to the food and drink simply marvellously, they distribute the tea and wine which I give them. If things continue thus, if their ardour doesn't cool, then our hospitals will be like the real thing.' Still, a bad beginning was very difficult to repair. In Simferopol the patients were still housed in stables and there was no straw available for mattresses so old, half-rotten, urine- and pus-sodden hay was dried and re-used. Pirogov worried about how the Sisters would manage in Sevastopol. In Simferopol they lived in a nice apartment and had a carriage, but in Sevastopol there were no such luxuries. They would have to live in barracks among the seriously ill patients and wear heavy soldiers' boots in order to make their way through the deep, clayey mud.[1] But there were other more immediate problems. Only four days after the first Sisters arrived, they had worked with such enthusiasm that they wore themselves out, and some succumbed to typhus. Two were so ill he feared they might not recover. He sent five Sisters to Bakhchiserai and the rest to Sevastopol. The Bakhchiserai Sisters also immediately fell ill with typhus, and one subsequently died. On the positive side there were no reports of the much feared love affairs with officers, but Pirogov had nevertheless taken the precaution of not sending Sisters to look after the military cadets. This seemed all the more sensible because few cadets were seriously wounded. By mid-January not one of the first group of Sisters was working in the military hospitals because those who were well were sent off to nurse the sick Sisters. Pirogov waited eagerly for the second party of Sisters of Mercy to arrive in Sevastopol. The roads were blocked with snow and he thought it would be some time before they could reach the besieged city. By the time they arrived, three Sisters from the first group had died and Stakhovich was so ill that Pirogov feared she might soon die too.

As in all the other armies, inability to transport patients out of Sevastopol was the medical department's worst problem: patients accumulated in the Sevastopol hospitals, often remaining for entire days and nights on the floor without mattresses or linen. Furthermore, when there was transport it consisted of the open, unsprung peasant carts which brought in supplies. They jostled the men so badly that they caused more injury, and even the slightest wounds became more serious. With no warm clothes or blankets the men had a seven-day journey to Perekop, and at night they slept in the open in the fields or in unheated Tatar huts. Sometimes they had to go three days without

Doctor-directed nursing

food.[2] Watching these men enduring in silence what seemed to him humanly unendurable made Pirogov feel he should be able to endure any deprivation. With no way of transporting the men to hospitals outside the town, he began establishing new hospitals in Sevastopol. He made the heavily protected Nicholas and Alexander Batteries; into hospitals and used the homes of two merchants, Orlovskii and Gushchin, as hospitals for gangrenous patients and those with suppurating wounds. He assigned the second group of Sisters to Sevastopol, where they did day and night shifts at the Assembly of Nobles, the Nicholas Battery, and the two private homes. Then, sending the Assembly of Nobles' sick and post-operative patients to the Nicholas Battery, he temporarily made the Engineers' Business House the main dressing station so that the Assembly could be properly cleansed and aired.

Pirogov now divided the Sisters into three functional groups: surgical nurses, or those responsible for dressings and what is now called direct nursing care; pharmacists; and housekeepers. The surgical nurses saved the doctors a great deal of time in the operating room, did dressings, and also helped the feldshers make the dressings. The pharmacists took complete charge of the medicines, seeing that they were distributed accurately to the patients. They also supervised the feldshers, who could not always be trusted. The housekeepers managed the servants, linen, and kitchen. In the field hospitals, however, each Sister had to be responsible for all three of these duties – housekeeping, pharmacy, and surgery. Another major and time-consuming job for the Sisters was taking care of the soldiers' money. In the hopeless cases the Sisters ascertained the final wishes of the men, including to whom their money and possessions should be sent on their deaths.[3] It was rare that a soldier came into the hospitals without any money so the Sisters collected a great deal of cash. Hübbenet believed that by May and June the Sisters on the ship side (the eastern side of the town) where he was then working were managing a sum of up to 60,000 roubles which the soldiers had given them.[4] When the British soldiers rifled the pockets and boots of the dead and dying Russian soldiers after the Battle of the Alma some men collected as much as £20.[5] Many soldiers preferred to carry their money with them rather than giving it to their officers for the safe-keeping fund because the officers so often stole it. The Sisters also bought many supplies with their own money.

The Sisters take over

In the Kherson hospital the pharmacy Sisters instigated an investigation into the dishonest conduct of their pharmacist, leading him to kill himself. 'One less crook,' Pirogov commented. While the housekeeping Sisters did an excellent job with the soldiers' possessions, the linen, and the servants, they were less successful in the kitchens where food was stolen wholesale.[6] This was probably because they could not be there all the time, while the pharmacy Sisters could lock the drug cupboards when they went into the wards.

Up until Pirogov assigned these roles to the Sisters, essentially placing them in charge of hospital administration, he had worked smoothly with the chief army doctors, but now he encountered fierce resistance. The chief doctors realized immediately what the Sisters' administration would mean for their incomes and lifestyles. They claimed Pirogov was exceeding his powers, and it was only through the energetic support of General Osten-Sacken and Prince Vasilchikov, chief of staff under both Menshikov and Gorchakov (who succeeded Menshikov), that the Sisters were able to retain full control of hospital administration. A few days after Bakunina's team of Sisters arrived Pirogov merged them with the second group and made Bakunina the Head Nurse. It was difficult to find a place where the Sisters could live in the devastated town. Bakunina's team stayed first with families, then in a former church, and when the bombardments became continuous, in the well-fortified Nicholas Battery which was half barracks, half redoubt. The Sisters lived in the basement where gunpowder was stored and several cannons faced the sea.[7] Bakunina would become the anchor of the nursing team, conscientiously managing everything with tact and energy. She was an unmarried 45 year old woman who came from an aristocratic background. Her father was governor of St. Petersburg and she was a cousin of the anarchist Mikhail Bakunin who was at that moment in the Peter and Paul prison. Pirogov described her as a woman of uncommon character who carried herself as befitted a lady of her years and education and who always commanded respect.[8] All that the commissariat had previously held back and which they still tried to withhold was now available for the patients and could no longer be used for personal gain by dishonest staff. At last doctors' orders were punctually and accurately carried out, but the senior army doctors were very angry and complained to their superiors that the Sisters were interfering women.[9]

Doctor-directed nursing

Hard work and typhus soon took its toll on the new Sisters' health. Within a month almost all had been stricken with typhus and two more died. On 21 February/4 March the Sisters from the first team who started in Simferopol arrived in Sevastopol. Barely recovered and still weak, Pirogov sent them to work under Hübbenet's direction in the hospital on the north side. On 4/16 March the Assembly of Nobles, thoroughly cleansed and aired, reopened, replacing the Engineers' House as the main dressing station.[10] The ballroom now held up to 100 army cots with green bedside tables, 'all very clean and tidy,' Bakunina wrote. The billiards room was an operating room and there were two more rooms full of cots. Now only the dressing station on the ship side and the naval hospital at Fort Michael had no Sisters, and when the fourth party of Sisters arrived on 28 March/9 April Pirogov sent them to these two hospitals.[11]

Following the Battle of Inkerman there was a lull in the artillery battle. One British officer described the siege as going very tranquilly: we just sit in the trenches, he said, and don't shoot at the Russians because we have no guns and they are not shooting at us. The Russian artillery was quiet because it had so little ammunition, but the Russians were not idle: they were beginning their underground operations which successfully wrecked the French mining corridors in January.[12] They were also energetically pursuing their sorties. They lost many men in these sorties; the French could not tell how many because the Russians did not abandon their men – they always carried their wounded and dead back into the city.[13] As the French pushed their saps towards the Mamelon the Russians retaliated with even more ferocious sorties. Tolstoy, who took part in at least one sortie himself,[14] gives a wonderful description of a sortie as seen from inside the city. First one saw thousands of tiny, constantly flaring points blazing along the whole length of the line and heard the terrible crackle of small-arms fire above the din of the artillery. Then came hundreds of voices shouting hurrah as the soldiers attacked. When the small-arms firing stopped it meant that the men were fighting hand-to-hand, and then came crowds of soldiers back into the city carrying men on stretchers or supporting the wounded by the arms as the rumble of artillery continued and the small-arms fire restarted.[15] For the Russian medical department the sorties meant constant work, mostly at night because the Russians usually sent the men out twice a day at 9 p.m. and 5 a.m. when the French were changing the guard.[16] Captain Goodlake, who worked in no man's land in charge of the British sharpshooters, said the French and Russians fought every day. He thought the Russians 'licked' the French on every occasion.[17] Military historians tend to think that the Russian sorties accomplished very little apart from losing a great many men, but this was certainly not the feeling of men like Herbé, Loizillon, or Montaudon who experienced the attacks.

When the French shifted their primary target from the Flagstaff and Central Bastions to the Malakhov in February, the Russians responded by building the White Works and the lunette the French called the Mamelon. Then they built trenches and rifle pits in front of the lunette from which Russian marksmen, who were armed with the few modern rifles the army had, efficiently shot the French sappers. The Mamelon was only 1,200 feet from the French lines, and together with the White Works enfiladed the French trenches and batteries, completely blocking them from advancing their trenches towards their new goal, the Malakhov. As the allies ramped up their artillery attacks Pirogov noted that few casualties resulted from the stronger cannonades. The real danger came from the sharpshooters with their Minié rifles,[18] and this was equally true for the allies.

Pirogov now had an establishment of ten doctors and twenty Sisters. The hospitals were less filthy than when he first arrived, although there were still not enough mattresses or linen and the soldiers sometimes had to lie for three weeks on the same dirty mattresses in the same dirty clothes. The Sisters were working diligently but he regretted that 'they have in their midst, just like the military officers in the general headquarters, their own share of plotting and scheming.'[19] Infighting and backbiting among the Sisters became a major problem but Pirogov was nevertheless able to keep them working efficiently. He now had seven hospitals on the south side of Sevastopol of which only one, the Nicholas Battery, was completely bombproof as well as out of reach of the bombs, and he considered its sanitary condition detestable. On the north side there were another 3,000 sick and wounded in old, humid barracks and also 1,500 sick sailors. There was only about one doctor to 100 patients, which was inadequate with the press from the sorties,[20] and gangrene was becoming more common which Pirogov believed to be due to the unsanitary, overcrowded conditions in the hospitals.

In early March four more doctors fell sick and Pirogov himself became too ill with stomach trouble to be able to work. Much to his delight, Menshikov was so sick he had to resign. In the meantime Count Osten-Sacken and Prince Vasilchikov, who were both supportive of Pirogov and his nurses, were in charge of the garrison. When Pirogov considered himself completely recovered he began making plans to leave the Crimea. He would have come home sooner, he told his wife, except for two things. First, ten doctors said they absolutely would not stay without him and would leave when he did. Second, his five years' service would be complete in May and nothing could convince him to stay beyond then. He had done everything he could for Sevastopol and now someone else should take up the burden.[21] When he came to the Crimea he already knew the fate which awaited the Russian and allied wounded, but he had hoped he would be able to make some improvement. Given the nature of the Russian military administration he now believed improvement was impossible: 'disorder, Slavic lack of concern, short-sightedness – all ineradicable,' he lamented. He was facing the same problems Scrive would face the following winter: he could not convince the administration that he would need many more beds, in his case if the enemy launched a new action. They ignored him, 'believing that something would surely turn up to solve the problem.' How could one think about the death rate or success of treatment when the men were crammed together and no one cared about their shelter, beds, or basic cleanliness, he asked.

Pirogov was also very concerned about what would happen to the Sisters when he left, and they themselves also worried about being left on their own. He needed to write to the Grand Duchess. As long as he was in Sevastopol the Sisters were treated with kid gloves but he feared that would not be the case when he left. What worried him the most was the infighting and mean tricks they played on each other. The Grand Duchess' influence might protect them, but only as long as she refused to listen to Stakhovich, who was writing to Elena Pavlovna complaining about Pirogov and especially Bakunina of whom she was intensely jealous. Pirogov had brought himself almost to tears pleading with the Sisters' chaplain and also with the senior Sisters to help

The Sisters take over

him stop the fighting, but without success. Furthermore, the Sisters in the Kherson hospital had put themselves in a very dangerous position when they insisted on the investigation of their pharmacist. Pirogov admired their bravery but believed the commissariat would surely seek revenge.[22]

He also worried about his patients. The number of sick grew after every sortie and skirmish, there were not enough doctors, nor enough medicine or wine, and quinine was running out. The army was reaping the consequences of the six months Menshikov had ignored its health, and if there were another major engagement Pirogov did not know where he could put the wounded.[23] On 8/20 March 1855 Gorchakov took command, bringing with him his able staff. He appreciated Pirogov's work and visited the hospital, where he made a point of awarding medals to whichever patient Pirogov pointed out to him. At first optimistic, Gorchakov soon decided that if the enemy had 'a little sense and decisiveness' defeat was inevitable: Menshikov's blunders made victory impossible.[24] It is a tribute to the Russians' fighting ability that, while Gorchakov was convinced that there was no possibility of winning, the British thought the Russians were getting stronger and stronger. It seemed to one British officer in March that the Russians were thrashing the French.[25]

On the nights of 2/14, 3/15, and 5/17 March, the Russians launched fierce attacks on the French trenches resulting in horrific amounts of work for Pirogov's team. Pirogov was feeling quite discouraged when he wrote to his friend Dr Seidlitz describing his work in Sevastopol. He could be killed at any moment he told Seidlitz, and the closeness of death was making him more pious. He had long since stopped being appalled by the blood, pus, and oozing wounds that he lived with, but what he found most depressing was that 'in spite of all my efforts and devotion things are not going better. I tell my younger colleagues not to lose courage; I repeat ceaselessly to them that they must not despair but wait for time and better results,' but he himself really felt very dispirited. While he thought something could be done for those with intermittent fever (probably malaria), he did not think there was any treatment which could prevent the fatal results of typhus, pneumonia, epidemic scurvy, and dysentery. This had been his experience in his fifteen years in the St. Petersburg hospitals and it was the same here except on a colossal and somewhat more deadly scale. Mortality in

271

Doctor-directed nursing

St. Petersburg was three out of five, and in Sevastopol three and a half or three-quarters to five. He kept careful statistics although he thought that was dangerous because he knew they could be fatal to his reputation as a surgeon. 'Our art,' he wrote sadly, 'is in an imperfect state.' He hoped someday there would be an invention which would make wounds heal in twenty-four hours. When he had asked one doctor whether his wounds healed by first or second intention the doctor had replied, 'By gangrene.' Pirogov currently had thirteen to fourteen doctors working under him. Each operated according to his own particular method but the results were the same for everyone.

Petechial typhus was reigning in Sevastopol and also in Simferopol and the patients suffered from choleraic diarrhea and gangrene as well. Typhus smote everyone – doctors, Sisters, volunteer nurses, orderlies, and feldshers. Six out of the twenty Sisters in Simferopol had died, and of Pirogov's sixteen doctors, seven were currently ill. He wanted to separate patients with typhus, choleraic dysentery, and gangrene, but with floods of new patients constantly pouring in it was impossible to keep the different diseases separate. He also wanted to keep the fresh post-operative patients away from contact with contagious diseases but with such a rush of patients all coming in at the same time that also was not feasible. The hospitals in other towns – Perekop, Kherson, Nicolaev – were all full. Pirogov was writing in the midst of a major bombardment and it took him three separate nights to complete his letter.

He was pleased that his system of triage was working very efficiently. He had organized a kind of mass assembly line for major surgery. He had timed the amount of time the amputations took, watch in hand, and found that with the help of inexperienced assistants fifteen doctors working on three operating tables could carry out ninety amputations in six hours and fifteen minutes. Following a sortie the surgeons could do all the most important operations within a day and a half. Hopeless cases – those with head injuries with loss of brain tissue, abdominal wounds with internal intestinal lesions, and other mortal wounds – were given narcotics to lessen their suffering, and sent to Gushchin's. The lightly wounded were dressed by feldshers under the supervision of one or two doctors and were then sent back to their regiments. Then the surgeons were able to focus their attention on the third group, those that they hoped to save. He

The Sisters take over

divided this group into two: men who needed immediate surgery and those whose operations could wait for the next day or later. Those who could wait he sent to a hospital where the Sisters looked after them. Then he began diagnosing those who needed immediate surgery. 'Attention!' he wrote to Seidlitz as a bomb crashed nearby, 'The bombardment has become violent. We are going to have three sorties tonight which will result in hundreds of wounded.' He thought the bombs not very effective. When the enemy shot 2,000 bombs into four or five redoubts they killed only twenty and wounded only sixty. In peacetime human life had a certain value, he commented, but in wartime it had none – it was only worth so much trouble and cost. Last night, he said, we lost 400 killed and 1,800 wounded but in two days we had all attended to.[26] Finally, Pirogov told Seidlitz that unless he were killed before then, he would soon be leaving the Crimea. He regretted that seven or eight good surgeons were going with him and he also regretted having to give up the direction of the Sisters of the Exaltation of the Cross. 'I am glad to have guided their blessed activity but it is the soldiers who have most appreciated it,' he wrote.[27]

The surgeons were able to work so quickly in part because, as well as helping with the bandaging, a number of Sisters became expert at ligating arteries, enabling the surgeons to move on to the next case without closing the wound. 'With bombs falling all around them,' Hübbenet wrote, 'they worked calmly and coolly tying off the squirting arteries,' and the arteries really were squirting because hemostats had not yet been invented. Hübbenet mentioned one Sister in particular, Sister Bartschewskaja, who was in his operating room from early in the morning until late at night, skillfully ligating arteries. He believed that, once they had overcome their fear of blood, women were better than men at this work because they knew how to sew and the flexibility of their hands seemed more suited to this delicate handiwork. Hübbenet praised without reservation the Sisters themselves, their courage and sacrifice, and their great efficiency. Shouldering the difficulties, privations, and danger with rare strength and heroism they assisted at the most difficult operations and, he said, were a proof of Pirogov's excellent instruction.[28]

Both Pirogov and Hübbenet thought the Sisters who had the most difficult job were those who worked with the hopeless cases. In Gushchin's and Orlovskii's houses Sisters Grigoryeva, Bogdanova, and Golubtsova devotedly cared for those whose wounds had become gangrenous or who had other conditions which were not only hopeless but dangerous to other patients. They gave analgesics to ease pain, either prescribed by the doctors or prescribed by themselves, for they were very experienced in this kind of work. Those who have not experienced it cannot imagine the horrors, Pirogov wrote, that were the lot of these particular Sisters and their patients. 'Death at every step in all of its different forms: repulsive, terrifying, and moving; all of this can disturb the soul of even the most experienced doctor, gone grey in the fulfillment of his duties.'[29] Hübbenet was equally full of admiration for his Sisters who cared for the dying. In his hospitals Sister Blagowetschtschenkaja was in charge of these cases whom she tended with what Hübbenet called self-sacrifice and Christian love. She was also more exposed to mortal danger than any of his other Sisters because she worked in a building which was not fortified or protected in any way. The care of fatal cases, Hübbenet said, 'requires nerves of steel which women rarely possess,' and is the most unrewarding kind of nursing, demanding the highest religious commitment, which this Sister had.[30]

On the night of 10/22 March, the Russians launched their largest and most famous sortie which Pirogov considered one of the great feats of Russian arms. General Khrulev with 5,000 men captured and destroyed the French saps and even penetrated the main trenches, from which he had great difficulty recalling his enthusiastic men.[31] The Russians were elated by their success but the casualties were colossal. Thousands of wounded arrived, first at the Alexander Battery where there were not enough hands or doctors to perform operations so many had to be transferred to the main dressing station at the Assembly of Nobles. Bakunina and her Sisters worked around the clock, assisting at operations, doing dressings, settling the men after their surgery, giving them drinks and medicine, and keeping a sharp eye out for changes in their medical condition. The most serious amputation cases were sent to the Engineers' House where Sister Travina was in charge. Because she had a smaller number of patients she knew each man well and carefully observed changes in wounds and looked after individual needs. Following treatment in the Assembly of Nobles the other wounded were transferred to the Nicholas Battery which had been transformed into a hospital for

The Sisters take over

600 men. Bakunina was in charge of the Sisters who worked there as well as those in the Assembly of Nobles.[32] Two weeks later Pirogov wrote to his wife that almost half the doctors as well as Bakunina and another Sister were ill. 'If there is anything good in all of this chaos, it is the Sisters of Mercy,' he said. If it hadn't been for them the patients would have been lying in the dirt and lapping up dishwater instead of hearty soup. 'I myself,' Pirogov continued, 'am extremely proud of their work; I defended the idea of introducing the Sisters into the military hospitals against the idiotic attacks of old duffers, and it was my view of the truth that came to be a reality.'[33]

The beginning of the end: the Second Bombardment and the fall of the White Works and the Mamelon

On Easter Sunday 28 March/8 April the allies began the Second Bombardment which Pirogov described as 'a terrifying day of bombing.' This bombardment would continue for more than ten days and was far worse than the First Bombardment in October because the allies had succeeded in getting their batteries so much closer to the Russian bastions.[34] The Russians had slightly more cannon than the allies but the allies had superior caliber guns, far more mortars, and a much larger supply of gunpowder and projectiles. As a result most of the time the allies were firing two to three shots for each Russian shot and the Russians were losing about three times as many men.[35] But despite the superiority of the allied fire, as in the First Bombardment, when the Second Bombardment finished the Russians still held all their advance positions and the allies could not follow through with the hoped-for final assault on the city.[36] 'The northern side remains, as before, completely open to us,' Pirogov wrote to his wife on 30 April/12 May, 'and prices on foodstuffs and other supplies have not risen at all.'[37]

When the bombardment started on Easter Sunday the Russians could hardly answer the allied fire because they had so few gun cartridges, but by the next day they had solved this problem by opening infantry cartridges to make up charges for their guns. They were now able to respond vigorously,[38] and when they started firing the tremendous racket instantly awakened Pirogov and his colleagues. The windows of our house shook and it seemed as if hundreds of smiths

275

Doctor-directed nursing

were hammering on its walls, he told his wife. We jumped up, dressed hastily, and raced at full speed to the hospital. Soon the entire hall began to fill with terrible casualties; torn off arms, legs ripped off up to the knee and to the waist were being carried next to the wounded on their stretchers. The soldiers were devoted to Pirogov because of the kind and respectful way he treated them; they also naively believed him a miracle worker. An often-told story is that stretcher-bearers brought a headless corpse to the dressing station. 'Can't you see he has no head?' the admitting doctor asked. The soldiers answered, 'Never mind, your Honor, the head is following on the next stretcher. Mr Pirogov will find some way to stick it back on, and our brother-soldier will still be of some use to us!'

The Second Bombardment produced a crisis situation for the medical department: 7,000 patients in Sevastopol with no transport to evacuate them, 6,000 in Simferopol, and infection was rampant. Pirogov spent almost all day and night at the Assembly of Nobles, where he slept. There ten doctors and eight Sisters toiled tirelessly in twenty-four-hour shifts, operating on and bandaging patients.[39] In the midst of these incredibly frantic times Stakhovich's jealousy of Bakunina and spiteful behavior towards her became so intense that to make the nursing team function more effectively, Bakunina resigned her head nurse position and placed Sister Lode in charge. Nevertheless, Pirogov noted, Bakunina retained her well-established moral authority over her Sisters. In order to understand how difficult the circumstances were, Pirogov wrote, you must picture:

> the dark southern night, the lines of stretcher carriers by the dim lamplight, heading towards the entrance of the Assembly, barely able to make a pathway for themselves through the crowds of wounded on foot choking the doors. Everyone is streaming there to receive aid and to give aid, everyone wants help quickly, the wounded loudly demand bandaging or an operation, the dying ask a final respite, and all want relief of their suffering. How could this be managed without effective and stern measures, without the tireless actions that made space available and the hands that provided immediate aid!

With rockets tearing up the earth and bombs bursting all around him Lt. Yani, the director of the excellent stretcher-bearer squad, stood at the entrance to the Assembly. He efficiently kept a constant stream of stretcher-bearers moving along the bloody track which marked the

The Sisters take over

way into the building. The enormous ballroom no longer held clean, tidy beds with green bedside tables but continuously filled and then emptied as the wounded were set down on their stretchers in long rows on the parquet floor which was covered almost two inches deep in clotted blood.

Pirogov described teams of doctors, feldshers, and orderlies moving constantly up and down the rows of men, who were as white as sheets from loss of blood and shell shock. The moans and cries of the wounded, the bursting of the bombs, the death rattles, and the orders of those in charge mingled together and echoed through the hall. 'Patients were carried in and out to various commands, "to the operating table", "to a cot", "to Gushchin's", "to the Engineers", "to the Nikolaevskii Battery",' Pirogov wrote. 'Among the soldiers' greatcoats there flitted everywhere the white veils of the Sisters as they gave the wounded wine and tea, helped with dressings, and collected money and personal items for safe-keeping.' In the billiards room three teams of surgeons operated on three bloody tables; amputated limbs lay in piles on the floor or were tossed into tubs. Despite constant airing the room reeked of blood, chloroform, and sulphur. A sailor who was nicknamed 'the living tourniquet' because he was so adept at compressing arteries could barely keep up with the calls for assistance from the doctors. The feldsher Nikitin applied plaster casts to those limbs which could be saved. Bakunina distinguished herself in charge of the operating room, standing ready with a bunch of ligatures in her hand. With bombs and rockets flying overhead and landing all around them Bakunina and her Sisters found what Pirogov described as 'courage, so not in keeping with the nature of women, but which so distinguished these Sisters to the very end of the siege. It was difficult to decide what is more amazing,' he thought, 'their cool composure under fire. Or the utter selflessness of their devotion in fulfilling their responsibilities.' At night they worked by the light of a tallow lamp. Without the tirelessness of the doctors, the diligence of the Sisters, and the efficiency of the transport corps leaders, Pirogov believed, such effective help could not have been delivered to the soldiers. He was very proud of the professional way his triage system worked, quickly assigning the wounded to the appropriate places and caregivers. He considered triaging the wounded at the bandaging stations the principal test of medical efficiency.[40]

Doctor-directed nursing

During the Second Bombardment when Tolstoy was stationed in Bastion IV he visited the hospitals and dressing stations frequently. He described the same ballroom scene but from a different viewpoint, that of a layman. 'The large, high ceilinged chamber, lit only by the four or five candles the surgeons used on their rounds of inspection was literally full,' he wrote, and the air was laden with the characteristic thick, heavy, stinking fetor produced by the fevered breathing of several hundred men combined with the sweat of the stretcher-bearers. Pools of blood were visible wherever there was an empty space and the men were so closely packed together on their stretchers that they smeared each other with their blood. A blood-curdling scream now and again broke the murmur of groans, sighs, and death rattles. Surgeons in their rolled-up shirtsleeves knelt beside wounded men, and despite the terrible groans and entreaties of the sufferers, probed wounds or turned over severed limbs which still held on by a thread. 'Try to put a brave face on it, colonel, or else I'll have to stop,' one doctor urged an officer with a fractured skull as he picked at his head with a kind of hook. 'Ah! AH! Stop it! Oh, for the love of God, be quick, be quick, for the love of … A-a-ah!' the colonel screamed. A soldier with a shattered leg cried, 'Oh – oh, father in heaven, father in heaven!' begging to be left alone. 'Ivan Bogayev, private, 3rd company, S–– Regiment, compound fracture of the thigh!' shouted his surgeon from the far corner of the room to a doctor who sat at a small table next to the entry door recording the admissions. 'Perforation of the chest … Sevastyan Sereda, private,' called out another doctor. 'What regiment? … Don't bother writing it down,' he corrected himself as the private began emitting the death rattle, 'he'll be dead in a minute. Take him away.' A group of about forty stretcher-bearers waited silently at the doorway to take patched-up casualties to the hospitals or corpses to the chapel. Now and then, Tolstoy wrote, one would heave a deep sigh.

But if Tolstoy was more impressed by the sufferings of the men than by Pirogov's medical efficiency and ability to save so many more men than in the days before triage, he saw the Sisters in exactly the same way as Pirogov – quietly and efficiently working their way through the wounded, alleviating their suffering:

The Sisters with their calm faces that expressed not the futile, morbidly tearful kind of sympathy that might have been expected of women, but an active, no-nonsense and practical concern, strode to and fro among the wounded men, bearing medicine, water, bandages and lint, their uniforms flashing white against the soldiers' blood-stained shirts and greatcoats.[41]

For the ten days that the bombardment lasted each day more than 400 casualties were brought into the Assembly of Nobles, and the surgeons performed thirty amputations every day. Even so, Pirogov still thought the damage to the bastions minimal. At night the soldiers were able to rebuild the embrasures which had been destroyed, although this was very costly in manpower because allied mortar fire and sharpshooters were active all night and killed so many of the men who were doing the repair work.[42] The allies of course had the same problem. Evelyn Wood reported that the embrasure for one of his guns was destroyed three times and had to be rebuilt under fire.[43]

The constant encroachment of the enemy's batteries upon the Russian bastions made it necessary to frequently move the wounded to different buildings which, it was hoped, would be less vulnerable to the shelling. The bastions in Sevastopol were made of stone and solidly roofed with iron so that 68 lb. shot (the heaviest the allies had) and 24-pound rockets made little or no impression on them.[44] But makeshift hospitals in private homes or the Assembly of Nobles had no such roofing and could not withstand the lethal bombardment of the allies. The fourth party of Sisters were living with their patients in the Alexander Battery when it became too dangerous for the patients to remain there. At the height of the bombardment Stakhovich and Sisters Chupati and Baroness Budberg distinguished themselves moving the patients under fire to the Paul Bastion, a process which took three days. The Second Bombardment finished on 8/20 April but the team in the Assembly of Nobles had to work constantly day and night looking after casualties from the horrific trench battles which followed, and cholera began to strike again.

In May, General A. J. J. Pélissier, a more aggressive and ruthless general than General François Canrobert, the previous commandant, took command of the French army; he and Raglan immediately began planning an attack on the Malakhov. The French were also pressing the Russians hard on the western end of the line, at Bastions IV and V where great trench battles were fought on 10/11 May

Doctor-directed nursing

and 22/23 May. Both sides fought ferociously, with the trenches changing hands several times, but the French finally gained control. Pirogov estimated 10,000 Russian soldiers were ultimately engaged. Two thousand Russians were wounded and 800 killed. The soldiers thought the French casualties were four times as great.[45] (The French soldiers thought the Russian losses were twice as great as theirs, but in fact they were almost the same: Scrive reported that there were 2,000 French wounded and 700 killed.[46]) With the wounded arriving all through the night as well as in the day, the doctors and Sisters were almost totally exhausted physically. Worn out from night shifts, performing operations, and changing dressings, the doctors and nurses tried to take short naps on a bench or a cot in a waiting room, only to be awakened by the bursting of bombs and the cries of newly arrived wounded men.[47] 'It was impossible not to notice the exceptional endurance of Pirogov in these unforgettable and horrific days,' one of Pirogov's staff doctors remembered. 'When we assistants would return to the bandaging station after a short rest early in the morning, I recall that we would often find Nikolai Ivanovich there, performing an operation with the help of the feldsher, the watchman, and a Sister of Mercy.'[48]

When in May convalescent soldiers had to be evacuated to make room for new admissions, 400 wounded were taken across to the north side and dumped into soldiers' tents. There were four men in each small tent, and there was hardly room to sit – 'people without arms, without legs, with fresh wounds, right on the ground, all together on the same foul straw mattresses,' Pirogov wrote. He was outraged. 'When the regiment commander wants to arrange a dinner,' Pirogov told his wife, 'he is able to transform these same tents into a banquet hall, but for the wounded he doesn't find it necessary: just let four legless soldiers lie in one tent. And when they begin to die, then it's the doctors who are at fault for the high death rate.' Almost an entire month before the Second Bombardment began, he had 'pleaded, shouted, written official reports to the commander in chief (Prince Gorchakov), that it was necessary to remove the wounded from the city, to arrange for tents outside of the city, and to transport them there,' but they refused to do anything.[49] Now, after three days of steady rain, the Sevastopol clay soil was sticky, viscous mud which adhered to everyone's boots, making them as heavy as 16

The Sisters take over

kilogram weights. There were no trenches around the pitiful number of ragged tents and no plank beds. The men lay in the mud and the feldshers who tended them sank into it up to their knees.[50] The Sisters went back and forth to the soaking wet tents in heavy soldiers' boots and they also sank into the thick mud as they knelt down to care for the men. They did few dressings because it was more important to give the men hot tea and wine to warm them and prop up their spirits, and there was not time to do both.[51]

Pirogov complained again to one of Gorchakov's staff officers but this officer just pretended not to understand what Pirogov was talking about. It is the doctors who are always said to be at fault, Pirogov declared. The doctors were at the mercy of the military leaders. Nevertheless, he believed the doctors did have to shoulder some of the blame if they remained silent about these abuses. His complaint bore fruit. Prince Gorchakov himself visited the tents and castigated the general staff doctor who took him around. The prince then instituted a scrupulous investigation, after which arrangements for the patients were much improved. They were given cots with double mattresses but, Pirogov pointed out, so much damage had already been done that the terrible loss of life continued for another two weeks. If he had accomplished any good for the soldiers, Pirogov said, he succeeded only by using 'force, with lots of noise and harsh words, this is not much fun.' The army doctors had no sense of Pirogov's humanitarianism; the only motivations he thought they recognized were personal grudges or interests. The 120,000-man Southern Army had arrived and there were now so many soldiers in the city that they had to bivouac in the streets. Now it was even more difficult for the doctors because they had to deal with two sets of army administrators, both replete with intriguers. All the doctors were discouraged and wanted to leave with Pirogov. It was not the work or the long hours that terrified them, but rather the sense of helplessness trying to deal with such corrupt administrators. Pirogov had not slept for two days and nights after the tremendous trench battles at Bastions V and VI and was utterly exhausted as he slowly prepared to leave.[52]

On 25 May/6 June the French opened a cannonade on the White Works and Mamelon, and the next day, after a tremendous fight, captured them. The French, who always under-reported their losses, claimed 3,000 men lost, the Russians 2,500. Gorchakov was very

Doctor-directed nursing

discouraged. He reported that his men had fought very well but were defeated because they were so terribly outnumbered. Furthermore, he was so short on gunpowder that if he made even a moderate response to the heavy allied fire he would exhaust his supplies in ten days.[53] When they seized the White Works, the French captured two Russian surgeons with their nurses. Both surgeons spoke French and lived with the French doctors while waiting to be exchanged. One had a head injury and could not work but the other, an admirable surgeon, directed a special service for the Russian wounded. The Russian nurses astounded the French. They were so skilled at ligating arteries and doing dressings that they never had a single case of secondary hemorrhage. Secondary hemorrhage, one of the most frequent and most feared complications of military surgery, typically occurred between the fifth and twenty-fifth post-operative days. When it took place in larger arteries it was so sudden and so profuse it quickly became fatal.[54] Surgeons used silk, horsehair, or catgut ligatures – of course not sterile – and they left them long so that the thread could act as a drain for the pus but, of course as we know and they did not, the ligatures also acted as wicks for secondary infection which increased the risks of hemorrhage.[55] One of the many advantages of Pirogov's plaster casts was that they prevented secondary infection.

With the French in control of the Mamelon, allied bombs and shells now fell all over the south side of the city, and reached the north side as well as the ship side. The Assembly of Nobles and Pavlosky Point were under particular threat of destruction while round shot and rockets had been falling in the courtyards of Gushchin's and the Engineers' houses for some time. The staff therefore decided to transfer the patients from the Assembly to the Nicholas Bastion, which was heavily reinforced and the furthest removed from allied rifle fire. Excess patients in Pavlosky Point were to be sent to the heavily protected Michael Battery on the north side. In the meantime Pirogov evacuated most of the convalescent wounded out of the city to two tent hospitals, one near the village of Belbek, about 6 kilometers from Sevastopol, and the other on the Inkerman Heights, 3 kilometers away. The Sisters were given the choice of remaining on the south side or moving to the safer north side. Sister Bakunina insisted on staying with her nine Sisters at the Assembly of Nobles until all of the wounded had been moved to the Nicholas Bastion. There they

The Sisters take over

remained until the Russians evacuated the south side on 27 August/8 September.[56]

With the Mamelon and White Works in allied hands the allies began a massive bombardment, the Third Bombardment, on 5/17 June. The next day was Waterloo Day, the great Russian victory. The French attacked first and were driven back by murderous fire from the bastions and the steamers in the bay. The British had to run across an open field of 800 yards to attack the Redan. As soon as the troops climbed out of the trenches they were assailed by the most lethal grapeshot that one commander had ever seen. Only a few men reached the abatis in front of the bastion. It was a total massacre. The British reported 1,570 men lost, and the French 3,338, but their losses are thought to have been more like 6,000. A few British soldiers reached houses on the outskirts of the town, and bursting through the door of one expecting to find Russian soldiers, they found instead three Sisters of Charity tending their patients. The Sisters kept working quietly and never raised their heads when the soldiers entered. When the soldiers were ordered to withdraw, out of respect for the Sisters, they left that house alone.[57]

The assault was such a disaster that the chief engineers in both armies recommended raising the siege if the fortress held out until winter.[58] The Russians were elated by their smashing victory but they had lost almost 5,000 men repulsing the assault.[59] Midshipman Wood noted that few of the skilled Russian naval gunners were still alive in June and were replaced with infantry soldiers who were much less competent.[60] The Russians suffered two more great losses in June. Totleben, who was accustomed to ride calmly through all the batteries every day giving orders and directions for the work to be done on them that night, was severely wounded in the leg on 8/20 June. He was out of commission for several weeks, and during this time his plans for more and heavier guns, two new batteries on the rear flanks of the Malakhov, and a mine system in front of it were not carried out.[61] Then on 28 June/10 July, while inspecting the batteries, Nakhimov was hit in the face by a bullet and died two days later.[62] Pirogov was in Sevastopol during the bloody fight for the White Works and the Mamelon but he and a number of his surgeons, physically and mentally exhausted, left for St. Petersburg five days before this great Russian victory. Not one of the Sisters left with the surgeons. Pirogov

Doctor-directed nursing

did not entrust them to another doctor, but rather placed the community under the direction of Count Osten-Sacken who continued to take a constant and sincere interest in their work. On the south side, the Sisters continued to work efficiently but Bakunina wrote that after Pirogov left, 'we worked just as uninterruptedly, just as conscientiously, but there was not the same liveliness, vivacity, the same spiritual involvement!'[63] On the north side and at the Belbek and Inkerman, Stakhovich was personally in charge and, without Pirogov's oversight, managed very badly.

Over the summer of 1855 the Russians were unable to return more than one shot for every four the enemy fired, and casualties increased. Hübbenet was appalled by the gruesome wounds the modern rifles inflicted. There were men with their intestines hanging out in front, or ripped out from the back, causing spinal paralysis. These men could still speak and would live for a few more hours. Hübbenet thought the worst of all were those who were hit in the face so that they no longer looked like a human being. Their faces were 'a bloody mass of tangled flesh and bone – no eyes, nose, mouth, cheeks, tongue, chin or ears to be seen,' and yet they were able to stand on their feet and move and wave their arms about so he thought they still had a certain level of consciousness. On 5/17 and 6/18 June alone 4,000 more casualties were brought into the Assembly. It was so crowded that sometimes the wounded were laid on top of each other. At the Paul Battery there were another 5,000 wounded lying on the bare floors of wharves and stores. At this point all the Sisters had been withdrawn from this bastion because it was under constant rifle fire from the Mamelon. In any case, there were so many patients that there was no place for the Sisters to live, so both the wounded and the surgeons had to do without their help.

Conditions in Sevastopol deteriorated rapidly. The Nicholas Battery became the location of the main dressing station as well as almost all the administrative, medical, and commercial activities in Sevastopol. The headquarters of Count Osten-Sacken, duty watches, a church, barracks, a shop, a bandaging station, a hospital, and the pharmacy run by N. P. Korvovskii, who provided medicines throughout the siege, were all in the battery. Supplies of food and water ran low, cholera increased, as did desertion.[64] Previously it was rare for a Russian to desert; deserters were usually soldiers from ethnic minorities, such as Hodasevich who deserted to join the allied Polish legion,[65] but now Russians were deserting because they were starving. There were rumors in August that there were mutinies in Sevastopol which the Russian officers had put down brutally.[66] The Russian High Command felt that despite the great victory on Waterloo Day, defeat was inevitable. Khrulev, who was the most aggressive of the Russian generals, as well as Osten-Sacken, Totleben, and Vasilchikov all recommended withdrawing to the north side, a move which would have saved thousands of lives. They argued that the allies had such superiority in fire power and the Russians were sustaining such terrible losses in manpower that this was the only sensible policy. A Russian attack on the allies would be suicidal because the allied position was basically impregnable.[67] It is all the more interesting that, despite the progress the French in particular were making pushing their saps closer and closer to the walls of the city, the allied soldiers remained impressed with the strength of the Russian defense. For example, on 10 August Captain Hawley wrote from the British camp that the Russians had found a way of shooting 34-pound shot right into the British camp and beyond.[68] Loizillon reported fierce Russian resistance in August. The Russian steamers fired on the French every night, and even at the end of August, when Russian firepower was markedly diminished, they invented a new kind of mortar which shot bombs, grenades, and grapeshot, causing many losses.[69]

Tsar Alexander II, who succeeded his father on his death in February, and the Ministry of War were pressing Gorchakov to make one last offensive effort. He agreed with his generals that it was folly to attack an enemy who so outnumbered him and was entrenched in such solid positions. Nevertheless, dutifully on 4/16 August he launched an attack on the all but impregnable French and Sardinian position along the steep slopes of the Tchernaya River. Before the battle began, fourteen Sisters were sent from the Belbek camp to the Tchernaya to help establish a field hospital. The battle was a horrible disaster, as noted previously. The Russians lost approximately 8,000 men – eleven generals, 2,273 men killed, almost 4,000 wounded, and 1,742 missing. Most of the missing were deserters who had taken advantage of the early morning fog to run away. The Sisters worked with surgeons and feldshers doing dressings, assisting at operations, distributing linens, warm drinks, wine, and so forth. There was no time to change their clothes, and it was only after sixteen days when all the wounded had been transported to hospitals in Bakhchiserai and Simferopol that they were able to bathe in the sea and return to their camp at the Belbek.[70] As Sevastopol became riddled with rifle fire as well as bombs and shells, the tent hospitals on the Belbek and Inkerman Heights gradually became the main hospitals. After receiving initial medical treatment the wounded from the north and south sides were transferred to these much safer hospitals. Many Sisters from the first, second, and fourth parties, as well as a newly arrived fifth party of Sisters, were moved to the Belbek hospital where they were housed in tents and Tatar huts.[71]

Sevastopol was taking a terrible bombardment. Morton, the American doctor who was working for the Russians, pointed out that the allies surrounded the city on three sides and their ships covered half of the fourth side. Hence they could concentrate their fire on one point while the Russian fire had to diverge in all directions. 'When our men are off duty they are nearly exposed to the same danger as when on, because the bombs and cannon balls are whizzing and bursting all over the city all the while,' he said. As a result, he thought by the summer of 1855 almost half as many soldiers in Sevastopol were killed when they were off duty as when they were on. When the French soldiers went off duty they went back to their camp which was beyond the range of the Russian guns.[72] In 'Sevastopol in August' the two fictional Kozeltsov brothers, who die heroically in the final assault, went to the hospital in the Nicholas Battery to visit a comrade named Martsov. A bomb had blown one of Martsov's legs off while he was off duty asleep in his room.

As the brothers entered the first ward they were overcome by the loathsome, cloying hospital miasma. Two Sisters of Mercy approached them. One, about 50 years old with black eyes and a severe expression, was carrying a pile of lint and dressings and was giving instructions to a young apothecary's assistant. The other Sister was a very pretty girl of about 20 with a pale, delicate, fair-complexioned face. The elder brother asked where Martsov might be. The Sister told the younger nurse to take the two brothers to him and then left with the apothecary's assistant. Volodya, the younger brother, stared in horror at the wounded men. Seeing that these dreadful results of war were new to him the young nurse asked his brother, '"I suppose he hasn't been out

The Sisters take over

here very long."' Kozeltsov explained Volodya had only just arrived, at which the nurse suddenly burst into tears. "'Oh God, God!" she cried, with despair in her voice. "When is all this going to stop?"' Martsov was in the officers' ward, his yellowish face displaying the expression of one trying not to cry out in pain. His undamaged leg, clad in a sock with the toes twitching convulsively, protruded from under the blanket.

> 'Well, and how are you today?' asked the nurse as with her delicate fingers, on one of which Volodya noted a gold ring, she raised the wounded man's slightly balding head and straightened his pillow for him. 'Here are some friends of yours who've come to see you.' 'I'm in pain, of course,' said the patient testily. 'Leave me alone, I'm all right.'

Martsov did not recognize Kozeltsov; he said a man forgets everything when he is in hospital. "'God, how it hurts! ... I wish it could all be over," he moaned giving his leg a jerk and covering his face with his hands. "You'd better leave now," said the nurse in a low voice; there were tears in her eyes. "He's in a very bad way."'[73] It is noteworthy that Tolstoy, who so dedicated himself to telling the truth,[74] depicted the Nicholas Battery hospital in these last few days on the south side of the city as well ordered and functioning smoothly despite the deteriorating conditions in Sevastopol.

Notes

1 Pirogov, *Sevastopol Letters*, p. 80.
2 Ibid, pp. 85–6, 90, 96, 99–100; Pirogov, 'Historical Survey,' pp. 31–2.
3 Pirogov, 'Historical Survey,' pp. 32–3, 40.
4 Hübbenet, *Russian Wounded*, p. 21; Curtiss, *Crimean War*, p. 462.
5 Peard, *Narrative*, p. 64.
6 Pirogov, *Sevastopol Letters*, pp. 125–6, 162.
7 Pirogov, 'Historical Survey,' pp. 33–4; Soroka and Ruud, *Grand Duchess*, p. 207.
8 Soroka and Ruud, *Grand Duchess*, p. 204; Pirogov, *Sevastopol Letters*, pp. 158, 161; Rappaport, *No Place for Ladies*, p. 115.
9 Malis, 'Editor's Introduction,' pp. 13–14; Bessanov, 'Russian Nurses.'
10 Pirogov, 'Historical Survey,' pp. 33–4.
11 Malis, 'Editor's Introduction,' p. 17.
12 Curtiss, *Russian Army*, p. 339.
13 Calthorpe, *Letters from Headquarters*, pp. 218–19, 233.

Doctor-directed nursing

14 Tolstoy, *Diaries*, vol. 1, p. 101.
15 Tolstoy, 'Sevastopol in May,' pp. 222–3.
16 Robinson, *Diary*, p. 309.
17 Goodlake, *Sharpshooter*, pp. 111–12.
18 Ibid, pp. 51–2; Curtiss, *Crimean War*, pp. 425–6, 428–9.
19 Pirogov, *Sevastopol Letters*, p. 102.
20 Pirogov, 'Pirogof à Sebastopol,' p. 43.
21 Pirogov, *Sevastopol Letters*, pp. 106–7, 109–12, 119.
22 Ibid, pp. 125–6; Soroka and Ruud, *Grand Duchess*, p. 212.
23 Pirogov, 'Pirogof à Sebastopol,' p. 40.
24 Curtiss, *Russian Army*, pp. 346–7; Pirogov, *Sevastopol Letters*, p. 119.
25 Gordon, *Gordon's Letters*, pp. 26–7, 29; Alan, *Crimean Letters*, pp. 91–2.
26 Pirogov, 'Pirogof à Sebastopol,' pp. 39–40; Sorokina, 'Russian Nursing,' pp. 59–60.
27 Pirogov, 'Pirogof à Sebastopol,' pp. 41–4.
28 Hübbenet, *Russian Wounded*, p. 7.
29 Pirogov, 'Historical Survey,' p. 35.
30 Hübbenet, *Russian Wounded*, p. 49.
31 Curtiss, *Russian Army*, p. 347.
32 Pirogov, 'Historical Survey,' pp. 34–5.
33 Pirogov, *Sevastopol Letters*, p. 124.
34 Pirogov, 'Historical Survey,' pp. 35–6.
35 Curtiss, *Crimean War*, pp. 428–30.
36 Curtiss, *Russian Army*, pp. 346–7.
37 Pirogov, *Sevastopol Letters*, p. 129.
38 Wood, *Midshipman*, p. 69.
39 Malis, 'Editor's Introduction,' p. 22; Pirogov, *Sevastopol Letters*, pp. 123, 127–9.
40 Pirogov, 'Historical Survey,' pp. 37–9.
41 Tolstoy, 'Sevastopol in May,' pp. 228–9.
42 Pirogov, *Sevastopol Letters*, p. 129; Curtiss, *Crimean War*, p. 430.
43 Wood, *Midshipman*, pp. 69–70.
44 Clifford, *Letters*, p. 83.
45 Pirogov, 'Historical Survey,' p. 39; Pirogov, *Sevastopol Letters*, p. 141; Curtiss, *Crimean War*, p. 431.
46 Scrive, *Relation*, p. 202.
47 Pirogov, 'Historical Survey,' p. 37.
48 Malis, 'Editor's Introduction,' pp. 18–19.
49 Pirogov, *Sevastopol Letters*, pp. 132–5.
50 Malis, 'Editor's Introduction,' p. 22.
51 Pirogov, 'Historical Survey,' p. 41.
52 Pirogov, *Sevastopol Letters*, pp. 132, 138–41.
53 Curtiss, *Russian Army*, pp. 349–50.

The Sisters take over

54 Baudens, *Souvenirs*, p. 43; Macleod, *Surgery in the Crimea*, pp. 139–40.
55 Gabriel, *Between Flesh and Steel*, pp. 135–6.
56 Malis, 'Editor's Introduction,' pp. 23–4; Pirogov, 'Historical Survey,' pp. 41–2.
57 Clifford, *Letters*, pp. 236–7.
58 Figes, *Crimean War*, pp. 364–71.
59 Ibid, pp. 373–4; Curtiss, *Russian Army*, pp. 350–1.
60 Wood, *Crimea in 1854*, p. 290.
61 Hodasevich, *Within Sebastopol*, p. 106; Curtiss, *Russian Army*, pp. 352–3. Figes gives a different date, 22 June/4 July.
62 Figes, *Crimean War*, p. 378.
63 Malis, 'Editor's Introduction,' p. 24; Pirogov, 'Historical Survey,' p. 42.
64 Pirogov, 'Historical Survey,' pp. 42–4; Figes, *Crimean War*, pp. 376–80.
65 Hawley, *Letters*, p. 48.
66 Figes, *Crimean War*, pp. 379–80.
67 Curtiss, *Russian Army*, pp. 351–2.
68 Hawley, *Letters*, pp. 72–3.
69 Loizillon, *Campagne*, pp. 176, 179–80.
70 Figes, *Crimean War*, pp. 380–4.
71 Pirogov, 'Historical Survey,' pp. 46–7.
72 Margrave, 'Dr John W. Morton,' p. 23.
73 Tolstoy, 'Sevastopol in August,' pp. 285, 287–8.
74 Tolstoy, 'Sevastopol in May,' p. 255.

14

The reorganization of the community

The fall of the south side of Sevastopol

The Battle of the Tchernaya made it clear that the south side of Sevastopol would have to be abandoned so the Russian engineers built a pontoon bridge from Fort Nicholas across to the north side to enable the evacuation.[1] Ten days after it was finished, on 25 August/5 September, the last bombardment began, demolishing large sections of the bastions. On one night alone 1,000 wounded were admitted to the hospitals. The gunfire had been so relentless that the Russians were unable to repair their severely damaged embrasures. For example, in the Malakhov only eight of the sixty-three cannons and mortars were in working order on the morning of 27 August/8 September. Although their guns were barely able to reply because their reserves of gunpowder and projectiles were so low, the Russians put up a tremendous fight. The allies made twelve different attacks on the batteries and bastions, and again and again the Russians repulsed them. Only the French attack on the Malakhov was successful. Having repulsed eleven out of the twelve assaults, the soldiers believed they had won an even greater victory than that of 18 June. In the dressing stations and hospitals there were triumphant shouts of victory. The men said beating the enemy so thoroughly was worth having an arm or leg amputated. The French generals were pleased to have taken the Malakhov but reported 10,000 men lost in the assault, and it was probably more, considering their standard under-reporting. Pélissier expected it would be a long and costly campaign to take the rest of the bastions and was not certain he could hold the Malakhov if the Russians tried to retake it as he expected them to do. At the end of the long, terribly exhausting day, Clifford lay down on

The reorganization of the community

his bed with his clothes on feeling more low-spirited than he ever had before because the British had failed to capture their objective, the Redan. The conduct of the officers had been beyond all praise, but many an officer dashed alone over the parapet to certain death because his men would not follow him. Many soldiers ran away, and although Clifford and a colleague beat them with their swords trying to get them to return to the fight, the Russian musketry and grapeshot was so fierce that the men still fled. 'Sevastopol will never give in,' Clifford thought to himself as he lay down, 'until we have fought for every inch of ground.'[2]

On the Russian side, Gorchakov had lost 12,913 men and knew it would be impossible to retake the Malakhov or to maintain the defense of the other severely damaged bastions and batteries. With the Malakhov in their hands, the allies could turn their heavy guns on the inner defenses of Sevastopol. At 5 p.m. he therefore issued orders to evacuate the south side of the city, and at 7 p.m. the move across the pontoon bridge began. Russian officers and soldiers were appalled because they so genuinely believed they had won a decisive victory. At first many troops refused to withdraw, thinking it was some kind of betrayal; the sailors, who considered Sevastopol their town, for which they had fought so valorously, were outraged.[3] 'The first reaction of every Russian soldier on hearing this order was one of bitterness and incomprehension,' Tolstoy wrote.[4] Nevertheless, the evacuation proceeded. Totleben and Vasilchikov had planned it carefully. Five regiments manned barricades in the city in case the enemy tried to pursue, and volunteers, of whom Tolstoy was one, remained in the bastions keeping up the fire to prevent the allies from learning the army was retreating across the bridge.[5] The allies were aware of heavy movements of Russian troops during the night but did not realize they were evacuating the city so they maintained only desultory firing. Still, there were shells flying and bombs dropping around them as the Sisters assisted their patients over the bridge.[6] Crossing the bridge was in itself a major exploit. The wind, which did not seem especially strong on shore, was violent and buffeting out on the bay, making the bridge pitch and sway as waves hissed across its boarded surface, and the Sisters met troops rushing across in the opposite direction to support their colleagues in the bastions.[7]

Doctor-directed nursing

In these last days when the allied artillery was reaching the Russian ships in the bay, the Sisters were injured more often. Sisters Smirnova and Budberg were both badly wounded by glass fragments from a window shattered by a blast. Smirnova almost lost her eyesight and Budberg was buried in glass fragments. One of her amputee patients immediately rushed to extract her.[8] As she crossed the pontoon bridge, weighed down with the possessions of the community and the money belonging to the soldiers, Sister Budberg nearly fell into the bay. Bakunina was the last of the Sisters to leave the south side. By 8 a.m. the next morning the crossing was complete. The last defenders were ordered to leave the bastions and set fire to the town.[9] 'Each man, on arriving at the other side of the bridge,' Tolstoy wrote four months later,

> took off his cap and crossed himself. But this feeling concealed another – draining, agonizing and infinitely more profound: a sense of something that was a blend of remorse, shame and violent hatred. Nearly every man, as he looked across from the North Side at abandoned Sevastopol, sighed with a bitterness which could find no words, and shook his fist at the enemy forces.[10]

On arrival in the city British Lt. Colonel Hamley reported finding two thousand desperately wounded men in the Assembly of Nobles. Scrive, however, said there were only 500 his doctors attended, and on 10 September the Russians sent one of their steamers under a flag of truce to collect those who were still alive.[11] Curtiss, who worked from Russian sources, supported Scrive's number: the Russians reported 500 hopeless cases left in the city with a feldsher who had been given a letter for the allies.[12]

On the north side the Russians were in a secure position on high ground overlooking Sevastopol with their heavy guns covering the bay and the lower reaches of the Tchernaya. Their fire was so strong that the allies could not house troops in the south side of the city. They therefore decided to wait until the spring to attack the north side. As a result, the fighting almost completely stopped after 8 September, but of course wounds and disease continued to take many lives and kept the doctors and Sisters very busy.[13] The Sisters' main activities were now concentrated in the tented hospitals at the Belbek and Inkerman Heights. At the Inkerman Heights, where most of the

292

The reorganization of the community

wounded from the final assault were, the doctors were performing up to eighty or a hundred operations every day. The Sisters were hard pressed distributing dry linen, hot drinks, and wine. The weather was windy, cold, and rainy and often they had to dress the wounded in the open air in the rain, on their knees on the wet ground or in the mud.[14]

The reorganization of the community

Although he had sworn he would never return to the Crimea, Pirogov's humanitarianism got the better of his resolve. After a rest of two months he returned with a team of doctors. He went to the encampment on the Belbek, and from there traveled about to the various hospitals in Simferopol and Bakhchiserai. The allies did continue to bombard the north side but without inflicting very much damage; only about four or five men were wounded or killed each day.[15] However, if there were fewer major injuries and deaths, Pirogov was very distressed when he saw the way Stakhovich had managed her two large tent hospitals while he was away. There were 13,000 patients, 7,000 wounded and 6,000 sick with bowel disease. Their lightweight tents were unbearably cold at night and they did not have enough blankets. Sheepskin coats had been sent but were still in the stores. Pirogov went to the storerooms himself and was disgusted to find double tents and 400 blankets as well. He attributed the failure to give out these much needed items to sheer laziness. He had them distributed immediately. There were now more Sisters per patient than ever before because a fifth party of Sisters had arrived in the summer, but the Sisters' pharmacy was in disorder and the patients were still in dirty linen although there was an ample supply of clean shirts in the stores. Stakhovich told Pirogov she had asked for linen and other supplies but the hospital administrators ignored her. Pirogov was very angry. He told her she should have continued demanding the supplies until she got them; it was not her business to care whether she made someone angry – she was not in the Crimea to earn popularity with the commissariat and staff bureaucrats.[16]

The Grand Duchess, to whom Stakhovich continued to spitefully and dishonestly complain about both Pirogov and Bakunina, sent Ekaterina Aleksandrovna Khitrovo, the head of the Compassionate Widows of Odessa, to the Crimea hoping she could sort things out.

Doctor-directed nursing

Khitrovo arrived on 5/17 September and proved a godsend. With less surgery to do, Pirogov now turned his attention to the Sisters. 'I have taken up the affairs of the Sisters with great energy,' he wrote to his wife on 9/21 October. During the day he was busy with the patients and giving lectures to the doctors but he met every evening, sometimes until 1 a.m., with Khitrovo, Bakunina, and one of the new Sisters, Elisaveta Kartseva. 'Having now entered into all the details,' Pirogov told his wife that some of the Sisters were unable to perform well unless he or the capable senior Sisters were supervising them. He learned that all the infighting and intrigues which had gone on for so long originated with one person only, Head Directress Stakhovich. She offended Pirogov's senior doctor and used her Sisters as mere servants, encouraging them to treat her with obsequiousness. She could give the appearance of efficiency, Pirogov said, but in reality she behaved like a fishwife and was capable of nothing but making a lot of noise and creating intrigues. Pirogov had never had real confidence in her but had hoped that with time she would improve. Now he could see that she 'looked at everything from her own selfish point of view and wanted only to shine with her own self-importance.'

Pirogov temporarily removed Stakhovich and her whole first party of nurses from the hospitals and asked Elena Pavlovna's permission to replace her. Realizing that Pirogov wanted to fire her, Stakhovich did everything she could to convince the Grand Duchess to maintain her position. Pirogov found it hard to believe that Elena Pavlovna would take Stakhovich's tales about Bakunina seriously, but apparently she did. If she refused to let him replace Stakhovich despite all the hard evidence from Khitrovo and himself, he was determined to abandon the community. A few days later Stakhovich was doing so much yelling that he thought she was losing her mind. Finally the Grand Duchess agreed to dismiss her and on 20 October/1 November she and her first group of Sisters left. Khitrovo, who became Superior several days previously, was a very able and popular manager. She did not make the Sisters call her 'Excellency' as Stakhovich had done, was quite prepared to take shifts herself, and was not ashamed to roll up gauze and do dressings. Pirogov suggested that she be called Senior Sister rather than Head Directress, a title he considered too bureaucratic. He established a committee consisting of Khitrovo, Bakunina, and Kartseva, the Sisters' chaplain, and himself who made all the decisions about the nursing. Kartseva, whom he placed in charge of the Simferopol hospital, had it back on its feet in seven days. In the hospitals where the Sisters worked the nursing was running beautifully, but the corruption and theft persisted. Every night when Pirogov and the new committee met, among other things, they devised traps to catch what Pirogov called 'the hospital crooks.' Pirogov thought the nursing was constantly improving while nothing else was.[17] Sadly Khitrovo did not last very long. In early February 1856 she contracted typhus and died. Bakunina agreed to take on her position for a year.

Between October and December 1855 Pirogov visited nearly seventy hospitals.[18] He found the standing problem from the beginning of the war, transporting the wounded from the crowded Crimean hospitals to hospitals on the mainland where the soldiers could complete their convalescence, was as bad as ever. It took the peasant carts six days to reach Perekop and two more if they went on to Kherson or Nikolaev. As in the preceding winter the carts often became bogged down in the mud on the dirt roads and the men suffered terribly. There was no straw or hay to put down in the carts so the men were laid, three or four on each cart's bare wooden floor and covered with bast mats.[19] The mats protected them from the hot sun in the summer but provided little warmth in the cold weather. The men desperately needed sheepskin coats and blankets, but although the government provided the commissariat with millions of roubles, misappropriation and theft meant few men got the necessary items; worse still, they were not even given enough water on the trip. In the bitter winter weather they shivered all night in the cold in the open carts under the sky.[20] Pirogov therefore suggested that the Sisters now make transport their central concern.[21] He placed Bakunina and a team of Sisters in charge of convoys of 300–500 patients, with full responsibility for prescribing medicines, doing dressings, and providing the men with shelter, food, and clothing.[22] There were not enough Sisters to accompany every convoy, but on those they did, they prepared food and warm drinks for the men, helped find shelter in peasant huts at night, and dressed their wounds. Bakunina and her nurses shared all the same traveling and housing arrangements as the soldiers. Wearing heavy soldiers' boots with a coarse peasant's sheepskin, they trudged through the mud and all the other hardships of life

Doctor-directed nursing

on the road. 'The trials of the road, nights in the villages, constant care of the sick – are nothing to her [Bakunina], a woman of uncommon character,' Pirogov wrote. 'I must say, women are accommodating/flexible!' He found it comforting that there was still a moral power which was above the intrigues and gossip that Stakhovich fostered; one just needed to know how to employ the moral power, something Bakunina was very good at, as was Pirogov himself. By the end of October there were few new wounded in the hospitals although there were still many sick with bowel disease and fevers. However, their number was rapidly declining as they were being regularly moved out to convalescent hospitals. Pirogov thought that soon he would have very little to do apart from his nightly meetings with the senior Sisters. On 3/15 December he left the Crimea envisioning a great future for the Community of the Exaltation of the Cross.[23]

It is noteworthy that although Pirogov was the main organizer, leader, and teacher of the Sisters in the Crimea, there were also highly competent Sisters in Perekop and Kherson and in the naval hospital in Simferopol where he never worked. For example, in Kherson Sister Shchedrina exercised what Pirogov called 'tireless devotion, uncommon efficiency and extraordinary self-sacrifice.' She integrated the Sisters into the hospital staff under the direction of Dr Gebhart.[24] After the war Dr Paltsev, then Chief Doctor of the Moscow Military Hospital, described his experience working with Shchedrina and her Sisters:

> If distribution of medicines and care had been handled by the feldshers and other hospital staff, not by nurses, then the patients would not have had even a half of the prescribed medicines, food and wine, while the staff (feldshers and servants) would have been constantly drunk. It was only owing to the nurses' indefatigable toil that the hospital in Kherson had only 400 patients by September 1857, while the number of them in 1856 exceeded 5,000 and the total majority of them recuperated.[25]

The different legal status for Russian women and the contributions of the Sisters

There can be no question that the Sisters of the Exhaltation of the Cross had the most difficult and dangerous nursing work of all the nurses in the Crimean War, and that they were enormously successful. There were for a time serious problems with the Head Directress, but she was replaced by the highly competent Khitrovo and, on her death, the equally able and very experienced Bakunina. The community's enormous success hinged on three factors: first, the Grand Duchess' daring idea of sending women to the front; second, Pirogov's willingness to accept women, his vast experience working with military patients, and his administrative and teaching talents; and third, the courage and ability of the Sisters themselves. The Grand Duchess' humanitarianism and her salons with their important political and intellectual contacts gave her the ideas and competency to work together with Pirogov in establishing the sisterhood.

The corruption, graft, and inefficiency in the government bureaucracy vitiated many of the Tsar's efforts to improve conditions for his army. But at the same time, the autocratic nature of his government made it possible for the Grand Duchess to start Pirogov organizing the highly effective team of nurses and doctors within twenty-four hours of conceiving the plan. It would have been impossible for a sister-in-law of Napoleon III or Queen Victoria to unilaterally, within twenty-four hours, send a civilian doctor as chief surgeon and director of an unprecedented female nursing unit to their armies, especially when the army strongly opposed both the plan and the director. Also one must keep in mind Geoffrey Best's point that there were stark contrasts among the officers in the army. There were many dishonest men in the commissariat but in the Crimea it was headed by a highly competent man of integrity, General Zatler, who had double mattresses, blankets, tents and so on right on site in Sevastopol, and once the Sisters took over the administration, they saw that they were properly distributed. When Pirogov went into the stores at the Belbek camp he did not find the ridiculous amounts of chloroform and purgatives, or cosmetics, dainties, and gynecological instruments which Slade found in the Ottoman stores, and Russian purveyors did not have the power to sell officers' positions as did the Ottoman commissaries. Tents and blankets, although not enough, were there as well as the sheepskin coats the men needed. Kartseva could not have turned the hospital in Simferopol around in seven days if there had not been adequate stores. There were numerous dishonest pharmacists but there were also men of integrity like N. P. Korvovskii.

Pirogov was an exceptionally fine teacher. Throughout the war he demonstrated developments in the healing of wounds, judging when surgery was indicated, ways of performing operations, and post-operative treatment. Hübbenet thought it was his excellent teaching that was responsible for much of the Sisters' success. An equally fine administrator, Pirogov organized the surgical supplies, of which there was an abundance, and of course he introduced triage.[26] Using the Sisters as the chief administrators, he completely reorganized the administration of the military hospitals, recognizing the need for all parts of the medical department to work together. He exercised what he called his moral influence with difficult nurses such as Stakhovich. At least when he was there, she and her Sisters were able to do excellent work such as transferring patients from the Alexander Battery to Pavlosk Point under direct rifle fire. He was prepared to use night watchmen as assistants in the operating room when more qualified people were not available and he worked well with Lt. Yani and his stretcher-bearers. Hübbenet pointed out that although Pirogov did not have a commission in the army, his international reputation and his backing by a member of the imperial court gave him the authority to overcome some of the worst shortcomings and abuses in the military hospital system. There was less of what Hübbenet called 'social evil and abuse' because Pirogov introduced measures to control this and he could ignore bureaucratic red tape because martial law was in effect.[27] Finally, Pirogov fully appreciated that nursing was more than simply implementing doctors' orders precisely, and spent hours with the senior Sisters teaching them better nursing practices and some medical procedures as well as working out better nursing policies.

These top Russian doctors would undergo radical changes in their view of women. When the first party of Sisters arrived Pirogov noted immediately that their presence and sympathetic care brought vivacity to the hospital. This did not surprise him but both Hübbenet and Pirogov were astonished by the Sisters' courage, coolness, and perseverance under fire, which Pirogov initially thought so uncharacteristic of women and so amazing. At first Hübbenet believed the degree of resignation and nerves of steel which working under fire required was something women rarely possessed. He was to be astounded by the Sisters' efficiency, strength, daring, self-sacrifice, and heroism, which he said 'would give honor to the bravest soldier.'[28] Tolstoy expected

The reorganization of the community

to see the futile, morbidly tearful kind of sympathy which he had thought typical of women, but found instead 'an active, no-nonsense and practical concern' for the patients.

Why were these Sisters of Mercy so unlike the stereotypical delicate, submissive ladies from whom no one expected physical courage, who needed to be protected, to remain in the haven of the home expressing tearful sympathy and attending to trivial details? Why was Pirogov in October 1854 willing to place heavy responsibilities, of a kind these women had never experienced before, on their shoulders, and as well as patient care, give them the administration of hospitals with thousands of beds? And why were these ladies willing to accept such a heavy charge? As well as living in a different political environment, upper-class Russian women had a somewhat different social position from that of their peers in Western Europe. Russian family law restricted all classes of women, perhaps even more than did family law in the West, but Russian women were in a better position in relation to property ownership. In Britain, her husband became the owner of all of a woman's property the day she was married. By contrast, from the mid-eighteenth century Russian property law gave women the right to own, buy, sell, and administer real estate independently of their husbands. Moneyed Russian women made good use of these legal privileges, proving themselves just as competent in land administration as men. By the nineteenth century women participated in roughly 40 percent of all real estate transfers and, on the eve of the emancipation of the serfs in 1861, owned as much as a third of private property in Russia as well as serfs and urban real estate. Indeed, foreigners commented on the number of houses women owned in the cities. In short, Russian real estate law recognized women as the equals of men, giving them very considerable power within the family, and for noblewomen, an important role in the economic life of provincial society.[29] For example, while he was in the Crimea Pirogov's wife was searching for an estate to buy, and he gave her power of attorney and arranged to have his salary sent to her.[30]

Because women were less confined to the private sphere, there was not the same degree of separation between public and private life as in the West. Noblewomen in particular, because of their greater wealth, but also upper middle-class women, enjoyed more freedom in the public arena. Tsar Nicholas's father, Paul I, who disapproved

299

of the Empresses Elizabeth and Catherine the Great, removed women from the line of succession, pronouncing that the principal sphere of action for a royal lady should be the home rather than the court or the state. The very conservative Nicholas had tried to encourage the cult of domesticity which his father wanted to promote, but in the case of noblewomen, exhortations to concentrate on motherliness fell largely on deaf ears. The adulation of motherhood and the importance of not earning a salary which existed in Britain did not carry the same weight with upper-class Russian women. In the earlier nineteenth century Pirogov's mother and sisters considered earning money more acceptable than a state scholarship. Women tended to use their ability to deal in real estate to keep property within the family. For Russian noblewomen, Michelle Marrese wrote, 'a good mother was one who, above all, looked after the financial interests of her children even if she neglected their physical care.'[31]

In addition to women having a space in the public sphere, the women's movement in Russia was well underway by the time of the Crimean War. Philanthropy had always been an important activity for noblewomen and charitable activities brought elite women into an increasingly wide-ranging involvement in public life. Elena Pavlovna was typical in becoming very involved in philanthropic activities. In the 1840s the new lay sisterhoods and salons like those of the Grand Duchess were another expression of the women's movement. Social critics began attacking the restraints on upper-class women and criticizing serfdom; by the 1850s elite women were attending boarding schools, reading scholarly journals, and publishing poetry and short stories as well as managing real estate.[32] Class did play a major role, as illustrated by Stakhovich's fatuous efforts to make herself into a great lady, but class was not as rigidly defined as in Britain. It would have been unthinkable for Florence Nightingale to travel unchaperoned under the same conditions as the common soldiers, in open peasant carts, and sleeping in Tatar hovels at night. It would have been even more unthinkable for the Daughters of Charity to travel with the soldiers. The Russian Sisters of Mercy were prepared to accept so much more responsibility than the female nurses in the other armies, and Pirogov and his doctors were prepared to give it to them, at least in part because upper-class women were used to taking responsibility in one public area.

The reorganization of the community

Pirogov did not consider the dreadful infighting and mean tricks the Sisters played on each other a characteristic of women, but thought them equally characteristic of the military commanders. Over the course of the war he dramatically revised his earlier view of women, later writing:

> The results of participation of women in the war prove at any rate that up to now we totally ignored the admirable gifts of women. These talents clearly demonstrate that the 'woman problem' had every right to be posed at the time of the Crimean Campaign ... Opponents of emancipation of women affirm that there are great differences between the sexes, such as the brain which is smaller in the female, etc. This should not be relied on; it holds no water. If a woman is brought up and educated properly she is just as capable as a man to adopt scientific, artistic and social culture. However, it is essential that she should not relinquish her 'womanhood' as a result of her new status.[33]

This of course was a big if. Unlike the excellent nursing educations Pirogov and his doctors gave their Sisters, few other women at that time had such advantages. Many factors contributed to the Sisters' success but the most important cause of their brilliant performance was their own courage and willingness to undertake an entirely new and very dangerous field of action. Pirogov and his doctors enabled them by not worrying about the Sisters exceeding their proper sphere, as British doctors did. Rather they gave these very able women a scope of practice which was wider than that of modern nurse practitioners and allowed them to use their abilities to the fullest. As a result, a larger number of soldiers were successfully treated.

Notes

1 Figes, *Crimean War*, pp. 380–5.
2 Clifford, *Letters*, pp. 257–60.
3 Curtiss, *Crimean War*, pp. 455–8; Curtiss, *Russian Army*, pp. 355–9.
4 Tolstoy, 'Sevastopol in August,' p. 332.
5 Curtiss, *Crimean War*, pp. 457–8.
6 Pirogov, 'Historical Survey,' p. 47; Figes, *Crimean War*, pp. 392–4.
7 Tolstoy, 'Sevastopol in August,' p. 284.
8 Pirogov, 'Historical Survey,' pp. 46–7; Soroka and Ruud, *Grand Duchess*, pp. 213–14.
9 Figes, *Crimean War*, pp. 392–4.

Doctor-directed nursing

10 Tolstoy, 'Sevastopol in August,' p. 333.
11 Hamley, *Campaign*, pp. 322–3; Scrive, *Relation*, p. 231.
12 Curtiss, *Crimean War*, p. 457.
13 Ibid, pp. 458–9.
14 Pirogov, 'Historical Survey,' pp. 47–8.
15 Pirogov, *Sevastopol Letters*, pp. 145, 152–6.
16 Ibid, pp. 147–9.
17 Ibid, pp. 151, 154, 156–60, 162–3.
18 Soroka and Ruud, *Grand Duchess*, pp. 214–16.
19 Bast was a material made from the inner bark of trees, most often the lime tree, similar to the bamboo fibre which is now often used for towels and blankets.
20 Curtiss, *Crimean War*, pp. 464–5; Pirogov, *Sevastopol Letters*, pp. 149, 155.
21 Pirogov, 'Historical Survey,' p. 48.
22 Soroka and Ruud, *Grand Duchess*, pp. 215–16.
23 Pirogov, *Sevastopol Letters*, pp. 163–5, 170; Fried, 'Pirogoff in the Crimean Campaign,' pp. 534–5.
24 Pirogov, 'Historical Survey,' p. 46.
25 Bessanov, 'Russian Nurses.'
26 Hübbenet, *Russian Wounded*, p. 7.
27 Ibid, p. 28; Malis, 'Editor's Introduction,' pp. 8–9.
28 Hübbenet, *Russian Wounded*, p. 7.
29 Marrese, *Woman's Kingdom*, pp. 1–3, 101, 117, 144–5.
30 Pirogov, *Sevastopol Letters*, pp. 158, 161, 164, 166, 168.
31 Marrese, *Woman's Kingdom*, p. 202.
32 Ibid, pp. 199, 202–3, 241–2; Clements, *Women in Russia*, pp. 66–7, 94–5, 115–18.
33 Fried, 'Pirogoff in the Crimean Campaign,' p. 534.

Conclusion:
Transcending the limitations
of gender

Of the three systems of nursing discussed here, there can be no question that the government-imposed method with all its political ramifications was the hardest to apply, and that Florence Nightingale faced the greatest challenge of any of the directors of military nursing services. Even Pirogov, who met with so much resistance from dishonest military staff and the bureaucracy, had a less complex job because he had the backing of the court and, with the important exception of Stakhovich, the support of his nurses. Other British lady superintendents such as Martha Clough in the Highlanders' regimental hospital, Mother Francis Bridgeman who reported directly to Hall at the Balaclava General Hospital, or Eliza Mackenzie in Therapia, had very much easier positions. They were not trying to build a foundation for a permanent female military nursing service, nor were they in such sensitive political situations. Despite being lionized for her nursing work in the war, after the war Nightingale met strong resistance in her efforts to establish a female nursing corps in the army. Nevertheless, in 1861 she managed to introduce a small group of six nurses with Jane Shaw Stewart as superintendent at the military hospital in Netley. The British army nurse corps would develop slowly from this small beginning, but Nightingale herself had no legitimate control over the new military nurses although she could exercise some moral influence.

The religious sisterhoods provided topflight nursing services, but in a secularizing world they would later find it difficult to recruit enough women to provide services on the scale they did in the Crimean War. The Piedmont-Sardinian Daughters of Charity continued their military nursing in the new united Italy through World

Conclusion: Transcending the limitations of gender

War II but in the other countries religious Sisters fared less well after 1856. Mother Francis Bridgeman, who ran such excellent nursing services in Koulali and Balaclava, had no interest in making military nursing a permanent part of her order's mission, and in fact said she would not undertake such a project again. In France the Daughters of Charity carried on their military nursing under the Second Empire, but when the anti-clerical Third Republic was established religious nursing Sisters came increasingly under attack, and in the first decade of the twentieth century the government removed them from public hospitals.

Doctor-directed nursing was very successful although it was much less innovative in Britain than in Russia. In the British hospitals at Smyrna, Renkioi, and Therapia doctors directed competent lady superintendents who had little or no training in nursing. The doctors followed the model of the civilian hospitals in which they had worked at home, with the one major difference that upper-class rather than lower middle-class ladies served as matrons. Unlike the old-style matrons, these ladies did some nursing themselves but they still thought of nurses as basically a kind of specialized domestic servant. While the secular lady nurses lacked clinical experience, they were used to giving orders to their domestic staffs and brought those management skills to the hospitals. The patients and doctors were immensely appreciative of the better housekeeping, cooking, laundry, and supervision of the nurses. The female nurses also added vivacity and variety to ward routine, which the soldiers enjoyed after living for months in an all-male society. However, the Victorian concept of woman's mission and women's lack of intellect and ability to govern would severely limit the development of nursing, particularly in the English-speaking world. Those who worked with military nurses understood the difference that nursing education and clinical experience made, but the public did not have the opportunity to actually physically see the difference between trained and untrained nurses. The general public's idea of ladies as motherly people who were innately good nurses and therefore needed no special training or education undermined the move which nursing was beginning to make toward professionalism. By contrast, the barely literate working-class nurses saw nursing differently. They were becoming aware of their expertise and body of knowledge and demanding that

Conclusion: Transcending the limitations of gender

it be recognized. However, the strong British sense of class prevailed, and because they were working-class women, those in authority continued to see nurses as servants. It was the class-structured British model, made glamorous by the socially elite Nightingale, which would become the transnational archetype after the war.

In Russia the Sisters of the Exaltation of the Cross took over military hospital administration, exercising a great deal of autonomy, successfully overcoming corrupt services in every area except the hospital kitchens, delivering first class nursing care, and working closely with the doctors, taking on a very wide scope of practice. Under the direction of the extraordinarily brilliant and gifted Pirogov, the Russians developed an innovative and much more efficient system of nursing, using triage and teaching less professionally qualified people to take on important jobs. The French used this Russian model for their dressing soldiers, taking the most talented convalescent soldiers and soldier nurses available and training them to perform specific nursing and medical procedures.

After the war the doctors who worked with the Russian Sisters were anxious to see them continue their military hospital management. However, entrenched corruption in the Russian bureaucracy defeated efforts to continue the model of a hospital governing committee including senior nurses which Pirogov developed in the Belbek and Inkerman hospitals. The fact that Pirogov, reputedly after a fight with the Minister of War, abandoned medicine and left the profession after the war meant the Sisters lost their most powerful advocate in government efforts to improve military hospitals. Disgusted and tired of having to effect change 'by force, with lots of noise and harsh words,' Pirogov entered the field of education. In the end female nurses were accepted in some military hospitals but not in the management positions they held during the war. The Sisters felt demoted and furthermore, when it was no longer a case of a national emergency, it became difficult to recruit the same caliber of individual; there was not the same sense of mission or the excitement of wartime nursing. Another factor was that after the war the Grand Duchess wanted to make the sisterhood a more traditional religious order, which both Pirogov and Bakunina thought would be counter-productive. Bakunina therefore resigned as Head Sister. The sisterhood continued, albeit with a lay female superior, nursing in the

Conclusion: Transcending the limitations of gender

1877–78 Russo-Turkish War, and ultimately becoming the basis for the Russian Red Cross.

Pirogov and Nightingale, the two outstanding directors of nursing in the war, make an interesting contrast. They shared many characteristics and positions. First, they could never have accomplished all that they did if they had not both had powerful political and financial support. It was the Grand Duchess who first had the daring idea of using women at the front, who financed the Sisters of the Exaltation of the Cross, and who secured the imperial fiat for Pirogov to direct the medical and nursing services in the Crimea. Nightingale enjoyed the support of Palmerston, the Home Secretary and then from February 1855 Prime Minister, and Newcastle and Panmure, the Secretaries for War. As Secretary at War, Herbert did not carry the weight of a prime minister or cabinet member but he was an accomplished politician and gave Nightingale strong support and advice. As financial officer for the army under the Aberdeen government he provided generous funding which continued under the Palmerston government. Both directors of nursing had powerful intellects, were multilingual, widely traveled, and internationally oriented. Both were humanitarians who were thoroughly committed to their patients. Both were gifted and experienced administrators – what used to be called 'systems thinkers,' people who appreciated that the whole organization had to work collaboratively if it were to function well. Finally, both fought powerful opposition from the organizations in which they were working. Pirogov had a free hand with the doctors he selected himself, but faced severe opposition from the corrupt army doctors and some of the purveyors and apothecaries. Nightingale struggled with purveyors, Hall and some of his doctors, as well as with many army officers. At the same time she did not enjoy full support from her employer, the War Office.

There were also very significant differences between the two individuals, in part because they came from two distinct cultures. Nightingale was so strongly motivated by the prevailing sense of class that she was prepared to make Mary Stanley and Jane Shaw Stewart superintendents although she was fully aware of their major failings, and even worse in Stanley's case, of her unwillingness to accept Nightingale's supervision. She made women like Tebbutt and Wear, whom she considered incompetent, superintendents simply

Conclusion: Transcending the limitations of gender

because they were ladies. In planning for the future, Nightingale saw a nursing hierarchy which reflected the earlier nineteenth-century social structure. Pirogov, on the other hand, was accustomed to women like his mother and sisters who were prepared to work for a living, and his wife to whom he gave power of attorney to deal with his financial affairs while he was in the Crimea. As in the British nursing corps and the Daughters of Charity, all classes were represented in the Community of the Exaltation of the Cross, but Pirogov was not particularly concerned with class. He never mentioned it as a qualification, or even referred to it except to say that Bakunina conducted herself as a lady and Stakhovich (also a lady) as a fishwife. He also pointed out that the most poorly educated Sisters were some of the most courageous, nursing the soldiers on the bastions.

Nightingale thought of the doctors as 'our masters' and the nurses as their 'trained instruments.' For her an excellent clinical nurse was one who, like Ruth Dawson, obeyed doctors' orders precisely. Pirogov also wanted nurses who, unlike the local untrained women, would carry out orders precisely but he saw a much wider field for his Sisters. They reported to the doctors but they ran the hospital administration and had far greater autonomy and a much wider scope of practice than the British nurses. Nightingale's idea of an excellent nurse as one who promptly and precisely obeyed doctors' orders was not unreasonable given that the biggest shortcoming of the old nurses was their failure to implement doctors' orders. However, it was a far cry from the way Pirogov and the French and Piedmontese army doctors conceptualized nurses. For them practical considerations transcended gendered roles. It was not a case of imposing an ideology of separate spheres but one of who was able to do the job best: men who had the physical strength and training to work on the battlefield and to turn and lift wounded men, and women who were excellent and experienced hospital administrators or who nursed the wounded and sick under direct fire. In the French case, gendered constructions of nursing as feminine work made it difficult to recruit men to the male nursing corps. In the Russian case, Russian doctors did not worry about women exceeding their proper sphere; when women proved they had the courage and nerves of steel to nurse patients under fire they were surprised but very pleased to have these new capabilities. Pirogov also had the major advantage of knowing a great

Conclusion: Transcending the limitations of gender

deal more about medical and nursing treatment than did Nightingale. She relied heavily on Roberts, whose knowledge of nursing and patient care was immense but, compared to leading doctors, knew little of the principles underlying treatment. Pirogov was hence better able to teach and train his nurses and feldshers. If there can be no question that Nightingale faced the most difficult challenge, there can also be no question that the French, Piedmontese, and Russian nurses, who nursed on the battlefield where they could save the most lives, provided the best nursing services in the war.

A persistent theme in the story of the Crimean War nurses is the way the upper classes looked down on them and what they considered their menial and repulsive work. Nightingale was an exception in that she admired nursing skills, but hospital nurses had historically been the lowest rung of the hierarchical ladder of domestic service, and this would be one of the most difficult obstacles nurses faced as they struggled to define their place in the armies and in society as a whole. In the Crimean War nurses were becoming assistants to the doctors, which today would be a major step up from work as charwomen. However, nineteenth-century doctors did not command the respect which they now do either. In Turkey doctors were a despised profession, and in Russia they were not highly regarded. Russian doctors were predominantly civil servants of non-noble origin who worked in low-ranking positions. Pirogov sought the greater independence and esteem which he believed doctors in Western Europe commanded, and they did command more than Russian doctors, but leading Western European doctors did not feel they received the respect they deserved. Scrive and Chenu believed the French army had little respect for its doctors and regretted that the medical department did not have the standing of the other two scientific branches of the army, the artillery and the engineers. In Britain younger sons of the nobility did not go into medicine as they did into the army, navy, church, or sometimes law, and army officers looked down on their medical colleagues. Doctors were not raised to the peerage. When Lister was made a baron in 1897 the medical profession was pleased, but less so when they saw that Lister was being recognized more for his scientific achievements than his medical accomplishments.[1] If doctors did not command much respect, nurses commanded almost none. Becoming assistants to doctors gave them little change in social status in

Conclusion: Transcending the limitations of gender

mid-nineteenth century Britain. In Russia Prince Menshikov thought they would spread syphilis among the soldiers. 'Mere' nursing was a constant theme when nurses were being discussed. Kinglake found it hard to believe that ladies would nurse, 'simply nurse,' soldiers. Bishop Delaney told Bridgeman she 'could not undertake the mere task of nurse tending unaccompanied by the higher functions' of her position. Grant, who proudly thought Catholic nuns exceeded all other nurses, told Moore 'if you are reduced to mere *Nurses*' Nightingale would have more authority over the nuns than he was prepared to give her. Although the French military doctors were so heavily dependent on their trained soldier nurses, Chenu said even the doctors did not treat them with respect, and this was also true of the higher-ranking nurses themselves, the non-commissioned officer nurses, who looked down on the nurses who were privates and corporals.

Nevertheless, thanks in part to laudatory press coverage, the idea of secular ladies as military nurses almost immediately became accepted transnationally. Caring for enemy patients was another transnational concept which all five armies shared. The Russians, French, Piedmontese, and Ottomans did not differentiate between their own soldiers and those of the enemy, giving all the same care. The British, however, as Bell noted, usually treated their own soldiers first, placing Russian patients second. Bell grieved the way Russian prisoners were treated after Inkerman. The idea of trained nurses for the armed forces became transnational among military doctors who had worked with trained nurses, but it failed to transfer to the general public. Doctors from many countries at the Geneva Convention in 1864 unanimously agreed that untrained volunteer women were unhelpful. They were keenly aware of the difference that experienced nurses made in the caliber of patient care but they lost their case. Six years later in the Franco-Prussian War the Red Cross used untrained volunteer lady nurses. Few other people differentiated between trained and untrained nurses. For example, Kinglake believed it was because ladies were involved that Nightingale was successful, a mistaken idea that did cross national frontiers. Other ideas crossed borders but failed to be implemented. McGrigor was unable to convince his superiors to introduce a French-style ambulance corps. Nightingale thought Pirogov's division of the nurses into

Conclusion: Transcending the limitations of gender

three classes was one which the British should follow but that did not happen either. Raglan's wish to establish a corps of muleteers with cacolets and litters was unsuccessful.

The Crimean War demonstrated that nursing was becoming a knowledge-based practice. It is striking how much difference it made when doctors and nurses were willing to teach neophytes, whether educated ladies, dressing soldiers, or British and Turkish orderlies. Even more striking is the transnational humanitarianism of the nurses, who came from all classes and five different backgrounds. Despite all the restrictions and obstacles these men and women faced, all managed to relieve some of the sufferings of their patients. Even the Ottoman doctors, who at best could only offer kind words and a bit of the simplest nursing care, eased their patients' sufferings. However, the military medical departments which were most successful, the Russian, French, and Piedmont-Sardinian departments, were those in which the nurses transcended gendered constructions and their competencies rather than their sex determined their roles.

Note

1 Reader, *Professional Men*, p. 150.

Glossary

Blister: It was believed until later in the nineteenth century that open sores or blisters allowed morbid materials to escape from the body. Hence it was standard for doctors to create open sores artificially with chemicals, or sometimes surgically, which they called blisters. Blisters were usually dressed with poultices.

Comminuted fracture: A fracture resulting in crushed, crumbled, or pulverized bone.

Compound fracture: The bone is broken in more than one place, or the pieces of bone protrude through the skin.

Contusion: A bruise; an injury in which the skin or another part of the body is damaged but not broken. Broken capillary veins produce the bruising.

Debridement: Removal of foreign objects or dead or damaged material (slough), especially from wounds.

Diaphoretic: A drug which increases perspiration.

Erysipelas: A disease of the skin which turns it bright red (also known as St. Anthony's Fire).

Fomentations: Treatment now known as soaks, usually with some medicine added.

Gangrene: Necrosis or death of bone and/or tissue, usually surrounded by healthy parts. In bone the dead part is called sequestrum, while in tissue it is known as slough.

Healing:

> **By first intention**: A wound is said to heal by first intention when the edges can be approximated and it closes without infection, leaving very little scar tissue.

> **By second intention**: Granulation tissue is formed to fill the gap

Glossary

between the edges of the wound, creating a significant scar. This form of healing is slower, and if the granulation forms first at the top it has to be opened and kept open so it can drain.

By third intention: Healing of an ulcer, wound, or cavity by filling with extensive granulation tissue, resulting in the formation of a large scar.

Hospital gangrene: A sloughing ulcer which spreads very rapidly.

Purulent infection: Another term for pyemia.

Pyemia: A form of septicemia due to pus-forming organisms in the blood, which produce multiple abscesses of a metastatic nature in the viscera.

Secondary infection: This is not a nineteenth-century term. It now means infection caused by a different organism than that causing the primary infection.

Septicemia: Previously known as blood poisoning, septicemia is now defined as the presence of pathogenic material in the bloodstream.

Slough: The separation of dead from living tissue; the dead or damaged tissue which is cast off.

Suppurating: This is a term which is no longer used. It means producing pus, as most wounds did in former times. There were two types. 'Laudable' or 'benevolent' pus, a thick cream-colored odorless liquid, was widely believed by surgeons to be a normal and necessary part of the healing process. But if the pus became watery, blood-tinged, and foul smelling it was considered 'ill-conditioned' and an unfavorable sign. After the Crimean War, when micro-organisms had been discovered, surgeons identified benevolent pus with a staphylococcus infection and ill-conditioned pus with the more dangerous streptococcus.

References

Archives

Boston University Nursing Archives (Howard Gottlieb Archival Research Center):
  LeMesurier Papers
  Nightingale Collection
British Library Additional Manuscripts:
  Nightingale Papers
Buckinghamshire Record Office:
  Verney Papers
Collected Works of Florence Nightingale, online at www.uoguelph.ca/~cwfn/, and sixteen-volume publication edited by Lynn McDonald (Waterloo, ON: Wilfrid Laurier Press, 2001–12)
Columbia University School of Nursing
  Nightingale Collection
Convent of Mercy, Bermondsey, London
Convent of Mercy, Dublin
Convent of the Community of St. John the Divine, Birmingham
Florence Nightingale Museum
Leeds County Record Office:
  Lady Charlotte Canning Papers
Leicestershire Record Office:
  Raglan Papers
London Hospital
London Metropolitan Archives:
  Charing Cross Hospital
  Guy's Hospital
  Nightingale Collection
  Nightingale Training School
  St. John's House
  St. Thomas's Hospital
  Westminster Hospital

References

London School of Economics:
  Booth Collection
Ministry of War, Turin
National Archives, Kew Gardens:
  Hawes Papers
Pusey House, Oxford
Royal College of Nursing
San Salvario Convent of the Daughters of Charity, Turin
United Kingdom House of Commons Sessional Papers 1854–55 (*Parliamentary Papers*)
Wellcome Institute:
  Nightingale Papers
  Queen's Nursing Institute Collection
Wiltshire Record Office:
  Herbert Papers

Primary sources

Alan, Major-General William, *Crimean Letters from the 41st (The Welch) Regiment, 1854–56*, ed. W. Allister Williams (Wrexham: Bridge Books, 2011).

Baudens, M. L., *La Guerre de Crimée: Les Campements, Les Abris, Les Ambulances, Les Hôpitaux, etc. etc.* (Paris: Michel Lévy Freres, 1858).

Baudens, M. L., *Souvenirs d'une Mission Médicale à l'Armée de l'Orient* (Paris: Imprimerie J. Claye, 1857).

Bazancourt, Baron de, *Cinq Mois au Camp Devant Sébastopol* (2nd edn, Paris: Amyot 1855).

Bell, Major-General Sir George, *Soldier's Glory, Being 'Rough Notes of an Old Soldier'*, ed. Brian Stuart (Tunbridge Wells: Spellmount, 1991).

Blackwood, Lady Alicia, *A Narrative of Personal Experiences and Impressions during a Residence on the Bosphorus during the Crimean War* (London: Hatchard, 1881).

Bonham-Carter, Henry, *Is a General Register for Nurses Desirable?* [pamphlet] (London: Blades, East & Blades, 1888).

Bridgeman, Mother Mary Francis, 'An Account of the Mission of the Sisters of Mercy,' in Maria Luddy, ed., *The Crimean Journals of the Sisters of Mercy 1854–56* (Dublin: Four Courts Press, 2004), pp. 121–246.

Bushby, Henry Jeffreys, *A Month in the Camp Before Sebastopol* (London: Longman, Brown, Green and Longmans, 1855).

Buzzard, Thomas, *With the Turkish Army in the Crimea and Asia Minor* (London: John Murray, 1915).

Calthorpe, Somerset, *Letters from Headquarters or, The Realities of the War in the Crimea by an Officer of the Staff* (2nd edn, London: John Murray, 1858).

References

Chenu, Jean-Charles, *Rapport au Conseil de Santé des Armées sur les Résultats du Service Médico-Chirugical* (Paris: Wiesener, 1865).

Cler, (General) Jean Josephe Gustave, *Reminiscences of an Officer of Zouaves*, translated from the French (New York: D. Appleton, 1940; originally published 1860).

Clifford, Henry, *Henry Clifford V.C.: His Letters and Sketches from the Crimea* (London: Michael Joseph, 1956).

Cobb, Peter G., 'Pusey, Edward Bouverie (1800–1882),' *Oxford Dictionary of National Biography* [online] [www.oxforddnb.com/view/article/22910, accessed 13 March 2017].

Codman, John, *An American Transport in the Crimean War* (New York: Bonnell, Silver & Co., 1896).

Croke, Sister Joseph, 'Diary October 1854 to May 1856,' in Maria Luddy, ed., *The Crimean Journals of the Sisters of Mercy 1854–56* (Dublin: Four Courts Press, 2004), pp. 63–117.

Dallas, Lt. Col. George Frederick, *Eyewitness in the Crimea: The Crimean War Letters (1854–56) of Lt. Col. George Frederick Dallas*, ed. Michael Hargreave Mawson (London: Greenhill Books, 2001).

Davis, Elizabeth, *The Autobiography of Elizabeth Davis*, ed. Jane Williams (London: Hurst & Blackett, 1857).

Dodd, George, *Pictorial History of the Russian War 1854-5-6 with Maps, Plans, and Wood Engravings* (Edinburgh and London: W. & R. Chambers, 1856).

Doyle, M., 'Memories of the Crimea,' in Maria Luddy, ed., *The Crimean Journals of the Sisters of Mercy 1854–56* (Dublin: Four Courts Press, 2004), pp. 1–61.

Duberly, Fanny, *Mrs Duberly's War: Journal and Letters from the Crimea, 1854-6*, ed. Christine Kelly (Oxford: Oxford University Press, 2007).

Engels, Friederich, *The Condition of the Working Class in England*, ed. David McClellan (Oxford: Oxford University Press, 1993).

Godman, Temple, *The Fields of War: A Young Cavalryman's Crimea Campaign*, ed. Philip Warner (London: John Murray, 1977).

Golding, Benjamin, *An Historical Account of the Origin and Progress of St. Thomas's Hospital, Southwark* (London: Longman, Rees, Orme & Brown, 1819).

Goodlake, Captain Gerald, *Sharpshooter in the Crimea: The Letters of Captain Gerald Goodlake, V.C.*, ed. Michael Springman (Barnsley, South Yorkshire: Pen and Sword Military, 2005).

Goodman, Margaret, *Experiences of an English Sister of Mercy* (London: Smith Elder, 1862).

Gordon, General Charles, *General Gordon's Letters from the Crimea, the Danube and Armenia*, ed. Demetrius C. Boulger (London: Chapman and Hall, 1884).

Graves, Robert James, *Clinical Lectures on the Practice of Medicine*, ed. Dr Nelligan (2nd edn, Dublin: Fannin, 1848).

References

Greig, David, *Letters from the Crimea: Writing Home, A Dundee Doctor*, ed. Douglas Hill (Dundee: Dundee University Press, 2010).

Guthrie, G. J., *Commentaries on the Surgery of the War in Portugal, Spain, France and the Netherlands with Additions Relating to Those in the Crimea* (6th edn, London: Henry Renshaw, 1855).

Hamley, E. Bruce, *The Story of the Campaign of Sevastopol* (Edinburgh: William Blackwood & Sons, 1855).

Hawley, R. B., *The Hawley Letters: The Letters of Captain R. B. Hawley*, ed. S. G. P. Ward (London: The Society for Army Historical Research, 1970).

Heath, Admiral Sir Leopold George, *Letters from the Black Sea During the Crimean War 1854–55* (London: Richard Bentley and Son, 1897).

Herbé, Jean François Jules, *Français & Russes En Crime: Lettres D'un Officier Français À Sa Famille Pendant La Campagne D'orient* (Primary Source Edition, Paris: La Librairie Nouvelle, 1892).

Hodasevich, Captain K., *Within Sebastopol: A Narrative of the Campaign in the Crimea, and of the Events of the Siege* (Driffield, UK: Leonaur, 2008; reprinted from London: John Murray, 1856).

Hübbenet, Christian, *Die Sanitäts-Verhältnisse der Russischen Verwundeten während des Krimkrieges in den Jahren 1854–56 [Russian Wounded]* (Memphis, TN: General Books LLC™, 2012).

Jameson, Anna, *Sisters of Charity, Catholic and Protestant and The Communion of Labor* (Boston: Ticknor and Fields, 1857).

Kinglake, Alexander William, *The Invasion of the Crimea: Its Origin and an Account of its Progress Down to the Death of Lord Raglan*, volume 4 (6 vols, New York: Harper, no date).

Kinglake, Alexander William, *The Invasion of the Crimea: Its Origin and an Account of its Progress Down to the Death of Lord Raglan*, volume 7 (9 vols, Edinburgh: Blackwood, 1891).

Lake, Colonel Atwell, *Kars and our Captivity in Russia* (London: Richard Bentley, 1856).

Lancet, 'Surgery of the War,' *Lancet* (16 December 1854) Vol. 64, No. 1663, p. 24.

Lancet, 'The Medical Officers of the Turkish Contingent,' *Lancet* (2 February 1856) Vol. 67, No. 1692, p. 136.

Lawson, George, *Surgeon in the Crimea*, ed. Victor Bonham-Carter (London: History Book Club, 1968).

Loizillon, Henri, *Campagne de Crimée: Lettres écrites de Crimée par la Capitaine d État-major à sa famille* (Paris: Ernest Flammarion, 1895).

Longmore, Surgeon-General T., *A Manual of Ambulance Transport* (2nd edn, London: Harrison and Sons, 1893).

Longmore, Surgeon-General T., *Gunshot Injuries: Their History, Characteristic Features, Complications and General Treatment* (London: Longmans Green, 1877).

References

Longmore, Surgeon-General T., *The Sanitary Contrasts of the British and French Armies during the Crimean War* (London: Charles Griffin & Co., 1883).

Macleod, George, 'Notes on the Surgery of the War,' *Lancet* (January 1856) Vol. 67, pp. 984–1001.

Macleod, George H. B., *Notes on the Surgery of the War in the Crimea with Remarks on the Treatment of Gunshot Wounds* (London: Churchill, 1858).

Malis, Iu. G., 'Editor's Introduction,' in Nicholas Ivanovitch Pirogov, *Sevastopol'skiia pis'ma 1854–55 [Sevastopol Letters]*, ed. Iu. G. Malis (St. Petersburg: Izdanie Russkago Kirurgicheskogo Obshchestva, 1907), pp. 3–28.

Masquelez, M., *Journal d'un Officier de Zouaves* (Paris: Librairie Militaire, Maritime et Polytechnique, 1858).

Montaudon, General Jean Baptiste, *Souvenirs Militaires: Afrique – Crimée – Italie* (Paris: Librairie C.H. Delagrav, 1898).

Nicol, Martha, *Ismeer or Smyrna and its British Hospital in 1855* (London: James Madden, 1857).

Niel, Le Général, *Siège de Sévastopol* (Paris: Librairie Militaire, 1858).

Nightingale, Florence, *Florence Nightingale: The Crimean War*, ed. Lynn McDonald, Collected Works of Florence Nightingale, volume 14 (Waterloo, ON: Wilfrid Laurier Press, 2010).

Nightingale, Florence, *Florence Nightingale's Spiritual Journey: Biblical Annotations, Sermons and Journal Notes*, ed. Lynn McDonald, Collected Works of Florence Nightingale, volume 2 (Waterloo, ON: Wilfrid Laurier Press, 2001).

Nightingale, Florence, 'Introduction of Female Nursing into Military Hospitals (1858),' in L. Seymer, ed., *Selected Writings of Florence Nightingale* (New York: Macmillan, 1954), pp. 1–119.

Nightingale, Florence, *Notes on Nursing: What It Is and What It Is Not* (London: Harrison & Sons, 1859).

Nightingale, Florence, *Notes on the Health of the British Army*, in *Florence Nightingale: The Crimean War*, ed. Lynn McDonald, Collected Works of Florence Nightingale, volume 14 (Waterloo, ON: Wilfrid Laurier Press, 2010), pp. 575–888.

Pack, Colonel Reynell, *Sebastopol Trenches and Five Months in Them* (London: Kirby & Endean, 1878).

Panmure, Lord, *The Panmure Papers Being a Selection from the Correspondence of Fox Maule, Second Baron Panmure, Afterwards Eleventh Earl of Dalhousie, K.T., G.C.B.*, ed. G. Douglas and G. Ramsay (2 vols, London: Hodder and Stoughton, 1908).

Parkes, E. A., *Report on the General Management and Formation of Renkioi Hospital* (Printed at the War Department April 1857), British Library Cup. 401 h 1.

Peard, Lieut. George Shuldham, *Narrative of a Campaign in the Crimea* (London: Richard Bentley, 1855).

References

Penney, Marjorie E., 'Letters from Therapia,' *Blackwood's Magazine* (1954) Vol. 275, pp. 413–21.

Pincoffs, P., *Experiences of a Civilian in Eastern Military Hospitals* (London: Williams and Norgate, 1857).

Pirogov, Nicholas Ivanovitch, 'Historical Survey of the Activities of the Sisters,' in *Sevastopol'skiia pis'ma 1854–55* [*Sevastopol Letters*], ed. Iu. G. Malis (St. Petersburg: Izdanie Russkago Kirurgicheskogo Obshchestva, 1907), pp. 29–51.

Pirogov, Nicholas Ivanovitch, 'Letters to his wife,' in *Sevastopol'skiia pis'ma 1854–55* [*Sevastopol Letters*], ed. Iu. G. Malis (St. Petersburg: Izdanie Russkago Kirurgicheskogo Obshchestva, 1907), pp. 57–171.

Pirogov, Nicholas Ivanovitch, 'Nicolas Pirogof à Sebastopol (1),' *Revue Scientifique* (January 1886) No. 2 (first published in *Revue historique russe*, August 1855), pp. 39–44.

Pirogov, Nikolas Ivanovitch, *Questions of Life: Diary of an Old Physician*, ed. Galina V. Zarechnak (Canton, MA: Watson Publishing International, 1991).

Radcliffe, J. N., 'The Turkish Hospital at Balaclava,' *Lancet* (5 January 1856) Vol. 67, No. 1688, pp. 7–9.

Reid, Dr Douglas A., *Soldier-Surgeon: The Crimean War Letters of Dr Douglas A. Reid 1855–56*, ed. Joseph O. Baylen and Alan Conway (Knoxville, TN: University of Tennessee Press, 1968).

Reid, Douglas Arthur, *Memories of the Crimean War January 1855 to June 1856* (London: St. Catherine Press, 1911).

Robinson, Frederic, *Diary of the Crimean War* (London: Richard Bentley, 1856).

Royer, Alfred, *The English Prisoners in Russia* (2nd edn, London: Chapman and Hall, 1854).

Russell, William Howard, *General Todleben's History of the Defence of Sevastopol 1854–55* (New York: D. Van Nostrand, 1865).

St. Vincent de Paul, *The Conferences of St. Vincent de Paul*, trans. Joseph Leonard (4 vols, Westminster, MD: Newman Press, 1952).

Sandwith, Humphrey, *A Narrative of the Siege of Kars and of the six months resistance by the Turkish Garrison under General Williams to the Russian Army* (London: John Murray, 1856).

Scrive, Le Dr G., *Relation Médico-Chirurgicale de la Campagne d'Orient* (Paris: Victor Masson, 1857).

Slade, Rear-Admiral Sir Adolphus, *Turkey and the Crimean War: A Narrative of Historical Events* (London: Smith Elder, 1867).

Small, E. Milton, ed., *Told from the Ranks: Recollections of Service during the Queen's Reign by Privates and Non-commissioned Officers of the British Army* (London: Andrew Melrose, 1897).

South, John Flint, *Facts Relating to Hospital Nurses* (London: Richardson Brothers, 1857).

References

Soyer, Alexis, *Soyer's Culinary Campaign. Being Historical Reminiscences of the Late War* (London: G. Routledge, 1857).

Steele, J. C., 'Statistical Account of the Patients Treated in Guy's Hospital during 1869,' in *Guy's Hospital Reports* (London: Churchill, 1871).

Steevens, Lieutenant-Colonel Nathaniel, *The Crimean Campaign with the Connaught Rangers* (London: Griffith & Farran, 1878).

Sterling, A. C., *Letters from the Army in the Crimea written in the years 1854, 1855, 1856* (published privately, 1856).

Sweetman, John, 'Maule, Fox, [*afterwards* Fox Maule-Ramsay], second Baron Panmure and eleventh earl of Dalhousie (1801–1874),' *Oxford Dictionary of National Biography* [online] [https://doi.org/10.1093/ref:odnb/18365, accessed 27 June 2019].

Taylor, Fanny, *Eastern Hospitals and English Nurses* (1st edn, 2 vols, London: Hurst and Blackett, 1856; 3rd edition, 1857).

Taylor, George Cavendish, *Journal of Adventures with the British Army* (2 vols, London: Hurst and Blackett, 1856).

Terrot, S., *Reminiscences of Scutari Hospital Winter 1854–55* (Edinburgh: Andrew Stevenson, 1898).

The Medical Chronicle or the Montreal Monthly Journal of Medicine & Surgery (1855) Vol. 1, No. 9.

Tolstoy, Leo, 'Sevastopol in August 1855,' in *The Cossacks and other Stories*, trans. D. McDuff and P. Foote (London: Penguin Books, 2006), pp. 256–334.

Tolstoy, Leo, 'Sevastopol in December,' in *The Cossacks and other Stories*, trans. D. McDuff and P. Foote (London: Penguin Books, 2006), pp. 185–202.

Tolstoy, Leo, 'Sevastopol in May,' in *The Cossacks and other Stories*, trans. D. McDuff and P. Foote (London: Penguin Books, 2006), pp. 203–55.

Tolstoy, Leo, *Tolstoy's Diaries*, ed. R. F. Christian (2 vols, New York: Charles Scribner, 1985).

Totleben, E. de, *Défense de Sébastopol* (2 vols, St. Petersburg: N. Thieblin, 1863).

Wood, General Sir Evelyn, *From Midshipman to Field Marshall* (5th edn, London: Methuen, 1907).

Wood, General Sir Evelyn, *The Crimea in 1854, and 1894* (London: Chapman & Hall, 1896).

Woods, N. A., *The Past Campaign* (2 vols, London: Longman, Brown, Green, and Longmans, 1855).

Secondary sources

Abel-Smith, Brian, *A History of the Nursing Profession* (London: Heineman, 1960).

Ackroyd, Marcus, Laurence Brockliss, Michael Moss, Kate Redford and John Stevenson, *Advancing with the Army: Medicine, the Professions, and Social*

References

Mobility in the British Isles, 1790–1850 (Oxford: Oxford University Press, 2006).

Armstrong-Reid, Susan, *The China Gadabouts: New Frontiers of Humanitarian Nursing 1941–51* (Vancouver: University of British Columbia Press, 2018).

Badem, Camden, *The Ottoman Crimean War (1853–1856)* (Boston: Brill, 2010).

Baumgart, Winfried, *The Crimean War 1853–56* (London: Arnold, 1999).

Beckett, Ian F. W., 'Wood, Sir (Henry) Evelyn (1838–1919),' *Oxford Dictionary of National Biography* [online] [www.oxforddnb.com/view/article/37000, accessed 27 November 2016].

Beddoe, Deirdre, 'Williams, Jane,' *Oxford Dictionary of National Biography* [online] [https://doi.org/10.1093/ref:odnb/29513, accessed 20 November 2018].

Bessanov, Yuri, 'Russian Nurses after the Crimean War,' *Journal of Nursing* [http://rn-journal.com/journal-of-nursing/russian-nurses-after-the-crimean-war, accessed 29 April 2018].

Best, Geoffrey, *War and Society in Revolutionary Europe 1770–1870* (Leicester: Leicester University Press, 1982).

Beyhan, Dr Mehmet Ali Ahmet Eryüksel, and Feyzullah Akben, eds, *Sağlik Ordusu/The Medical Forces* (2nd edn, Istanbul: Ajansfa, Ağustos 2010).

Bolster, Evelyn, *The Sisters of Mercy in the Crimean War* (Cork: Mercier Press, 1964).

Bostridge, Mark, *Florence Nightingale: The Making of an Icon* (New York: Farrar, Straus and Giroux, 2008).

Brooks, Richard, *The Long Arm of Empire: Naval Brigades from the Crimea to the Boxer Rebellion* (London: Constable, 1999).

Bynum, W. F., *Science and the Practice of Medicine in the Nineteenth Century* (Cambridge: Cambridge University Press, 1994).

Cannadine, David, *Class in Britain* (New Haven, CT: Yale University Press, 1998).

Cantlie, Neil, *A History of the Army Medical Department* (2 vols, Edinburgh: Churchill Livingstone, 1974).

Chadwick, Owen, *The Victorian Church* (2 vols, London: A. & C. Black, 1967).

Clements, Barbara Evans, *A History of Women in Russia* (Bloomington, IN: Indiana University Press, 2012).

Cobb, Peter G., 'Sellon, (Priscilla) Lydia (1821–1876), *Oxford Dictionary of National Biography* [online] [https://doi.org/10.1093/ref:odnb/25060, accessed 27 June 2019].

Colli, Colonel G., 'L'Organisation Sanitaire du Corps Expèditionnaire Sarde en Crimèe,' *Revue Internationale de la Croix Rouge* (October 1955), pp. 621–32.

Compton, Piers, *Colonel's Lady and Camp Follower: The Story of Women in the Crimean War* (London: Robert Hale, 1970).

Cook, Sir Edward, *The Life of Florence Nightingale* (2 vols, London: Macmillan, 1913).

References

Curtiss, John Shelton, 'Russian Sisters in the Crimea, 1854–55,' *Slavic Review* (1966) Vol. 25, No. 1, pp. 84–100.

Curtiss, John Shelton, *Russia's Crimean War* (Durham, NC: Duke University Press, 1979).

Curtiss, John Shelton, *The Russian Army Under Nicholas I, 1825–1855* (Durham, NC: Duke University Press, 1965).

Davidoff, Leonore, 'Class and Gender in Victorian England,' in Judith L. Newton, Mary P. Ryan and Judith R. Walkowitz, eds, *Sex and Class in Women's History* (London: Routledge, 1983), pp. 17–71.

Davis, Richard W., *Dissent in Politics 1780–1830: The Political Life of William Smith MP* (London: Epworth Press, 1971).

Digby, Anne, 'Tuke, Samuel (1784–1857)' *Oxford Dictionary of National Biography* [online] [https://doi.org/10.1093/ref:odnb/27808, accessed 27 June 2019].

Dock, L., and I. M. Stewart, *A Short History of Nursing from the Earliest Times to the Present Day* (4th edn, New York: G. P. Putnam's Sons, 1938).

Dossey, Barbara Montgomery, *Florence Nightingale: Mystic, Visionary, Healer* (Springhouse, PA: Springhouse Corp., 1999).

Duckers, Peter, *The Crimean War at Sea: Naval Campaigns Against Russia, 1854–56* (Barnsley, South Yorkshire: Pen & Sword Maritime, 2011).

Figes, Orlando, *The Crimean War: A History* (New York: Henry Holt & Co., 2010).

Fortescue, J. W., *A History of the British Army*, Vol. XIII 1852–1870 (London: Macmillan, 1930).

French, Roger, and Andrew Wear, *British Medicine in an Age of Reform* (London: Routledge, 1991).

Fried, B. M., 'Pirogov in the Crimean Campaign,' *Bulletin of the New York Academy of Medicine* (July 1955) Vol. 31, No. 7, pp. 519–36.

Frieden, Nancy Mandelker, *Russian Physicians in an Era of Reform and Revolution, 1856–1905* (Princeton: Princeton University Press, 1981).

Gabriel, Richard A., *Between Flesh and Steel: A History of Military Medicine from the Middle Ages to the War in Afghanistan* (Washington, DC: Potomac Books, 2013).

Gilley, Sheridan, 'Roman Catholicism,' in D. G. B. Paz, ed., *Nineteenth-Century English Religious Traditions: Retrospect and Prospect* (Westport, CT: Greenwood, 1995), pp. 33–56.

Goldie, Sue, ed., *'I Have Done my Duty': Florence Nightingale in the Crimean War* (Iowa City: University of Iowa Press, 1987).

Harrison, Brian, *Drink and the Victorians* (Pittsburgh, PA: University of Pittsburgh Press, 1971).

Harrison, Mark, 'Parkes, Edmund Alexander (1819–1876),' *Oxford Dictionary of National Biography* [online] [www.oxforddnb.com/view/article/21352, accessed 29 December 2016].

References

Helmstadter, Carol, 'Navigating the Political Straits in the Crimean War,' in Sioban Nelson and Anne Marie Rafferty, eds, *Notes on Nightingale: The Influence and Legacy of a Nursing Icon* (Ithaca, NY: Cornell University Press, 2010), pp. 28–54.

Helmstadter, Carol, 'Robert Bentley Todd, St. John's House, and the Origins of the Modern Trained Nurse,' *Bulletin of the History of Medicine* (1993) Vol. 67, pp. 282–319.

Helmstadter, Carol, and Judith Godden, *Nursing Before Nightingale 1815–1899* (Farnham, Surrey: Ashgate, 2011).

Hickey, Daniel, *Local Hospitals in Ancien Régime France: Rationalization, Resistance, Renewal 1530–1789* (Montreal: McGill-Queens, 1997).

Himmelfarb, Gertrude, 'Mayhew's Poor: A Problem of Identity,' *Victorian Studies* (March 1971) Vol. 14, pp. 307–20.

Hoppen, K. Theodore, *The Mid-Victorian Generation 1846–1886* (Oxford: Oxford University Press, 1998).

Hosking, Geoffrey, *Russia and the Russians* (2nd edn, Cambridge, MA: Belknap Press of Harvard University, 2011).

Humble, J. G., and Peter Hansell, *Westminster Hospital 1716–1966* (London: Pitman Publishing Co., 1966).

Jones, Colin, *Charitable Imperative: Hospitals and Nursing in Ancien Régime and Revolutionary France* (New York: Routledge, 1989).

Kagan, Frederick W., *The Military Reforms of Nicholas I* (New York: St. Martin's Press, 1999).

Kaufman, H., *Surgeons at War: Medical Arrangements for the Treatment of the Sick and Wounded in the British Army during the Late Eighteenth and Nineteenth Centuries* (London: Greenwood Press, 2001).

Kennedy, Dane, 'Sandwith, Humphry (1822–1881),' *Oxford Dictionary of National Biography* [online] [https://doi.org/10.1093/ref:odnb/24647, accessed 19 December 2017].

King, Lester S., *Transformations in American Medicine: From Benjamin Rush to William Osler* (Baltimore: Johns Hopkins University Press, 1991).

Lambert, Andrew, *The Crimean War: British Grand Strategy against Russia, 1853–1856* (Farnham, Surrey: Ashgate, 2011).

LaTorre, Anna, and Maura Lusignani, 'Nursing in the Sardinian-Piedmontese Army during the Crimean War,' *Professioni infermieristiche* (2013) Vol. 66, No. 4, pp. 237–42.

Laughton, J. K., revised by Andrew Lambert, 'Boxer, Edward (1784–1855),' *Oxford Dictionary of National Biography* [online] [https://doi.org/10.1093/ref:odnb/3096, accessed 26 June 2019].

Laughton, J. K., 'Slade, Sir Adolphus (1804–1877),' *Oxford Dictionary of National Biography* [online] [www.oxforddnb.com/view/article/25703, accessed 26 March 2017].

Lawrence, Christopher, 'Democratic, Divine and Heroic: The History and

References

Historiography of Surgery,' in Christopher Lawrence, ed., *Medical Theory, Surgical Practice: Studies in the History of Surgery* (New York: Routledge, 1992), pp. 1–47.

Lawrence, Susan C., *Charitable Knowledge: Hospital Pupils and Practitioners in Eighteenth-Century London* (Cambridge: Cambridge University Press, 1996).

Lewis, Michael, *The Navy in Transition 1814–1864: A Social History* (London: Hodder and Stuart, 1965).

Lloyd, C., and J. Coulter, *Medicine and the Navy 1200–1900* (4 vols, London: E. & S. Livingstone, 1963).

Luddy, Maria, ed., *The Crimean Journals of the Sisters of Mercy 1854–56* (Dublin: Four Courts Press, 2004).

Margrave, Tony R., 'Dr John W. Morton of Tennessee: An American Surgeon in the Crimea,' *The War Correspondent* (September 2015) Vol. 33, No. 1, pp. 22–3.

Marrese, Michelle Lamarche, *A Woman's Kingdom* (Ithaca, NY: Cornell University Press, 2002).

McDonald, Lynn, ed. *Florence Nightingale: The Crimean War* (Waterloo, ON: Wilfrid Laurier Press, 2010).

McLean, David, *Surgeons of the Fleet: The Royal Navy and its Medics from Trafalgar to Jutland* (London: I. B. Tauris, 2010).

Meehan, Brenda, *Holy Women of Russia* (San Francisco: Harper Collins, 1993).

Meynen, Nicolas, 'Les Hôpitaux militaires sous tentes et baraqués au XIXe siècle,' *Revue Historique des Armées* (2009) Vol. 254 [https://rha.revues.org/6543, accessed 10 May 2019].

Mikulinsky, S. R., 'Pirogov, Nikolay Ivanovich,' *Complete Dictionary of Scientific Biography* (2008) [www.encyclopedia.com, accessed 20 March 2015].

Mumm, Susan, *Stolen Daughters, Virgin Mothers: Anglican Sisterhoods in Victorian Britain* (London: Leicester University Press, 1999).

Murray, Elizabeth, 'Russian Nurses: From the Tsarist Sister of Mercy to the Soviet Comrade Nurse,' *Nursing Inquiry* (2004) Vol. 11, No. 3, pp. 130–7.

Nelson, Sioban, *Say Little Do Much: Nurses, Nuns and Hospitals in the Nineteenth Century* (Philadelphia, PA: University of Pennsylvania Press, 2001).

O'Brien, Susan, 'French Nuns in Nineteenth-Century England,' *Past and Present* (1997) Vol. 154, No. 1, pp. 142–80.

O'Malley, I. B., *Florence Nightingale 1820–1856* (London: Thornton Butterworth, 1934).

Prochaska, F. K., *Women and Philanthropy in Nineteenth-Century England* (London: Faber, 1988).

Ralston, David B., *Importing the European Army: The Introduction of European Military Techniques and Institutions into the Extra-European World 1600–1914* (Chicago: University of Chicago Press, 1990).

Rappaport, Helen, *No Place for Ladies* (London: Aurum Press, 2007).

References

Reader, W. J., *Professional Men: The Rise of the Professional Classes in Nineteenth-Century England* (London: Weidenfeld and Nicolson, 1966).

Roberts, M. J. D., *Making English Morals: Voluntary Association and Moral Reform in England 1787–1886* (Cambridge: Cambridge University Press, 2004).

Rochard, Jules, *Histoire de la Chirugerie Française au XIXᵉ Siècle* (Paris: J.-B. Ballière et Fils, 1875).

Rodger, N. A. M., *The Command of the Ocean: A Naval History of Britain 1649–1815* (New York: W. W. Norton, 2004).

Rodger, N. A. M., *The Wooden World: An Anatomy of the Georgian Navy* (New York: W. W. Norton, 1986).

Roxburgh, Sir Ronald, 'Miss Nightingale and Miss Clough: Letters from the Crimea,' *Victorian Studies* (September 1968) Vol. 22, pp. 71–89.

Scherpereel, Philippe, 'Gaspard Léonard Scrive, un pionnier de l'anesthésie et de la chirurgie de guerre' [http://www.philippe-scherpereel.fr/histoire6/index.html, accessed 26 November 2017].

Shepherd, John, 'The Civil Hospitals in the Crimea (1855–56)' *Proceedings of the Royal Society of Medicine* (March 1966) Vol. 59, No.3, pp. 199–208.

Shepherd, John, *The Crimean Doctors: A History of the British Medical Services in the Crimean War* (2 vols, Liverpool: Liverpool University Press, 1991).

Silver, Christopher, *Renkioi: Brunel's Forgotten Crimean War Hospital* (Sevenoaks, Kent: Valonia Press, 2007).

Simpson, F. A., *Louis Napoleon and the Recovery of France* (London: Longmans, 1960).

Smith, F. B., *Florence Nightingale: Reputation and Power* (London: Croom Helm, 1982).

Soroka, Marina, and Charles A. Rudd, *Becoming a Romanov: Grand Duchess Elena of Russia and Her World (1807–1873)* (Burlington, VT: Ashgate, 2015).

Sorokina, T. S., 'Russian Nursing in the Crimean War,' *Journal of the Royal College of Physicians in London* (January/February 1995) Vol. 29, No. 1: pp. 57–63.

Stanmore, Arthur Hamilton-Gordon, *Sidney Herbert Lord Herbert of Lea: A Memoir* (2 vols, London: Murray, 1906).

Stoff, Laurie S., *Russia's Sisters of Mercy and the Great War* (Lawrence, KS: University Press of Kansas, 2015).

Strachan, Hew, *Wellington's Legacy: The Reform of the British Army 1830–54* (Manchester: Manchester University Press, 1984).

Stuart, Vivian, *The Beloved Little Admiral: The Life and Times of Admiral of the Fleet The Hon. Sir Henry Keppel, G.C.B., O.M., D.C.L., 1809–1904* (London: Robert Hale, 1967).

Sullivan, Mary C., *The Friendship of Florence Nightingale and Mary Clare Moore* (Philadelphia, PA: University of Pennsylvania Press, 1999).

References

Summers, Anne, *Angels and Citizens: British Women as Military Nurses 1854–1914* (London: Routledge & Kegan Paul, 1988).

Sweetman, John, *War and Administration: The Significance of the Crimean War for the British Army* (Edinburgh: Scottish Academic Press, 1984).

Taylor, Gordon, *The Sea Chaplains: A History of the Chaplains of the Royal Navy* (Oxford: Oxford Illustrated Press, 1978).

Vogel, Morris J., and Charles E. Rosenberg, *The Therapeutic Revolution* (Philadelphia, PA: University of Pennsylvania Press, 1979).

Webb, R. K., *Modern England from the Eighteenth Century to the Present* (2nd edn, London: Unwin Hymans, 1980).

Westwood, J. N., *Endurance and Endeavour: Russian History 1812–1899* (4th edn, Oxford and New York: Oxford University Press, 1993).

Wiener, Martin J., *Reconstructing the Criminal: Culture, Law and Policy in England 1830–1914* (Cambridge: Cambridge University Press, 1990).

Williams, Thomas Jay, *Priscilla Lydia Sellon: The Restorer after Three Centuries of the Religious Life in the English Church* (London: SPCK, 1950).

Williams, Thomas Jay, and Allan Campbell, *The Park Village Sisterhood* (London: SPCK, 1965).

Wirtschafter, Elise Kimerling, *From Serf to Russian Soldier* (Princeton: Princeton University Press, 1990).

Woodham-Smith, Cecil, *Florence Nightingale 1820–1910* (London: Constable, 1950).

Worboys, Michael, *Spreading Germs: Disease Theories and Medical Practice in Britain, 1865–1900* (Cambridge: Cambridge University Press, 2000).

Index

Aberdeen, Lord 2–3, 37, 44, 86, 162, 306
administration
  of the British army 35–7
  of military hospitals 267, 270
Agamemnon (ship) 204
agrarian economies 9, 245
alcohol problem 83
  see also drunkenness
Alexander II, Tsar 285
Alma River and Battle 18, 20
American Civil War 9
amputations 252–3, 279
Anderson, Emily 88
Anderson, Kate 88
anesthesia 24, 154
Anglican Sisters 137–43
Armstrong-Reid, Susan 6
asceticism 139–40
assistant nurses 32

Bakunin, Mikhail 267
Bakunina, Ekaterina Mikhailovna 264, 267, 270, 274–7, 282, 284, 292–7, 305, 307
Balaclava, Battle of 20, 195
Baltic campaigns 10, 219
Barrie, Mary Gonzaga 95, 135–6, 142
Bashi-Bazouks 195

Baudens, M.L. 175, 177, 181–6, 195, 250
Baumgart, Winfried 8
Bazancourt, Baron de 8
bedsores 123–4, 167, 217
Bell, Sir George 14–24, 33–4, 200, 309
Bermondsey Sisters 132–7
Best, Geoffrey 246, 297
bleeding as a medical procedure 153–4, 179
blisters, 134, 215, 311
Blunt, John 195–6
Bolster, Evelyn 112
Bonaparte, Napoleon *see* Napoleon I
Bonham-Carter, John 41
Bostridge, Mark 84, 110
Bournett, Mary Ann 65, 68–71
bowel disease 25
Bowman, William 68–9
Boxer, Edward 210
Bracebridge, Charles and Selena 43, 49, 66, 71–2, 83–5, 114–15, 137
bribery 194
Bridgeman, Francis 63–4, 81–6, 88–9, 96, 103–28, 132–4, 137, 142, 189, 229, 240, 303–4
  advantages and disadvantages faced by 127, 133–4
  kindness to patients 128

326

Index

system of nursing espoused by 116–21
view of Nightingale's nursing 110–18
Brown, Caroline 239
Brunel, Isambard 235
Budberg, Baroness 279, 292
Bulgaria 4, 18, 53, 158, 193, 195
Burgoyne, Sir John 34
Bushby, Henry 204
Byron, Harriet Brownlow 138

Calthorpe, Somerset 204, 218
Campbell, Sir Colin 83, 88
Canning, Lady 240
Canrobert, François 279
cantinières 151
Cardwell reforms (1871) 34
Catherine the Great 3, 299–300
Cator, Susan 32, 76, 215
Caucasus region 5, 12
Cavour, Camillo 162, 165
Chadwick, Owen 132
Chalmers, Thomas 211
Chantal, Jean de 136
Chantal, Mary de 133
Charge of the Light Brigade 2
Charité Hospital, Berlin 252
Charity Commissioners 31
Chenery, Thomas 38–9
Chenu, Jean-Charles 155–8, 234, 308–9
cholera 16, 18, 25, 116, 134, 158, 163, 196, 214, 284
Clarendon, Lord 3, 42, 163
Clark, Sir James 241
Clarke, Elizabeth (nurse from University College Hospital) 239
Clarke, Miss (housekeeper at the Barrack Hospital) 90, 137
Clarke, Mrs (matron at Harley Street) 47–8, 65–6, 69, 90, 115, 137

class structure 6, 32, 40, 43–4, 65–71, 81, 85, 188, 206, 228–99, 300, 304–8;
see also lady nurses; working-class nurses
Clifford, Henry 14–15, 22, 150, 153, 205–7, 213, 290–1
Clough, Martha 83, 88, 96, 109, 140, 303
Codman, John 173
commanders-in-chief 35, 38, 194, 258
comminuted fractures 11, 311
commissariat functions 35–7, 157, 181, 184–6, 202, 206, 267, 271, 297
Commissetti, Antonio 164
commissions, purchase of 33–4
communications systems 12–13
compound fractures 252, 278, 311
'conservative surgery' 23–4
Constantinople 4
contusions 124, 311
conversion to Catholicism 112–13, 131, 135–6
Coote, Holmes and Mrs Coote 227–8, 230
Cordero, Countess 165–6
corruption 194–7, 248–50, 253, 295, 297, 305–6
Coyle, Mary Ann 65–71
Cranworth, Lady 216–17
Crimean Fever 232
Crimean War 1–9, 193, 310
British army's lack of preparedness for 3
causes of 6
deaths in 1
declaration of 4
maps of xiv–xvii
public attitudes to 1–2, 177
separate campaigns within 5
see also war aims

327

Index

Croke, Mary Joseph 103–4, 108–10, 122–3
Cronstadt 12
Cruveilhier, Jean 252
Cuffe, Fr 112, 136
Curtiss, John Shelton 245, 292

Danube, River 197
Daughters of Charity 49–50, 103, 132, 135, 146–50, 163–7, 185–8, 200, 217–18
Davidoff, Leonore 32
Davidson, John 202, 209–14, 218–20
Davis, Elizabeth 62, 90
Dawson, Ruth 76, 215–17, 307
Deas, David 211–17, 220
debridement 123, 311
desertion by soldiers 15, 35, 194, 246, 284–5
Devonport Sisters 49, 136, 139–41
Devonshire Square Sisters 47–8, 218
diaphoretics 25, 311
diplomacy 4, 8, 162
dismissal of individual nurses 64–7, 72, 76, 82–3, 93–4, 108, 210, 230, 238, 241
Dixon, Mary Bernard 82, 105, 107–8
Dock, Lavinia 81
doctors
    attached to the army 7, 16–19, 22, 25, 31, 33, 35–6, 38, 63
    attitudes to female nurses 105, 226, 267, 301
    nurses' obedience to orders from 42, 120–1, 231, 238, 241, 261, 267, 298, 307
    respect commanded by 308
    Russian 249–51, 298, 307–8
    shortages of 171–5, 183–5, 224, 255, 271
    sickness of 170, 178, 226, 270, 272, 275

subordination to military authority 83, 185–6, 281
    Turkish 196–200, 308
Dondukoff, Princess 188
Doyle, Mary Aloysius 93, 103–4, 114–17, 127, 134
Drake, Elizabeth 65, 68–70, 219
dress, nurses' 45–6, 228–9
drunkenness 15, 47, 52, 82–3, 93–4, 97, 111, 114, 151, 166
Duberly, Fanny 210
Duncan, Janet 239
Durando, Giacomo and Marcantonio 163

Eastern Question, the 3
Elmslie, Margaret 239
Enfield rifles 10–11
Engels, Friedrich 46–7
Erskine, Harriet 49, 140, 143, 218–20
erysipelas 24–5, 90, 311
expenses incurred by nurses 80, 92

Fagge, Emma 65, 68–71
Federovna, Maria, Empress 254–5
feldshers 250, 258, 260, 266, 272, 277, 281
female nurses
    maximum acceptable number of 82, 93
    resistance to 31–3, 38–45, 55–7, 61, 63, 86, 118–19, 146, 89, 212–13, 220, 226, 233, 237–8, 242, 256–7, 267
fever 16, 25, 171, 179, 226, 232, 271
Filder, James 36
floggings 15, 196, 246
food
    supplies of 13, 114–15, 177, 196, 284
    theft of 249–50, 267
fomentations 25, 56, 311
Foster, Theresa 45, 48

328

Index

France 3–6, 11, 146–7, 155–7, 177–8, 242
Franco-Prussian War 309
Frere, Elizabeth 48
frostbite 25, 159, 232
Fry, Elizabeth 47

gangrene 24–6, 124, 160, 173–4, 198, 269–74, 311–12
gendered constructions of nursing 155, 307, 310
    see also 'separate spheres'
Geneva Convention (1864) 158, 309
'gentlemanly' conduct of war 8
germ theory 12, 252
Godman, Temple 90
Goldie, Sue 84, 110
Golding, Benjamin 31, 39–40, 67
Goodlake, Gerald 178, 269
Goodman, Margaret 49, 117, 136, 141–3
Gorchakov, Prince 267, 271, 280–2, 285, 291
Grant, Thomas 49, 112, 134, 136, 309
Graves, Robert James 232
Greig, David 15
Grey, Mary 238
gunnery and gunshot wounds 10–11, 24, 247, 275, 283, 295
Guthrie, G. J. 153–4

Hall, Sir John 19, 43, 56, 63–4, 81, 87–9, 104, 108–10, 118, 121, 220, 225, 227, 235–6, 306
Hamley, Col. 292
Hardinge, Henry 35
Hawes, Benjamin 86
Hawkins, Elizabeth 74–5
Hawley, Capt. 285
hay shortages 13
head nurses 72–3

healing by first, second or third intention 124, 252–3, 272, 311–12
Hepburn, Marion 238
Herbé, Jean-François 9, 12, 148–50, 171–3, 176, 187–8, 269
Herbert, Elizabeth (Lizzie) 41, 49, 228, 230
Herbert, Sidney 35–6, 40–5, 49, 54–5, 71, 83–7, 106, 109, 115, 157, 225, 228, 306
Higgins, Ann 65–71
Himmelfarb, Getrude 32
Hodasevich, Capt. 12, 246–7, 260, 284–5
Hosking, Geoffrey 248–9
hospital locations, map of xvi
hospital ships 173, 208–9, 212, 214
hospitals, military and civilian 62, 68, 224–42
Hübbenet, Christian 258, 266, 268, 273–4, 284, 298
humanitarian movements 14
Hutton, Amy 116–17, 143, 240

ideological approaches to health care 122–3
illness amongst doctors and other medical staff 170, 226, 270, 272, 275
imperialism 6
industrial capacity 9, 12–13, 245
inflammatory fever 179
Inkerman, Battle of 20–1, 34–5, 63, 151, 188, 204, 259, 268
Irish nationalism 104
Irish Sisters of Mercy 49, 104–5
Italian unification 162

James, Sarah 238–9
Jameson, Anna 40
Jennings, Edward 50, 52
Jones, Colin 146–7

329

Index

Jones, Mary 65, 69–70, 219
Jowett, Benjamin 96–7

Kalashnikov (medical aide to Pirogov) 258
Kartseva, Elisaveta 294–5
Khitrovo, Ekaterina Aleksandrovna 293–7
Khrulev, General 274, 285
Kinglake, Alexander 80, 205, 242, 309
Kornilov, Vladimir 247
Korvovskii, N. P. 284, 297

ladies
  as distinct from working-class women 40–4
  myth of their transformative effect on nursing 80–1
  Nightingale's attitude to 71–3, 80–1, 85–6, 230
  payments to 91–2
  see also pay for nursing work
  position in relation to men 131, 138–9
  property law 299–300
lady nurses 48, 61–2, 65, 71–2, 80–1, 85–6, 93, 117, 121, 127, 214, 218–19, 224, 226, 231–4, 240–1, 304, 309
lady superintendents 85–6, 89–93, 147, 219, 224, 228, 230, 234, 237–41, 304–7
Lake, Colonel Atwell 188
Lancet, The 199
Land Transport Corps 37–8, 56
  see also Royal Waggon Train
Langston, Emma 49, 83, 140, 143, 218
Larrey, Baron Dominique Jean 155
laudanum, use of 17
Lawfield, Rebecca 67–70
Lawson, George 90, 215
LeFroy, John Henry 118, 233
LeMesurier, Charlotte 227

LeMesurier, Henrietta 224, 228, 230, 238, 241
Lister, Joseph 308
Loizillon, Henri 170, 178, 184, 269, 285
Longmore, Thomas 24–5, 157
Luddy, Maria 103
Lushington, Stephen 207

McAuley, Catherine 132
McGrigor, Sir James 33, 155, 309
Mackenzie, Eliza 115–16, 126, 211–14, 217–20, 303
Mackenzie, John 211
Macleod, George 124, 153–4, 188–9, 224–5, 231–4, 242
McLeod, Mrs and Abigail 88–92
malaria (intermittent fever) 16, 179, 271
male nurses 154–6, 187–9, 242, 307
Manning, Henry Edward 84
marines 204, 208, 218
Marrese, Michelle 300
Masquelez, Lt. 17, 149–50, 176, 187
matrons 39, 65–7, 72, 118, 229, 304
Maule, Lauderdale 37–8
medical comforts (extras) 19, 115, 232, 238
medical department of the army
  British 7, 19, 31–8, 126, 165, 185–6
  French 152–3, 156–8, 161, 165, 171, 174–7, 181–6, 308, 310
  Piedmont-Sardinian 163
  Russian 249, 268–9, 276, 298, 310
  see also Turkish military hospitals
medical department of the Royal Navy 209
Medical Staff Corps 56
medicine, military 23–6
Menshikov, Prince 247, 258–9, 267, 270–1, 309
Menzies, Duncan 52
mercenary soldiers 35

Index

Middlesex Hospital 211
Miller, Agnes 239
Minié rifles 10–11, 152, 199, 269
Moldavia 3
Moltke, Helmuth von 194
money belonging to soldiers, taking
  care of 266, 292
Montaudon, Jean Baptiste 149–52,
  187, 206, 269
Moore, Mary Clare 63–7, 83, 95–6,
  105–16, 122, 126–8, 132–7,
  142, 166
moral influence, power, reform 96,
  175–7, 296, 298
mortal wounds 272
Morton, Anne Ward 91, 94–6
Morton, John 11, 286
motherhood, adulation of 300
Mumm, Susan 132
muster-roll fraud 197

Nakhimov, Pavel 247, 283
Napoleon I 155, 157
Napoleon III 4–5, 159, 162, 177–8
Naval Brigade 38, 204–8, 214, 220
Nelson, Horatio 203
Netley military hospital 90, 303
Newcastle, Duke of 38–43, 225, 306
Newman, Anne 239
Nicholas I, Tsar 4, 249, 256–7, 261,
  297, 300
Nicol, Martha 224–5, 229, 232–4
Niel, Adolphe 159
Nightingale, Florence
  attitude to and standards expected
    of her nurses 45–6, 69–73,
    95–6, 216–17
  criticisms of 69, 84–7, 110, 118, 306
  diplomatic behaviour by 63, 67
  emphasis on propriety and raising
    the moral character of her
    nurses 47, 64, 67, 73–4, 83, 96,
    176, 217, 241

lack of clinical experience but
  respect for those who had it
  67–8, 96, 307–8
lack of status as an unmarried
  woman 42–3
legendary position with ordinary
  soldiers and the public at
  home 2, 63, 109–10, 146, 203,
  303
others' personal dislike of 104, 106
parentage and social position of
  41–3, 305
personal characteristics and
  mission of 96–7, 126, 137,
  306
politically-driven appointment of
  31, 40–1, 44–5, 303, 306
problems faced by 61, 63, 70–1,
  116, 120–2, 126–7, 303, 308
qualities looked for in a clinical
  nurse 90, 307
relations with army doctors 63, 71,
  87, 115
relations with ladies on her staff
  72–3, 80–1, 85–6, 230
relations with purveyors 63, 306
religious faith of 41, 131
sense of betrayal felt by 85, 95
supervisory control exercised by
  44, 54–5, 61–4, 75, 81–2, 87,
  94, 106–9, 112–13, 123, 126–7,
  241, 309
support for 306
views on the conduct of the
  Crimean War 6
views on military nursing 175, 180,
  184, 187, 240–1, 309–10
Nightingale, W. E. 41
Nikitin (feldsher) 258, 277
nurses
  appearance of working-class 45–6
  arriving parties of 61, 104–5, 226,
    264, 268, 293

Index

nurses (*cont.*)
  best of those working for
    Nightingale 94–6
  division of labour between 75
  shortage of 155, 183, 186, 255–6
  see also female nurses; male nurses
nursing
  comparison between different
    countries' services 308
  different systems of 70, 103, 120–8
  doctor-directed 241, 304
  histories of 2, 81, 203
  as a knowledge-based practice 310
  natural aptitude for 39, 80
  preparation for 26, 304, 309
  seen as a form of imperialism 6
  seen as a pastoral calling, with
    nurses as assistants to the
    chaplains 86
  systematic reform of 33
  three functional categories within
    266, 309–10

officer corps
  British and French 34, 206–7
  Russian 245–7
  Turkish 194–5, 197
orderlies 50–3, 56–7, 93, 114, 121,
    123, 186, 199, 212, 218, 231–4,
    237
Osten-Sacken, Count 8, 267, 270,
    284–5
Ottoman Empire and its troops 3–4,
    193–9
Our Lady of the Orphans convent
    (Norwood) 49, 82, 105–6,
    111
outcomes for patients admitted to
    the French army's medical
    department 161, 176, 182

Palmerston, Lord 2–3, 36, 41–2, 162,
    306

Panmure, Lord 37–8, 87, 162–3, 186,
    306
'Papal Aggression' 44, 104
Park Village Sisters 49, 139–40, 211
Parkes, Edmund Alexander 224,
    235–41
Parkes, Martha 237–41
Paul I, Tsar 299–300
Paulet, Lord William 74, 106
Pavlovna, Elena (Grand Duchess) 146,
    254–7, 261, 270, 293–4, 297,
    300, 305–6
pay for nursing work 48, 66, 80, 91–4,
    131, 188, 234, 240
Peel, William 207–8
Pélissier, A. J. 279, 290
Peninsular War 14, 16–17, 37
Percy, Baron Pierre-François 154,
    157, 185
pharmacists 266–7, 271, 284, 297
philanthropic work 56, 131, 254, 300
Pillans, Etheldreda 139, 143
Pincoffs, Peter 118–19, 127, 165–6,
    180
Pirogov, Nikolai 5, 200, 247–84,
    293–306
  contrasted with Nightingale 306–8
prisoners of war, treatment of 9, 174,
    185, 187–8, 309
Prochaska, Frank 92
Protestantism 44, 104, 113, 122,
    133–4, 137, 142
purulent infection 252, 312
purveyors 63, 157, 197, 202, 297, 306
Pusey, Edward Bouverie 139–41
pyemia 24, 252, 312

Raglan, Lord 14–15, 19–20, 34–5,
    54–5, 160, 163, 204, 233, 279,
    310
Rappaport, Helen 147–8
regimental hospitals 33, 50–1, 182–3
Register of Nurses 224

332

Index

Reid, Mary Ann 239
reinforcement of troops 22, 178
religious commitment and dissension
3–4, 44–5, 86, 96–7, 106, 122,
188, 234
religious nursing 7, 26, 74, 81, 103,
131, 186, 230, 303–4
reporting of war 2–3, 9, 14, 39, 86,
184, 186, 203, 240
requisitioning system 66, 88, 120–1
rifles, supply and quality of 10–12
Roberts, Eliza 32, 67–8, 72, 76, 83,
95–6, 118, 123, 125, 232,
239–40, 308
Roberts, Michael 96
Robinson, Frederick 199, 204
Roebuck Commission 36
Roman Catholicism 44–5, 81, 84–8,
106, 109, 112, 122, 131, 134–5,
142, 188
Ronan, Fr 84, 111–12, 136
Royal Navy 202–4, 214
advantages over the British army
206–7, 220
Royal Waggon Train 37–8
Russell, Lord John 162
Russian army 245–9, 268–72, 274–5,
284–5, 290–2, 297–8
Russian economy and society 9–10
Russian names, English equivalents
of xix
Russification 6
Russophobia 2
Russo-Turkish Wars 5, 193, 305–6

St Bartholomew's Hospital 45–6
St John's House 33, 47–9, 65–71, 92,
96, 115, 138, 211, 219, 238,
242
St Thomas's Hospital 31–2, 45, 134
St Vincent 146–8
Salisbury, Charlotte 72–3, 82–3, 87–8,
92, 96, 109

Sandwith, Humphry 193–4, 197–8
sanitary conditions 122–5, 166, 171,
188, 270
scientific medicine 31, 153–4
Scrive, Gaspard-Léonard 154–5,
157–61, 170–87, 242, 253, 270,
280, 292, 308
scurvy 26, 164, 170–1, 175, 180, 220,
271
sea power 10
Seacole, Mary 151–2
secondary infection 282, 312
Secretary *at* War and Secretary *of* War
35, 37
Seidlitz, Karl Karlovich 253, 271
Sellon, Lydia (and Sellonites) 49,
139–41
'separate spheres' ideology 6, 39–40,
63, 188, 213, 307
see also women
septicemia 312
serfdom 245, 254, 299–300
Sevastopol 1, 4, 9–10, 13–14, 19, 159,
161–2, 170, 247–8, 258, 261,
265–6, 269–72, 276–80, 283–6
fall of south side 174, 177–9, 183–4,
233
maps of xiv–xviii
successive bombardments of 20,
272–3, 275–9, 283, 286, 290–2
sexual relationships 46–7, 73–4
Shaftesbury, Lord 211
Shamil 5
Shaw Stewart, Jane 78 n47, 85, 89–90,
93–7, 142, 219, 303, 306
sickness
amongst doctors 170, 178, 226, 270,
272, 275
amongst soldiers 16–18
Silistria 4, 195
Simferopol 261, 264–5, 272, 276
sisterhoods 32–3, 47–9, 131–2, 138–9,
255–7

333

Index

Sisters of Charity 147–50, 158–9, 163–4, 166–7
Sisters of the Exaltation of the Cross 255–8, 264–8, 270–1, 273–87, 296–7, 305–7
  infighting amongst 269–70, 294, 301
Sisters of Mercy 47–9, 103–4, 111–12, 131–2, 165–6, 200, 256
Sisters of the Poor 138
Slade, Adolphus 150, 153–4, 167, 193–6, 297
sloughing off dead tissue 124, 180, 312
Smart, William 208–9
Smith, Andrew 33, 35–8, 53, 118, 225
Smith, F. B. 85
Smith, William 41
Smythe, Drusilla 227
social determinants of health 220
soldats militaires or *infirmiers* 154
soldats panseurs 183
sorties 9, 160, 170, 268–9, 273
Soyer, Alexis 51, 118
Stakhovich, Aleksandra Petrovna 257, 264–5, 270, 276, 279, 284, 293–300, 303, 307
Stanley, Mary 49, 61, 64, 80–8, 96, 105, 108–10, 116, 121, 136, 225, 228, 240, 306
Sterling, A. C. 55–6, 154
Stewart, Isabel 81
storekeeping 110–11, 115, 209, 213–14, 237–8, 293, 297
Storks, Henry 108, 233, 241
Struthers, Alexander 63
Summers, Anne 93
superintendents' reports 61
suppurating 124, 172–3, 252, 312

Tattersall, Mary 90–2
Taylor, Fanny 85, 88, 176–7, 228–9

Tchernaya, the, Battle of 171, 174
Terrot, Sarah Anne 49, 66, 135–6, 139, 142–3, 216, 236–7
tetanus 24
Thom, Anne 142–3
The Times 14–15, 42, 72, 86, 236
Tolstoy, Leo 247–9, 258, 268, 278–9, 287, 291–2, 298–9
total war 9
Totleben, Edouard 9–10, 12, 152, 159–60, 247, 283, 285, 291
training for military nurses 74, 304
transnational concepts 6–7, 127, 189, 242, 309–10
transportation of wounded soldiers 18–19, 53, 173–4, 295
Travers, Dorothy 50
trench warfare 9, 170, 279–80
  see also sorties
triage system 255, 272–3, 277–8
troop movements 12
  see also transportation of wounded soldiers
Tuke, Samuel 176
Turkish Contingent 199–200
Turkish military hospitals 196–8
Turkish public hygiene 226
Turnbull, Bertha 49, 95–6, 117, 136, 141–3
turnover of nurses 93–4
typhus and typhoid fever 26, 178–81, 198, 226–7, 265, 268, 271–2

Vaillant, Marshall 181
Vasilchikov, Prince Viktor 258, 267, 270, 285, 291
Velpeau, A.-A.-L.-M. 252
Vesey, Gertrude 218–19
Victoria, Queen 3, 165
victualing 203
  see also purveyors

Index

Villiers, Sir James 249, 254
Viney, Mary 239
volunteering
 philanthropic 92, 131, 156, 158, 224, 234, 240, 257, 309
 soldiers 34, 155

Wallachia 3
war aims 3–5
War Office's instructions to Nightingale 106–9, 120
Wear, Margaret 61, 64, 71, 89, 96, 109, 306–7
Wellington, Duke of 37
Westwood, J. N. 246
Wheeler, Elizabeth 49, 64, 72, 143, 213, 236–7
Whitty, Robert 112
Wiener, Martin 96
Williams, William 197–8
Wirtschafter, Elise 249

women
 supposed capabilities and role of 6, 39–40, 213, 298–9, 301, 304
 mission of 80–1, 92, 97, 187, 189, 242
women's movement 300
Wood, Charles 141
Wood, Lady Emma 215–17
Wood, Evelyn 204–8, 214–17, 279, 283
Woodward, Elizabeth 215
working-class nurses 46–7, 63–76, 81–3, 93–7, 111, 119, 142, 214, 218, 226–31, 240–2, 304–5
wounded men, number of xii–xiii
wounds 11, 24–5, 123–4, 284, 292–3
Wreford, Matthew 37

Yani, Lt. 276–7, 298

Zatler, General 297
Zouaves, the 10–11, 17, 150–3, 160

Printed in the USA
CPSIA information can be obtained
at www.ICGtesting.com
JSHW060536131124
73471JS00014B/619